CH00903631

Directions in
Nursing Research

Developments in Nursing Research

Series Editor
Jenifer Wilson-Barnett Professor and Head of Department of Nursing Studies, King's College, London University

Volume 1
Recovery from Illness
Jenifer Wilson-Barnett and Morva Fordham

Volume 2
Nursing Research: Ten Studies in Patient Care
Edited by *Jenifer Wilson-Barnett*

Volume 3
Psychiatric Nursing Research
Edited by *Julia I Brooking* Lecturer in Nursing Studies, King's College, London University

Volume 4
Research in Preventive Community Care
Edited by *Alison While* Lecturer in Nursing Studies, King's College, London University

Volume 5
Research in the Care of Elderly People
Edited by *Pauline Fielding* Director of Nursing Services, Whipps Cross Hospital, London

Volume 6
Nursing Issues and Research in Terminal Care
Edited by *Jenifer Wilson-Barnett and Jennifer Raiman* Education Adviser, Cancer Relief Macmillan Fund; Research Fellow, Department of Therapeutics, The London Hospital Medical College

Developments in Nursing Research Volume 7

Directions in
Nursing Research:
Ten Years of Progress
at London University

Edited by

Jenifer Wilson-Barnett

Professor and Head of Department of Nursing Studies,

King's College, London University

and

Sarah Robinson

Senior Research Fellow, Nursing Research Unit, King's College,

London University

and presented by past and present members of the Department

and of the Nursing Research Unit

SCUTARI PRESS
London

A division of Scutari Projects, the publishing
company of the Royal College of Nursing

First published 1989

British Library Cataloguing in Publication Data

Directions in nursing research: ten years of progress at
  London University.
  1. Medicine. Nursing
  I. Wilson-Barnett, Jenifer II. Robinson, Sarah, *1948–*
  III. Series
  610.73

ISBN 1-871364-21-3

Typeset by Dobbie Typesetting Limited
Printed and bound in Great Britain by The Alden Press, Oxford,
London and Northampton

List of Contributors

Christine Barnes Genetic Counsellor, South East Thames Regional Genetic Centre, formerly Research Associate, Nursing Research Unit, King's College, London University

Lynn Batehup Lecturer in Nursing Studies, King's College/Clinical Nurse Specialist, Camberwell Health Authority

Julia Brooking Chief Nurse Adviser/Senior Lecturer, Bethlem, Royal and Maudsley Hospitals/Institute of Psychiatry, London, formerly Lecturer in Nursing Studies, King's College, London University

Gillian Chapman Nursing Officer, Department of Health, formerly Lecturer in Nursing Studies, King's College, London University

Jessica Corner Lecturer in Nursing Studies, King's College, London University

Brenda de Carle Nurse Researcher, King's College, London University

Sally Farnish Health Visitor, Genetic Services, Leicestershire, formerly Research Associate, Nursing Research Unit, King's College, London University

Morva Fordham Lecturer in Nursing Studies, King's College, London University

Brian Gilchrist Lecturer in Nursing Studies, King's College, London University

Sheila Haverty Evaluation Officer, Department of Nursing Studies, King's College, London University

Jack Hayward Emeritus Professor, London University/Director of Nursing Research Unit, King's College, London University

Joanne Howard Sister, Coronary Care Unit, Norfolk and Norwich Hospital, formerly student in nursing studies, King's College, London University

Keith Jacka Statistician, Nursing Research Unit, King's College, London University

Sally Kendall Lecturer in Nursing, Buckinghamshire College of Higher Education, formerly Evaluation Officer, Department of Nursing Studies, King's College, London University

Judith Lathlean Independent Researcher in Nursing, formerly Research Fellow, Nursing Research Unit, King's College, London University

Andrée C Le May Specialist Nurse Research and Project Development, West Middlesex University Hospital, Isleworth, formerly postgraduate student in nursing studies, King's College, London University

David Lewin Director of Clinical Research, The London Hospital, formerly Research Associate, Nursing Research Unit, King's College, London University

Paul Lewis Midwifery Tutor, Queen Charlotte's Maternity Hospital, London, formerly student in nursing studies, King's College, London University

Jill Macleod Clark Senior Lecturer in Nursing Studies, King's College, London University

Julienne Meyer Postgraduate Student, King's College, London University

Edana Minghella Clinical Teacher, Maudsley Hospital/Postgraduate student, Institute of Psychiatry, London, formerly postgraduate student in nursing studies, King's College, London University

Heather Owen Research Associate, Nursing Research Unit, King's College, London University

Sally Redfern Senior Lecturer in Nursing Studies, King's College, London University

Sarah Robinson Senior Research Fellow, Nursing Research Unit, King's College, London University

Fiona Ross Lecturer in Nursing Studies, King's College, London University

Kate Seers Project Officer, Daphne Heald Research Unit, Royal College of Nursing, formerly postgraduate student in nursing studies, King's College, London University

Gillian Smith Independent Researcher/Trainee Psychotherapist, formerly Research Associate, Nursing Research Unit, King's College, London University

Pamela Smith Senior Nurse – Research and Development, Bloomsbury Health Authority, formerly postgraduate student in nursing studies, King's College, London University

Barbara Stilwell Nurse Practitioner/Researcher, West Lambeth Health Authority, formerly Nurse Researcher, King's College, London University

Christine Terrey Personal Secretary, Department of Physics, King's College, formerly secretary to Department of Nursing Studies, King's College, London University

Ann Tomlinson Freelance Lecturer in Nursing, formerly Evaluation Officer, King's College, London University

Sally West Information and Policy Officer, Age Concern, formerly postgraduate student in nursing studies, King's College, London University

Alison While Lecturer in Nursing Studies, King's College, London University

Jenifer Wilson-Barnett Professor and Head of Department of Nursing Studies, King's College, London University

Contents

Series Preface

This series, which began in 1982, has developed apace with the growing volume of nursing research produced in this country. Aimed to review research in specialist areas of nursing and to form a scholarly contribution to the literature, it draws on a wide range of expertise among chapter authors. Readers are encouraged to exploit the collective bibliographies and new research findings and to appraise critically this expanding body of knowledge in nursing.

Preface

Nursing research has been undertaken at King's College, London University, since 1977, the year when the Department of Nursing Studies and the Nursing Research Unit were established. Commissioned to celebrate the tenth anniversary of that development, this volume encompasses much of the research undertaken in the ensuing decade. Our purpose in asking our colleagues to write for this volume has been to produce a comprehensive record of a programme of research that has covered many aspects of nursing, midwifery and health visiting, and has employed a diversity of research methods.

The research undertaken at King's College has focused on four main areas of concern to the profession: monitoring and improving the delivery of patient and client care; exploring the views and experiences of patients and their relatives; evaluating and developing the educational preparation available at both basic and post-basic levels and investigating reasons for retention in and loss from the service through long-term follow-up studies of the careers of staff. As well as illustrating the diversity of subjects that we have studied, we have also tried to demonstrate how particular themes have been pursued over a number of years through a succession of projects, for example, recovery from illness, communication skills, developing experimental training schemes to prepare staff for new responsibilities, and the nature of interprofessional relationships.

Nursing, midwifery and health visiting require a diversity of clinical and interpersonal skills, and an innovative approach to the education of practitioners; consequently, it is necessary to deploy a wide range of research strategies in the study of both practice and education. This volume demonstrates the eclectic approach that the Department and Unit staff have adopted in this respect, with the use of many forms of descriptive, experimental and action research.

Our aim has been to produce a collection of studies that will be of interest to nurses, midwives and health visitors who work in practice, in education and in management. We hope it will also be of interest to members of other health-care professions and to health-care researchers. As editors we would like to thank all the authors who have contributed to the book, the various organisations who have funded the research programme at King's, and the editorial and production staff of Scutari Press.

Jenifer Wilson-Barnett
Sarah Robinson

King's College, London
September 1988

Chapter 1

Developments in Nursing Research at King's College, London University

Jenifer Wilson-Barnett and Sarah Robinson

Immense progress has been achieved in nursing research in the United Kingdom over the last 10 years. Each of the academic departments and research units has contributed to this, as have many others in practical care and educational settings. Over time, departments and units develop specific strengths and research traditions; these are influenced by current concerns in health care and the particular interests of staff, as well as by opportunities for funding.

The research presented in this volume comprises much of the work undertaken by staff at the Department of Nursing Studies and the Nursing Research Unit of King's College, London University (formerly Chelsea College). Its publication marks the tenth anniversary of the department and the unit, which was celebrated in October 1987. A comprehensive programme of research has been generated in this first decade, and although it has not been possible to include all of the studies undertaken in a single volume, the major directions we have pursued are all represented. We hope, therefore, that this volume will be of interest to many nurses, midwives and health visitors, as well as to members of other health-care professions and to health-care researchers.

NURSING STUDIES AND NURSING RESEARCH AT KING'S COLLEGE

The Department of Nursing Studies was established in 1977 under the leadership of Jack Hayward, the first Professor of Nursing at London University. From its inception, the department included the Nursing Research Unit, which is funded by the Department of Health and Social Security (DHSS), and collaboration between lecturing and research staff, in both research and teaching activities, has been very much a part of the history of nursing at King's College.

The department offers undergraduate degrees as well as masters' and doctoral programmes, and research undertaken by students at all these three levels is represented in the book. Other studies presented document the work of major research teams led by lecturing staff and funded by such organisations as the Health Education Authority, the Cancer Research Council and the DHSS. Research is a continuous process and the department feels that this should be reflected in its major activities. By having clinical teaching responsibilities, each member of staff is encouraging integration of research and practice whenever possible. They also benefit by being exposed to issues that are important to practitioners and that may suggest directions for future research.

Work in the unit is funded primarily by the DHSS and has, in the main, taken the form of projects that are broad in scope and large in scale. The unit team is multidisciplinary and its staff comprise nurses, midwives, social scientists and a statistician. Work in both the department and the unit benefits from collaboration with teaching and research staff from a diversity of disciplines within the university; these include education, physical and biological sciences, medicine and law.

RESEARCH DIRECTIONS

Identifying the strengths of any organisation is a difficult task but both the department and the unit have developed programmes of research and concomitant expertise in particular areas. Turning first to the department, then, psychological care and nurse–patient communications have been the focus of much research activity. Several of the first members of the department held major grants and published widely in this area. Not only did this area dominate in research, but it was also very well represented in the teaching programmes within the department. This type of work, as applied to aspects of health or specific illness and treatment, relies on a broad basis of psychological, biological and medical knowledge. As such, it is impossible to define discrete areas for nursing research. Health promotion work, for instance, both exploits communication skills and draws on information from social, political and physiological sources.

In more recent years, a human biology base for nursing practice has been developed as a primary focus for research in the King's College department. Work on hypothermia in the elderly and on the treatment of leg ulcers, for example, is in progress, although some previous studies on recovery from illness and surgery also relied on a certain level of knowledge of ergonomics and physiology.

Perhaps the third area of research in the department that builds on previous experience is that of developing and evaluating new roles or new challenges for nursing. Work on the nurse practitioner is a case in point, but many other studies are exploring additional demands on health professionals and the type of educational preparation they require to be successful. Another main concern is patient teaching, and a number of projects have developed not only teaching packages for patients but also programmes to help nurses, midwives and health visitors to develop skills in employing these programmes.

Professional education, interprofessional relationships, role development and careers have provided the main themes of the unit's work. Basic professional training has, for example, been the focus of both a longitudinal study of wards as clinical learning environments for student nurses and a study of the effects on student midwives' confidence of extending midwifery training from 12 to 18 months. Post-basic preparation for the roles of ward sister and staff nurse is the subject of a series of past and present projects, which has provided much valuable information for the profession. Data from unit evaluations of experimental schemes, for example, have been used by many health authorities in the development of their own schemes. A new project investigating the role of the ward sister and the implementation of the nursing process has just been initiated.

Interprofessional relationships have been another of the unit's main concerns. The early work on midwifery, for example, investigated the overlap of midwifery and medical responsibilities for normal maternity care. Unit research also demonstrates the advantage of developing a substantial database in particular areas. Thus, factors causing professional dissatisfaction identified in the midwifery research, such as role erosion and short staffing, have been further explored in the context of projects on midwives' career patterns. Career patterns is in fact an area that the unit is currently developing, with plans to follow up personnel who have already participated in unit projects and departmental courses, as well as recruiting new participants to a series of longitudinal follow-up studies. More recently, unit staff moved into another area of research, namely psychiatric nursing, with the first project focusing on the prevention and management of violence.

The unit was originally known as the Nursing Education Research Unit, but subsequently changed its title to the Nursing Research Unit in order to reflect more accurately the nature and scope of its research programme. Education and practice cannot be arbitrarily divided into discrete areas of research, as enquiries into educational strategies must also address issues of what kind of practice or particular role the learner or practitioners are being prepared for, or could develop in the future.

RESEARCH STRATEGIES

Staff of the department and unit have always adopted an eclectic approach to theoretical perspectives and research methods; these have become more diverse and complex as the programme of research has developed. Such a diversity is entirely appropriate, however, given the wide range of clinical and interpersonal skills that nurses, midwives and health visitors employ in the delivery of care, and the development in recent years of many new approaches to their professional education.

Much of the earlier work took the form of descriptive surveys. These employed questionnaires, and in some cases historical records, to obtain data from a range of settings on subjects about which little prior information existed. Subsequent descriptive work has adopted a more intensive approach, focusing on a small number of cases and attempting to gain a deeper understanding of professionals' and patients' views and actions, and the context in which they occur. Methods employed have included a range of attitude and psychometric scaling techniques, interviews and observation.

Many of the later studies have moved on from description to evaluation of innovations in both practice and education. Some of these have adopted a 'before and after' design, others have compared an experimental with a control group, and staff in the unit have employed an action research strategy to evaluate the impact of experimental training schemes. An increasing number of studies have used a triangulation strategy, combining different methods to enhance the validity of the data. This book, however, is not presented as a series of studies that purports to demonstrate how to do research. Nonetheless, each of the authors has been requested to describe their methods critically and to suggest directions for future research.

STUDIES INCLUDED IN THIS VOLUME

Attempting to categorise the diversity of work undertaken at King's College into groups of chapters is difficult. This diversity lies in the nature of nursing research itself, as its subject matter encompasses such a wide range of phenomena – from discourse of psychiatric nurses to assessment of patients' pain, from healing and flora of leg ulcers to evaluating care of the elderly in the community. Categorisation is especially difficult with a guiding philosophy of holism as opposed to separatism or division. The research undertaken does, however, fall into four major categories, each of which constitutes a section of the book. These are as follows:

1. The delivery of care.
2. Patients' and relatives' experiences and opinions.
3. Basic and post-basic education.
4. Career paths.

In the rest of this chapter the studies subsumed under each of these sections are briefly outlined.

The delivery of care: present practice and future directions

The first section of the book is concerned with descriptions of practice: how care is delivered at present and how it might be improved in the future. Two kinds of studies are included: first, those that focus on specific aspects of care, ranging from interactions between professionals and clients to the treatment of leg ulcers, and, second, those that examine the role that nurses and midwives fulfil in the health services.

In the first chapter Le May and Redfern explore the nature and frequency of touch between nurses and elderly people. As a fundamental component of non-verbal communication, touch may be particularly important for certain people at times of illness, yet little research to date has focused on its effect. This project is part of our ongoing programme of work on communication skills in nursing, which developed from Macleod Clark's early work in this area. The methodological problems involved in observing and recording interactions between nurses and patients are discussed by Le May and Redfern, as well as by authors of many of the other chapters in this volume.

While's study is an example of how information about practice can be obtained from secondary sources: in this instance from health visitors' records of events in the first 2 years of an infant's life. Analysis of these records demonstrated a strong relationship between home visiting practice and uptake of prophylactic measures, indicating the importance of personal contact in health promotion.

Chapman's work represents an attempt to understand the nature of the professional discourse of nurses, as constituted by their meetings and their written accounts, and the extent to which this discourse reflected the ideals of the therapeutic community in which they worked. Using techniques derived from literary criticism she demonstrates the richness of these data as a means of understanding how nurses perceive their work, and suggests that such data have been underused in nursing research in the past.

The importance of interdisciplinary collaboration and of sharing information with patients is demonstrated in Ross's study. This focused on discrepancies of knowledge about prescribed medication held by elderly patients, district nurses and general practitioners and examined the effect of a patient-held drug guide in reducing these discrepancies.

Gilchrist's contribution is obviously very different from the other chapters in this section. It deals with the very real problem of how to treat leg ulcers - a problem frequently encountered by nurses working in the community. Repeated microbiological and physical measures were taken to monitor healing of ulcers treated with a new kind of dressing. Trials of this kind require immense effort, but, as Gilchrist argues, not only are they essential if treatments and procedures are to be evaluated, but also nurses should take an active role in monitoring their work by initiating and carrying out such studies.

The nursing process is one of the most significant innovations in the profession in recent years, yet little is known about the extent to which it has been introduced into practice and of the difficulties that may have been encountered in its implementation. Hayward's chapter describes the process by which a working party undertook the task of documenting evidence on these issues and identifying priorities for research in this area. Drawing on documentation, previous research and the expertise of many professionals, this task was obviously a great challenge, but very much needed.

The final three chapters in this section are concerned with roles in health care, on the one hand with constraints that militate against role fulfilment, and on the other with opportunities to develop new and expanded roles. Robinson's work on the role of the midwife is an example of the former; her study demonstrates the extent to which opportunities for midwives to exercise their clinical judgment have diminished with increasing involvement of medical staff in normal maternity care. Developing the role of the nurse practitioner in general practice is the focus of Stilwell's work, while Minghella describes the introduction and evaluation of an expanded role for community psychiatric nurses in the management of parasuicides in the community.

The consumers' perspective: patients' and relatives' experiences and opinions

Perhaps it is a truism that nurses' care should be based on the preferences and wishes of those whom they serve, yet all too often research that attempts to document this finds considerable disparity between these wishes and the care provided. The second section of the book (Chapters 11-15) includes some of the work undertaken at King's College in this area. Brooking's chapter documents the extent to which British consumers are passive and fail to seek a degree of participation in their own health care. Whether nurses created this passivity and how they can rectify this for the benefit of patients and their families are important topics for debate. Seers's research demonstrates that nurses fail to assess pain on an individual basis for surgical patients, preferring routine approaches or standard regimes instead. Moreover, her study showed that nurses consistently and significantly rated patients' pain as lower than did the patients themselves.

Although the majority of patients taking part in West and Wilson-Barnett's study demonstrated an overall positive recovery from coronary surgery, their work identifies a group of patients who may be at risk of a poor outcome. They explore the feasibility of nurses assessing patients preoperatively and then providing extra support pre- and post-discharge for those identified as being at risk. Recovery from surgery is also the focus of Fordham's work, which was designed to investigate the relationship between physical fitness, work and leisure activities and the existence and treatment of an inguinal hernia. The combination of analytical strategies employed in this study demonstrates the importance of individual case histories in revealing findings that may be masked by group means and levels of statistical significance.

The final chapter in this section is concerned with those who suffer a stroke, many of whom will return home to be cared for by relatives. Hospital staff, however, often fail to involve these relatives in care during the period of the patient's hospitalisation, when skills could be taught and advice given. Batehup's research demonstrates this failure, despite the relatives' expressed wishes to be involved in this care and to prepare for the time when they will be the chief carer. Batehup maintains that relatives should be given the opportunity to participate in care if they wish to do so, and recommends the introduction of nurse specialists to provide teaching and support in this respect.

Preparation for practice: aspects of basic and post-basic education

The research described in this section of the book falls into two main sections. Chapters 16–20 are concerned with educational preparation for the role of staff nurse and sister and comprise analyses of basic and post-basic training schemes. Chapters 21–26, on the other hand, each focus on education for specific aspects of care of particular patient groups.

Turning first to basic nurse education, then whatever its future direction, the need for good clinical instruction and experience for the learner nurse will not diminish. This subject is tackled in the research reported here by Smith and Redfern and by Jacka and Lewin. Both studies investigate the learning environment of hospital wards using a strategy that combined observation, interviews and document analysis. Smith and Redfern's study comprised a cross-sectional study of first- and third-year students, whereas Jacka and Lewin undertook a cohort study of learners from the beginning of training to final qualification. The extent to which the affective component of nursing care was valued in practice and in teaching is the main focus of the former study; methods of monitoring the experience of individual learners is the focus of the latter. Both of these studies highlighted the importance of ward sisters in creating a conducive learning environment, a finding reported by many other researchers.

However, lack of preparation of ward sisters for this and other aspects of their role has also been a consistent research finding. This issue has been one of the main themes in the unit's programme of research and is represented in three chapters in this volume. Farnish identified those aspects of sisters' roles for which they felt the least well prepared, and Lathlean and her colleagues evaluated experimental training schemes for ward sisters. Concern also exists that newly registered nurses often feel inadequately prepared for their responsibilities, and that this is an important factor in poor retention rates. Consequently, experimental training schemes for these nurses have been introduced in some areas, and three of these were evaluated by Lathlean and her team.

Communication skills are at the heart of much nursing care, and a number of studies at King's College and elsewhere have investigated the teaching of such skills in basic, post-basic and degree courses. This development is represented in this volume by Macleod Clark and Tomlinson's work; this comprised an evaluation of integrating a communication skills teaching programme in schools of nursing, and a study of the extent to which nurse tutors are prepared to undertake teaching on this subject. Health education and promotion are increasingly recognised as important aspects of the role of nurses, midwives and health visitors. This is reflected in two chapters in this volume: Meyer's study of the introduction of a health education component in basic nurse training; and Macleod Clark et al's study of an educational programme designed to teach nurses, midwives and health visitors how to help their patients and clients to give up smoking.

The next two studies in this section report on the evaluation of teaching programmes designed to improve nursing skills in the care of particular groups of patients. In the first study, de Carle and Wilson-Barnett evaluated a ward-based teaching programme on the care of patients with a tracheal stoma, and in the second study Corner and Wilson-Barnett evaluated a workshop-based programme on the care of patients with cancer. Both studies were undertaken in response to earlier research, which indicated deficiencies in the psychological care provided for these patients. The tracheal stoma teaching programme was based on the premise that nursing should be taught where nursing is carried out, and was, therefore, ward based. It raises again the importance of the possession of teaching skills by practitioners, a topic explored in some of the earlier chapters.

The final chapter in this section is concerned with violence – a growing problem in many of the caring professions. As part of a wider study, Robinson and Barnes have investigated the provision of continuing education for nurses on the prevention and management of violence; their findings highlight various difficulties in the provision of relevant and appropriate courses on this subject.

Career paths of nurses and midwives

At a time of much concern about recruitment and retention of nursing and midwifery staff, the research on career paths described in the final section of the book is particularly timely. The first two chapters focus on midwives; one is a longitudinal study of the careers of midwives from the time of qualification until the present, and the other is a survey of the careers of male midwives. Both studies involved tracing midwives scattered worldwide and devised strategies for maximising response rates in this kind of research.

Two undergraduate students have contributed chapters in this section, demonstrating that research and publication can be achieved early on in nursing careers. The final chapter of the volume is in fact a report on a longitudinal study of the careers of all the King's and formerly the Chelsea graduates, the majority of whom have remained in nursing. Thus this study, like others of graduate nurses, indicates that a high level of education in nursing appears to be a worthwhile investment.

All the contributions in this volume arise from work that has been undertaken or directed by staff in one academic department of nursing studies over a decade. Advances and expansion in methods used and the continuation of work in certain areas are more evident of late. Major themes, developed through collaboration among staff, are evolving, and these are represented in this book. Many authors themselves view their research as part of an ongoing programme, learning about their area of study as well as the most successful research approaches. We hope that this progress will become apparent to the reader, who may share some of the authors' excitement and interests.

Section 1

The Delivery of Care: Present Practice and Future Directions

Chapter 2

Touch and Elderly People

Andrée C Le May and Sally J Redfern

This chapter focuses on one form of non-verbal communication that nurses can use as a powerful means of communication with patients – touch. We describe a research study designed to establish the nature and frequency of touch between nurses and elderly patients and the relationship of touch to patient well-being.

BACKGROUND

Touch is a basic need, which continues throughout life. Although an adult's need for touch may be less immediate than that of an infant or a child, situations can occur that increase this need. Sickness, danger and incapacity have been highlighted as reasons for adults to revert to earlier, more active states of tactile need and acceptance (Bowlby, 1958). Touch can communicate caring, empathy and reassurance as well as providing physical support, and is particularly important in nursing settings that are technologically sophisticated. Nurses who touch naturally emphasise the caring element of their role.

For the purpose of our research we adopted Watson's (1975) definition of touch as 'an intentional physical contact between two or more individuals'. Watson distinguished between two kinds of touch. 'Instrumental' touch is deliberate and necessary for task completion (e.g. taking a patient's pulse, or giving a patient a bed-bath), whereas 'expressive' touch is more spontaneous and affective and does not necessarily form part of a task (e.g. reassuring a patient by holding hands, or comforting a patient by putting an arm around his or her shoulder).

Despite the increased need for touch during illness, for example, studies have found that some patients may be deprived of expressive touch, particularly if they are impaired, dependent or elderly (Barnett, 1972; Watson, 1975; Goodykoontz, 1979).

Nurse–patient touch has been found to be effective in several patient-care settings. In intensive and coronary care units McCorkle (1974) found that if the nurse touched the patient's arm while talking to him or her, the patient was less tense and the value of the communication increased. McCorkle suggested that this might be because patients who received touch were more attentive and perceived the interaction as more meaningful, helpful and caring than did those who were not touched.

Whitcher and Fisher (1979) describe an experimental study that evaluated the effects of nurses touching patients during preoperative teaching on a patient's psychological and physiological responses. The touch intervention consisted of the nurse holding the patient's hand during the preoperative teaching. This was evaluated in several ways: by assessing the patient's satisfaction with preoperative instructions, measuring anxiety and the degree to which the patient liked the nurse, estimating the time the patient spent reading the preoperative literature, observing the extent to which touch was reciprocated, and measuring the patient's pulse and blood pressure. The results suggested that women in the touched group experienced more favourable reactions than men in either group and than women in the control group. The touched women were less anxious, demonstrated more positive preoperative behaviours (booklet reading, reciprocal touch and a greater liking for the nurse), and postoperatively their blood pressure levels were lower. The authors suggest that the men's negative responses may stem from having been socialised into believing that discomfort and dependency convey a lack of manliness and can only be exhibited by the very old or if under extreme stress. The touched person is seen to be of inferior status, and the toucher is dominant. Women may have more experience of touch from a variety of people and may, therefore, be more familiar with it.

Lorensen (1983) carried out a small study that focused on touching women in labour. She found that primiparous women in the experimental group responded more favourably than women in the control (usual care) group when given hugs and affectionate touches during their labour. These women had shorter labours and perceived the midwife as being helpful in relieving their discomfort. Touch, therefore, has a calming and comforting effect on patients in pain and is an effective means of communicating with patients in crisis.

The importance and effect of touch used by nurses caring for elderly patients has been studied by several authors. Touch can help old people to cope with bereavement, dependency and an altered body image, and it is a therapeutic form of non-verbal communication that can decrease sensory deprivation, increase reality orientation (Burnside, 1973) and, as Lorensen (1983) found, alleviate pain. Touch may also be one way of helping old people to recognise nurses who like them and are ready to listen and help them (Ernst and Shaw, 1980), and who promote trust and empathy (Hollinger, 1980). Touch may be the most effective way of communicating when other senses are impaired or declining.

Despite the advantages of touch it should be used with caution. The perceptive nurse recognises patients' needs for privacy and personal space, and considers individual differences in each person's need for and acceptance of touch. Touch may be misconstrued by both the toucher and the recipient. De Wever (1977) studied nursing home patients' perceptions of nurses' expressive touch and found that some people, especially some men, found nurses' touch uncomfortable. De Wever suggested that it may be more appropriate to use 'safe' touches, such as hand shakes, in these circumstances.

Other studies have emphasised the lack of expressive touch between health-team personnel and patients. Barnett (1972) found that registered nurses and junior student nurses used more expressive touch than senior student nurses and junior doctors. Patients who were less than 1 year old or aged between 26 and 33 years were more frequently touched than those aged between 6 and 17 or over 65 years.

The literature suggests that more attention should be directed towards exploring the use of touch, particularly expressive touch. Our study was designed to do this and we focused on one specific patient group that had been highlighted in earlier research as being deprived of expressive touch – elderly people.

THE STUDY

There were five aims to the study:

1. To record the amount and type of nurse–patient touch that occurred in different institutional environments for elderly people.
2. To identify individual characteristics that were associated with the use and acceptance of touch.
3. To establish whether nurses' attitudes towards the elderly were associated with their use of touch.
4. To determine whether patient dependency and well-being were associated with nurse touch.
5. To establish any relationship between nurses' expressive touch and patient well-being.

Patients were randomly selected from those consenting in each care setting. Eighty-six patients were included in the study from 10 care settings for elderly people (4 continuing care wards, 4 acute/rehabilitation wards, 1 day hospital and 1 private nursing home). The nurses (133) who interacted with the patients were observed and data concerning touch were collected.

Touch

Patient-focused observations of nurse–patient touch were made, using a time-sampling technique, during the day shift (7.15 to 21.30 hrs). As touches are often of very short duration and follow each other rapidly, a schedule was designed to facilitate fast, accurate recording of touch and its associated variables. This schedule consisted of the following items which were thought to be important to each touch episode:

1. *When* the touch occurred in each interaction.
2. The *duration* of the interaction.
3. The *length* of each touch within the interaction.
4. The *type of touch* – instrumental, expressive or undefinable – was recorded on a manikin in the *body area* touched.
5. The *response* of the recipient to each touch – silence, verbal or non-verbal communication – the essence of the verbal response and the type of non-verbal communication.
6. The *verbal communication*, if any, given by the toucher, and its nature.
7. The *task* or nature of the interaction.
8. The *patient's position* and the *nurse's position* during the touch.

Assessment of inter-observer reliability of the touch observation schedule was made on four occasions during the data collection. Reliability coefficients were calculated using the kappa coefficient (Cohen, 1960), and per cent agreement between the two observers. A kappa coefficient of $\geqslant 0.60$ was selected as an acceptable level of reliability (Cichetti, 1984), and a per cent agreement of $\geqslant 70$. Of the 10 schedule components, seven were consistently acceptable, with kappa coefficients greater than the criterion (when, duration, type of touch, body area touched, task, patient's position and nurse's position). The other three components (length of touch, recipient's response and verbal communication by toucher) were unacceptable, with kappa coefficients and percentage levels consistently below the criteria.

Table 2.1 Touches received by elderly patients during hours of observation

	Total 86 individuals		Continuing care wards 30 individuals		Day hospital 10 individuals		Acute rehabilitation wards 40 individuals		Nursing home 6 individuals		p
	n	%	n	%	n	%	n	%	n	%	
Instrumental touch	2275	88	1241	86	74	79	694	91	266	90	NS
Expressive touch	253	10	172	12	15	16	46	6	20	7	<0.001
Undefinable touch	62	2	30	2	5	5	19	3	8	3	
Total	2590		1443	(56)	94	(4)	759	(29)	294	(11)	
Touches per patient (mean)	30		48		9		19		49		

The numbers in parentheses refer to the percentage of all touches received in each setting.
NS = not significant.

These three unreliable components were difficult to assess, and despite rigorous training, they continued to be open to differing interpretations by the observers. Additional information was collected in the form of notes made after each interaction, which described the content, speed of touch and communication patterns observed. This information enabled a comprehensive description of the communication during the interaction to be made.

Touches from the nurse to the patient and from the patient to the nurse were observed and recorded. The patients gave 49 touches and received 2590. Of those they received, 2275 (88 per cent) were instrumental touches, 253 (10 per cent) were expressive and the remaining 62 (2 per cent) were undefinable (Table 2.1). The type of touch that nurses received from patients varied considerably from this, with 49 per cent (24) being expressive, 41 per cent (20) instrumental and 10 per cent (5) undefinable.

The amount and type of touch varied in the different settings, with patients in the two continuing care settings receiving, on average, the most touch (Table 2.1). Proportionately more expressive touch occurred in the four continuing care wards and the day hospital – 12 per cent and 16 per cent respectively. In the acute/rehabilitation wards and the nursing home most (90 per cent) of the touches were instrumental, and only 6–7 per cent were expressive.

The frequency of instrumental touch did not vary significantly between settings, but expressive touch did ($p < 0.001$), with more than expected occurring in the continuing care wards and the day hospital, and less than expected in the acute/rehabilitation wards and the nursing home.

From these results we can conclude that old people received more touch than they gave, and that the received touch was principally instrumental in nature. Undoubtedly nurses have to use a lot of instrumental touch in order to nurse patients, but the relatively low incidence of expressive touch, when compared with instrumental touch, does support earlier work by Barnett (1972) and Watson (1975).

Variables associated with touch

Biographical details were recorded for patients (e.g. age, reason for and length of admission, sex, ethnic group and occupation) and for nurses (e.g. sex, grade, age group and ethnic group), in order to identify individual characteristics that may have been associated with the use and acceptance of touch. Results indicate that there was a relationship between the amount of expressive touch patients received and their reason for admission, with patients admitted for 'social' reasons receiving more expressive touch than those admitted for 'medical' reasons ($p < 0.05$). There was also a relationship between the total amount of touch patients received and the length of time spent in hospital, with those who had been hospitalised for over 1 month receiving more touch than those admitted for shorter periods of time ($p < 0.05$). When nurses were considered, a relationship between the amount of touch they used and their age group was found, which suggested that older nurses (over 40 years) gave more touch than younger ones ($p < 0.05$).

In an attempt to look more closely at preferences for using and receiving touch, a photographic exercise was carried out to encourage nurses and old people to discuss their feelings about touch. Patients and nurses were individually shown pairs of monochrome photographs featuring a nurse and patient in communication. Each pair showed a similar interaction except for touch, which only occurred in one of the photographs. Subjects were asked to decide which photograph they preferred in each pair and to give reasons for their choice. This approach was taken to encourage patients and nurses to discuss their attitudes to communication and touch without questioning them directly.

Although no significant relationship was found between expressed preference for touch from the photographs and touch observed, some interesting points emerged. The patients' reasons for choosing the touch photographs varied, although 'touch' was the most frequently given reason (11.9 per cent). It was closely followed by other reasons not specifically related to physical contact, e.g. 'happy/cheerful' (11.6 per cent), 'smiling' (8.3 per cent), or 'better photograph' (6.5 per cent). Nurses, on the other hand, gave 'touch' as a reason for their choice more frequently than other reasons (31.7 per cent), with 'reassuring' (12.9 per cent) as the second most frequent reason. Another frequently occurring reason for choosing the touch photographs was that the patient looked 'happy/content' (12.6 per cent) or 'relaxed' (6.2 per cent).

Attitudes

Nurses' attitudes towards old people were assessed with the Kogan's (1961) Old People Scale, which is made up of 34 statements (17 positively phrased and 17 negatively phrased), for example: 'Most old people are cheerful, agreeable and good humoured' and 'Most old people are irritable, grumble and are unpleasant'. Subjects were asked the extent to which they agreed or disagreed with each statement. No significant relationship was found between the nurses' attitude scores and the amount or type of touch they used.

Dependency

Patient dependency was assessed with the modified version of the Crichton Royal Behavioural Rating Scale (Charlesworth and Wilkin, 1982). This 10-item scale is designed to assess patients' physical and mental ability, and it focuses on mobility, memory, orientation, communication, co-operation, restlessness, dressing, feeding, bathing and continence. Daily assessments were made of observed patients' dependency, based on information from the nurse-in-charge. Results suggest that more dependent patients (those with scores of 16 or above) received more touch than the less dependent, and similarly received more expressive touch, but the differences just failed to achieve significance ($p < 0.10$).

Well-being

A variety of approaches was used to assess patient well-being. The Affect Balance Scale (Bradburn, 1969), a 10-item scale which focuses on happiness and unhappiness, was completed by each patient, with the researcher's help if needed. The respondent was asked to answer 'yes' or 'no' to 10 questions relating to how she or he felt on that day, for example:

'Today have you felt:
1. Proud because someone complimented you on something you had done?
2. Upset because someone criticised you?'

Some earlier researchers have experienced problems in administering the Affect Balance Scale to elderly patients (e.g. Peace et al, 1979), so a short Well-being Scale was designed for the study (Le May and Redfern, 1987). This scale was developed with a sample of 'healthy' elderly volunteers, and it consists of five adjectives describing well-being – pleased, satisfied, happy, content and confident. Patients were asked to decide using a four-point scale (not at all, a little, quite a bit and extremely) how much they felt that way 'today'. The scale is being validated against the Affect Balance Scale, and preliminary analysis has shown a significant correlation between the Well-being Scale scores and the Positive Affect score of Bradburn's scale ($r = 0.56$, $p < 0.001$).

Patients' engagement levels were also assessed, using an adapted version of a technique developed by Felce et al (1980). These authors have suggested that the extent to which a patient is engaged in an activity may be an indirect indicator of well-being. Patients were observed individually and recorded as being engaged if they were pursuing an observable activity with another person or an object (e.g. reading, watching TV), were involved in daily living activities, or were purposefully moving about. One problem discovered with this technique is that any activity that cannot be observed (e.g. silent reminiscence) is classified as 'not engaged', when if patients were questioned about what they were doing, they might have been found to be actively engaged in thinking.

Felce et al's suggestion that engagement was a positive indicator of patient well-being was not supported in our study, as there was no significant relationship between engagement and well-being. Further work is necessary here, as the patients' desire for occupation in observable activities was not considered and may influence their well-being.

Although no significant relationship was found between the amount or type of touch patients received and their well-being ($p < 0.10$), the results do suggest that patients with low well-being scores received more expressive touch than patients with high scores. This might be because nurses recognised these patients as being unhappy and responded by giving them expressive touch, or because the patients needed something and called for a nurse, who responded with expressive touch. This is another area that needs further work, and could possibly benefit from more in-depth questioning of nurses and patients about touch in specific interactions.

CONCLUSIONS

Touch is a complex yet fundamental component of non-verbal communication, and this study has begun to explore touch between British nurses and elderly patients. Our study focused on developing a method for recording touch and its associated variables, and, by doing so, we have highlighted the need for further research. This should help us to understand the problems, as well as the benefits, of using touch in nursing practice.

If touch is to be studied in more depth, it would be beneficial to develop a simpler observation schedule, which could be used in conjunction with other recording devices (e.g. a small portable computer programmed as an event recorder, and a tape-recorder or a video-camera). Deeper questioning of patients and nurses about their perceptions and experience of touch is important if we are to learn more about use and acceptance of touch. This knowledge would help nurses to give appropriate touch as a skilled nursing intervention forming part of individualised nursing care.

This study has concentrated on one patient group, and replication of the study in other specialties would enable us to establish whether certain patients are deprived of expressive touch. In addition, a more detailed approach is needed to assess the effect of touch on patient well-being. The study described in this chapter forms a basis for future research in an area that is fundamentally linked to the caring role all nurses share.

ACKNOWLEDGEMENTS

This study was funded by the DHSS through a nursing research studentship awarded to Andrée Le May. We are indebted to the nursing and medical management who allowed us access, and to the nurses and old people who participated in the study.

REFERENCES

Barnett K (1972) A survey of the current utilization of touch by health team personnel with hospitalized patients. *International Journal of Nursing Studies*, **9**: 195–209.
Bowlby J (1958) The nature of the child's tie to his mother. *International Journal of Psychoanalysis*, **39**: 350–373.
Bradburn N M (1969) *The Structure of Psychological Wellbeing*. Chicago: NORC Aldine Publishing Co.
Burnside I M (1973) Touching is talking. *American Journal of Nursing*, **73**(12): 2060–2063.
Charlesworth A and Wilkin D (1982) *Dependency among Old People in Geriatric Wards, Psychogeriatric Wards and Residential Homes, 1977–1981*. Research Report No. 6, University of Manchester, Psychogeriatric Unit.
Cichetti D V (1984) On a model for assessing the security of infantile attachment: issues of observer reliability and validity. *The Behavioral and Brain Sciences*, **7**: 149–150.
Cohen J (1960) A co-efficient of agreement for nominal scales. *Educational and Psychological Measurement*, **20**(1): 37–48.
De Wever M K (1977) Nursing home patients' perception of nurses' affective touching. *Journal of Psychology*, **96**: 163–171.
Ernst P and Shaw J (1980) Touching is not taboo. *Geriatric Nursing* (New York), **1**(3): 193–195.
Felce D, Powell L, Jenkins J and Mansell J (1980) Measuring activity of old people in residential care. *Evaluation Review*, **4**: 371–387.
Goodykoontz L (1979) Touch: attitudes and practice. *Nursing Forum*, **18**(10): 4–17.
Hollinger L M (1980) Perception of touch in the elderly. *Journal of Gerontological Nursing*, **6**(12): 741–746.
Kogan N (1961) Attitudes towards old people. The development of a scale and an examination of its correlates. *Journal of Abnormal and Social Psychology*, **62**: 44–54.
Le May A C and Redfern S J (1987) A study of non-verbal communication between nurses and elderly patients. In: *Research in the Nursing Care of Elderly People*, ed. Fielding P. Chichester: John Wiley.
Lorensen M (1983) Effects of touch in patients during a crisis situation in hospital. In: *Nursing Research: 10 Studies in Patient Care*, ed. Wilson-Barnett J. Chichester: John Wiley.

McCorkle R (1974) Effects of touch on seriously ill patients. *Nursing Research*, **23**(2): 125-132.

Peace S M, Hall J F and Hamblin G R (1979) *The Quality of Life of the Elderly in Residential Care.* Research Report No. 1, Survey Research Unit, Polytechnic of North London.

Watson W H (1975) The meanings of touch: geriatric nursing. *Journal of Communication*, **25**(3): 104-112.

Whitcher S J and Fisher J D (1979) Multidimensional reaction to therapeutic touch in a hospital setting. *Journal of Personality and Social Psychology*, **37**(1): 87-96.

Chapter 3

Health Visiting Practice with Families with Young Children

Alison E While

The increasing cost of the curative services caused the Department of Health and Social Security (DHSS) to posit the view that curative medicine may increasingly be subject to the law of diminishing returns (1976). Indeed, McKeown (1976) argued that the burden of disease and the cost of curative services could be reduced through the redistribution of funds in favour of prevention.

The history of health visiting is one of an occupation specifically developed to provide a preventive home visiting service to children and their families. Both the Brotherston (SHHD, 1973) and Court (DHSS, 1976b) Reports laid great emphasis upon the value of preventive paediatrics, and particularly acknowledged the contribution of health visitors in this field. The reports identified developmental assessment as the means of recognising handicapping conditions at the earliest possible time and expressed the view that subsequent active management of the identified problem would reduce the detrimental consequences for the child. The value of infant immunisation lies in its very real contribution to child welfare and the prevention of ill-health. These prophylactic measures have had a striking effect on the control of infectious disease in the post-war period (Dick, 1978) and their cost-effectiveness is now well established. Health visiting has been identified as a means of persuading parents to accept prophylactic care and of educating parents in child care. Health visitor home visits were also seen as a means of providing health education to parents who did not attend child health clinics. The Black Report (DHSS, 1980) has further suggested that inequalities in health experience could be reduced through the development of community services and health education.

PREVIOUS HEALTH VISITING RESEARCH

Dingwall (1977a) demonstrated, in his study of a particular training course, that the implicit assumption that all previous professional knowledge is well integrated by the experience of health visitor training does not necessarily hold true. Indeed, he found that health visitor students may be presented with a series of conflicting perspectives, and, thus, it may be argued that the nature of the present training does not set out a coherent 'picture' of health visiting.

19

The acquisition of organisational and planning skills is considered fundamental in health visitor training (CETHV, 1982). In an exploratory study it has been suggested that, although health visitors were confident in their performance of tasks and saw the prevention of ill-health as important, they were vague about priorities (Bolton, 1980). The widely used terms 'at risk' and 'vulnerable' apparently encompassed such a wide variety of meanings that Bolton doubted whether they could be considered useful terms in the organisation of health visitor work, despite their status in health visitor training. Similarly, Robinson (1982) has contended that different health visitors may define their objectives according to fundamentally different criteria, while Dingwall (1977a) found that objectives and priorities set by health visitor fieldworkers and their managers do not necessarily coincide. Thus it seems that health visitors use discretion in deciding how they apportion their own resources in terms of home visiting and it may be argued that health visitors individually decide what they consider to be good practice.

The national statistics relating to health visiting are confusing, since there seems to be a variable definition of what counts as a 'case'. Robinson (1982) has further argued that the data derived from the collection of national statistics of health visiting activity are misleading because of differences in local interpretations of the requirements of activity recording. However, despite this limitation, the Central Statistical Office (1981) showed that most (60 per cent) health visitor contacts were with children aged under 5 years and their families. This was similar to the pattern of contact revealed by Dunnell and Dobbs (1982) in their national survey of community nurses.

A review of research in the field of health visiting during the 20 years 1960-1980 indicated that the majority of health visitor clientele were families containing young children (50-80 per cent of the clientele visited) (Clark, 1981). Perkins (1977), Fitton (1981) and Speakman (1984) also found a similar concentration upon families with children under 5 years of age. And, although home visits account for between a quarter and a third of the health visitors' time (Clark, 1981), no study has considered the amount of home visiting an individual client may receive. Indeed, this most important constituent of health visiting activity has only been investigated in terms of the number of home visits made by a health visitor during an average day or average week, the average duration of home visits, the proportion of 'no-reply' visits and the initiation of home visits. Clark (1981) concluded that most home visits are health visitor initiated, an analysis with which McClymont's (1983) more recent survey concurred, which supported the view that it is health visitors themselves who decide to whom they will allocate their time.

A potential measure of the effectiveness of health visiting in terms of promoting child welfare must be an examination of the relationship between health visiting and infant mortality and morbidity rates. Research in Sheffield suggested that it was possible to identify 'at risk' infants and their families who, when given intensive home visiting by health visitors, experienced much improved mortality rates (McWeeney and Emery, 1975). Protestos's (1973) research, which found that the 'at risk' population included a large proportion of non-utilisers of health services, suggested that the health visiting services may succeed in providing an 'outreach' service to those families, through individual education and support and mediation with other health service agencies. More evidence of the benefits of health visiting has been offered by MacQueen (1960) and the Wynns (1974). However, the assumption that health visiting alone may achieve such notable success in the field of infant mortality seems to disregard all the evidence that suggests that social circumstance has much influence upon child health status. A more recent study by Powell (1986) developed the Sheffield project further.

There has, however, only been one study (Butler, 1977) that has attempted to investigate whether health visitors spontaneously positively discriminate towards families in poor social circumstance. Butler suggested that, although the home visiting practice in his sample did not reflect a bias towards the lower social classes, home visiting positively discriminated towards the disadvantaged as identified by means of a Social Index (Osborn and Morris, 1979). It was notable, however, that Butler (1977) referred to a significance level of less than 0.01 when the data involved very large sample numbers.

RATIONALE FOR THIS STUDY

Despite the long history of health visiting in the field of preventive paediatrics, research evaluating the contribution of health visiting to child health is very limited. No research had previously examined 'normal' health visiting practice and related it to the uptake of prophylactic care. This research further examined what 'normal' health visiting practice was in the research area, in terms of how many home visits individual families could expect to receive in the first 2 years subsequent to an infant's birth.

METHODS AND DESIGN OF STUDY

The study was designed to provide data on a wide range of aspects of health visiting practice, thus highlighting problems and potential research areas. This descriptive study consisted of a systematic survey which focused on utilisation rates of child health services currently available within the National Health Service (NHS) and the contact of health visitors with families at the home.

A retrospective design was selected as the most appropriate to achieve the stated aims. The study benefited from this choice of design because it permitted two types of comparison to be made without the manipulation of a variable. First, it allowed for comparison of three sample groups (inner city, suburb and affluent suburb), which were selected in a similar manner and differed only in their location of residence, and, second, it allowed a comparison to be drawn between different utilisation levels of NHS provisions and aspects of the infant's social history.

The sample was drawn from a series of cohort months, and a census of health records relating to infants born in a selected cohort was undertaken. Thus, all children known to be resident in the selected geographical areas on their second birthday were included in the sample. The geographical areas were derived from local authority and district health authority boundaries.

A survey of health visitor records (home visiting and clinic records) permitted the gathering of data retrospectively. Data were collected by means of an interview with all health visitors practising in the selected geographical areas and holding records for infants included in the chosen birth cohort. The health visitors were thus able to control access to the records by the researcher and, in so doing, to maintain families' confidentiality.

The data collection instrument was a questionnaire consisting of 143 questions, which was designed to extract as much relevant information as possible from the records. The reliability of health visitor records as a data source has been explored in depth (While, 1987a) and, for the purposes of this study, were found to be a reliable source of data. The use of records as a data source was further justified because data extraction did not depend on decoding the record content. Rather, the records were perceived as providing a timetable of health events during the first 24 months of selected infants' lives, as known and recorded by health visitors.

The collected data were analysed by computer with use of the Statistical Package for the Social Sciences (Nie et al, 1975).

MAIN FINDINGS

The data revealed that inner city health visitors made more home visiting contacts than their counterparts in the suburbs. During the first 6 months of an infant's life, the difference between the areas was small; however, health visiting practice became significantly disparate when comparing visits in an infant's entire first year of life with visits in the second year of life (see Tables 3.1, 3.2 and 3.3). Access to families was not a problem in any of the geographical areas.

Table 3.1   Area of residence by health visitor home visiting during the first 6 months of infant life

Area of residence		Number of home visits			
		0 %	1-2 %	3-6 %	7-24 %
Inner City	(n=756)	4.2	31.8	50.6	13.4
Suburb	(n=127)	4.0	42.9	46.0	7.1
Affluent suburb	(n=97)	2.1	41.2	47.4	9.3

$\chi^2 11.231 01.6df. p = 0.0815$

Table 3.2   Area of residence by health visitor home visiting during the first year of infant life

Area of residence		Number of home visits			
		0-2 %	3-6 %	7-10 %	11-24 %
Inner City	(n=756)	21.6	46.8	23.1	8.5
Suburb	(n=127)	31.7	49.2	15.9	3.2
Affluent suburb	(n=97)	19.6	60.8	15.5	4.1

$\chi^2 18.893 16.6df. p = 0.0043$

Table 3.3   Area of residence by health visitor home visiting during the second year of infant life

Area of residence		Number of home visits			
		0 %	1-2 %	3-6 %	7-24 %
Inner City	(n=756)	10.8	47.9	33.9	7.4
Suburb	(n=127)	22.2	47.6	24.6	5.6
Affluent suburb	(n=97)	28.9	54.6	11.3	5.2

$\chi^2 44.385 29.6df. p = < 0.0001$

Table 3.4   Area of residence by home visiting to encourage uptake of
hearing test as percentage

Area of residence		Home visit %	No home visit %
Inner city	(n = 756)	66.4	33.6
Suburb	(n = 127)	57.4	42.5
Affluent suburb	(n = 97)	74.2	25.8

$\chi^2 7.10444. 2df. p = 0.0287$

Health visiting practice was very similar in the three localities regarding encouraging the uptake of the sixth week developmental assessment (95 per cent of infants were visited), the uptake of the first immunisation (85 per cent of infants), the uptake of the second immunisation (62 per cent of infants), the uptake of the third immunisation (55 per cent of infants) and the uptake of the measles immunisation (69 per cent of infants). Uptake of the hearing test was less encouraged through home visiting in the suburb than in the inner city, while the affluent suburb health visitors made more home visits to encourage uptake than did those in the inner city (see Table 3.4). The toddler developmental assessment was only a feature of inner city prophylactic provision and, therefore, home visiting of toddlers prior to this assessment only occurred in the inner city (69 per cent of infants were visited).

A home visit by a health visitor was found to enhance the uptake of the sixth week developmental assessment ($\chi^2 118.00288. 1df. p = <0.0001$). Furthermore, a home visit by a health visitor prior to the uptake of the first immunisation not only enhanced the uptake generally, but was also related to the increased uptake of the pertussis element ($\chi^2 27.68515. 2df. p = <0.0001$). The completion of the primary immunisation with the uptake of the third immunisation was not related to a previous health visitor home visit; however, general health visitor home visiting during the first 6 months of an infant's life ($\chi^2 59.03997. 3df. p = <0.0001$) and second year of an infant's life ($\chi^2 13.26516. 3df. p = 0.005$) was important to increased uptake. Health visiting practice was also found to be related to the uptake of the infant hearing test; of particular importance was general home visiting contact during early infancy ($\chi^2 52.23940. 3df. p = <0.0001$). Both general home visiting practice and a home visit prior to a toddler developmental assessment were significantly related to improved uptake levels in the inner city samples. Measles vaccination uptake in all three localities was lower than for the other immunisations, with only inner city infants reaching an uptake level in excess of 60 per cent. Among that group there was a weak relationship between health visiting practice and uptake levels.

Analysis of home visiting practice demonstrated that health visitors appeared to give priority to families with infants under 6 months of age who had also experienced adverse childbirth factors, rather than to families with poor social circumstances (While, 1986). The analysis of home visiting practice during the entire first year of infant life revealed the emergence of a different priority system, in which a selected number of social factors were associated with increased support, such as lower social class, council accommodation and receipt of social work assistance. However, throughout the first year of infant life, increased health visitor home visiting was also related to known morbidity as measured by infant hospital attendance. In contrast, the analysis of home visiting practice during the second year of infant life demonstrated an attempt by health visitors to compensate for social disadvantage. Thus, health visitors provided additional home visiting support to families with a variety of detrimental social attributes (While, 1986), although known infant morbidity as measured by hospital attendance continued to attract increased home visiting by health visitors.

DISCUSSION

The different health visiting practice in the three localities cannot be explained in terms of organisational differences, since none of the three districts had health visitor home visiting policies that expressly stated optimum visiting patterns, and all the health visitors had caseloads of similar size. The variation in home visiting patterns would seem, therefore, to reflect the selected performance of the health visitors themselves.

The findings suggested that there was a strong relationship between home visiting practice and the uptake of prophylactic care, such that health visitors are effective in promoting the uptake of prophylactic measures. Perhaps health visitor home visits provide the opportunity to persuade and reassure parents, with informed answers about particular health issues such as pertussis (While, 1987b). Furthermore, the value of general home visiting contact may rest upon the fostering of regular personal contact with a health visitor, which allows parents to extend their knowledge of the efficacy of prophylactic care, while also providing details of relevant service provisions for health service consumers and, thereby, facilitating access. Indeed, this study supported the assertion of Dingwall (1977b) that postal reminders are a poor substitute for regular personal contact in the field of health promotion.

The limited research in the field of evaluating the effectiveness of health visiting has produced favourable results. However, the Sheffield Study (Carpenter and Emery, 1974, 1977) and Powell's study (1986) provided considerably more contact for 'at risk' families with the health visiting service than was revealed in this survey of health records. Lauri's (1981) study was also based on a more frequent contact. However, it is noteworthy in this survey how few families received frequent, regular contact with their health visitor. The vast majority of families received six or fewer home visits during the entire first year of their infant's life, a similar finding to that of Butler (1977). This limited home visiting contact was unlikely to yield the therapeutic results suggested in the research studies. As in Butler's (1977) study, this survey revealed a dramatic decrease in home visiting to infants over 1 year of age, so that most families received minimal health visitor home visiting, of one or two visits, during the second year. It may be argued that such minimal contact with families is unlikely to sustain a full teaching programme that will enhance child health status.

According to Clark's (1981) review, health visitors spend at least a quarter of their time on home visits, the majority of which are to families containing young children. However, despite this concentration of resources upon the home visiting of such families, neither this study nor Butler's (1977) suggested that health visiting resources are able to sustain adequate home visiting practice for meaningful health promotion through frequent and regular contact of the type evaluated in the sudden infant death studies. Furthermore, frequent and regular support was found to promote successful breast feeding (Houston and Howie, 1981).

Findings from this survey reported elsewhere suggest that health visitors employ a variety of strategies to organise their home visiting practice (While, 1986). It appeared that the health visitors showed a preference for a medical model in the organisation of their practice with families with an infant aged less than 6 months. It was noteworthy that factors relating to childbirth and known infant morbidity, rather than factors associated with poor social circumstance, increased home visiting support. While (1985) argued that the health visitors used a medical model for the organisation of their work because they lacked an alternative framework. Analysis of home visiting practice during the entire first year of infant life suggested a move away from a medical model towards a consideration of the infant's social circumstance. However, the use of the Observation Register and other morbidity indicators continued to influence home visiting practice. It may, therefore, be argued that health visiting may not be fulfilling its potential, because not only is the extent of home support limited, but also the extra support was not wholly directed towards disadvantaged families who would benefit from an 'outreach' service. The analysis of home visiting practice during the second year of infant life revealed a more positive attempt to compensate for poor social circumstance, with health visitors offering greater support to families with a variety of adverse variables in their social history. The analysis, however, did not permit an understanding of why health visitors adopted a different strategy, and it may be argued that they either responded to the reduced prophylactic care uptake rates of disadvantaged families or that they adopted a model similar to Becker's Health Belief Model (1974) in the organisation of their work.

The limited amount of home visiting to families with infants in their second year of life is of special concern in view of the much reduced child health clinic attendance rates. The consequence must be a very limited amount of child surveillance and health promotion. Furthermore, the study revealed that many families even with children aged under 1 year received a minimal number of home visits. It is difficult to believe that health visitors were able to use their skills to the full and sustain a comprehensive teaching and support programme with this level of contact.

The use of a medical model for the organisation of home visiting in the early months of infant life may reflect the lack of an underpinning theoretical framework in health visiting, so that the health visitors returned to their nursing origins to assess need. Indeed, Dingwall (1977a) argued that student health visitors were not presented with a clear framework during training. The problem is perhaps further exacerbated by the lack of a definition of what constitutes good practice (Clark, 1983), so that health visitors vacillate between a relationship-orientated approach and a problem-orientated approach to practice. The dependence upon an apprenticeship model for practical training, during which a student health visitor may see only one model of practice that may not be the 'ideal' (Chapman, 1979; While, 1980), would seem to contribute to the 'problem' of health visiting.

Three areas of future research emerged from this study: a description of health visiting practice outside London, and especially rural health visiting practice, an investigation of how health visitors think they organise their home visiting practice, and the development of a health visitor priority scale instrument to aid health visitor practice.

REFERENCES

Becker M H (1974) The health belief model and sick role behaviour. *Health Education Monograph*, **2**(4): 409–419.

Bolton G (1980) Prevention: an exploratory study of health visiting in England, Wales and Scotland. *Health Visitor*, **53**(6): 203–206.

Butler N R (1977) *Family and Community Influences on 0–5's; Utilisation of Pre-school Day-care and Preventive Health Care.* Paper from a seminar on '0–5: a changing population, implications for parents, the public and policy makers', held at the Institute of Child Health, University of London on May 20 1977. London: Voluntary Organisations Liaison Council for Under Fives.

Carpenter R G and Emery J L (1974) Identification and follow-up of infants at risk of sudden death in infancy. *Nature*, **250**: 729.

Carpenter R G and Emery J L (1977) Final results of study of infants at risk of sudden death. *Nature*, **268**: 724-725.

Central Statistical Office (1981) *Social Trends II*. London: Her Majesty's Stationery Office.

Chapman V (1979) *An Exploratory Study of the Role of the Fieldwork Teacher*. Unpublished MSc Thesis, University of Surrey.

Clark J (1981) *What Do Health Visitors Do? A Review of Research 1960-1980*. London: Royal College of Nursing.

Clark J (1983) Educating health visiting practice. *Health Visitor*, **56**(6): 205-208.

Council for the Education and Training of Health Visitors (1982) *Rules, Regulations, Notes for Guidance and Syllabuses for Courses*. London: CETHV.

Department of Health and Social Security (1976a) *Prevention and Health, Everybody's Business: A Reassessment of Public and Personal Health*, Cmnd 7047. London: Her Majesty's Stationery Office.

Department of Health and Social Security (1976b) *Fit for the Future. Report of the Committee on Child Health Services*, Cmnd 6684. Chairman: Professor S D M Court. London: Her Majesty's Stationery Office.

Department of Health and Social Security (1980) *Inequalities in Health*. Report of a research working group. Chairman: Sir D Black. London: Department of Health and Social Security.

Dick G (1978) *Immunisation*. London: Update.

Dingwall R W J (1977a) *The Social Organisation of Health Visitor Training*. London: Croom Helm.

Dingwall R (1977b) What future for health visiting? Evidence to the Royal Commissions on the National Health Service. *Nursing Times*, **73**, June 2, Occasional Paper, pp. 77-79.

Dunnell K and Dobbs J (1982) *Nurses Working in the Community*. OPCS. London: Her Majesty's Stationery Office.

Fitton J M (1981) What health visitors say they do - a job description approach. *Health Visitor*, **54**(4): 159-162.

Houston M J and Howie P W (1981) Home support for the breast feeding mother. *Midwife, Health Visitor and Community Nurse*, **17**(9): 378-382.

Lauri S (1981) The public health nurse as a guide in infant child care and education. *Journal of Advanced Nursing*, **6**(4): 297-303.

McClymont A (1983) *Setting Standards in Health Visiting Practice*. A workshop for Health Visitors, Fieldwork Teachers and Nursing Officers (Health Visiting) in the Northern Region, June 1981-June 1982. Edinburgh: National Board for Nursing, Midwifery and Health Visiting for Scotland.

McKeown T (1976) *The Role of Medicine: Dream, Mirage or Nemesis?* London: Nuffield Provincial Hospitals Trust.

MacQueen I A G (1960) Evaluation of a scheme of health education. *Medical Officer*, **103**: 295-298.

McWeeney P and Emery J (1975) Unexpected postneonatal deaths (cot deaths) due to a recognisable disease. *Archives of Disease in Childhood*, **50**(3): 191-196.

Nie H H, Hull C H, Jenkins J G, Steinbrennen K and Bent D H (1975) *Statistical Package for the Social Sciences*. New York: McGraw-Hill.

Osborn A F and Morris A (1979) The rationale for a composite index of social class and its evaluation. *British Journal of Sociology*, **30**(1): 39-60.

Perkins E R (1977) *Community Nursing and Midwifery in the Sutton Area: Opportunities for Health Education*. Leverhulme Health Education Project, Occasional Paper No. 5, University of Nottingham.

Powell J (1988) Study on home visiting of babies in Gosport at high risk of sudden infant death. In: *Research in Preventive Community Nursing Care*, ed. While A E, pp. 147-164. Chichester: John Wiley.

Protestos C D (1973) Obstetric and perinatal histories of children who died unexpectedly (cot death). *Archives of Disease in Childhood*, **48**: 835-841.

Robinson J (1982) *An Evaluation of Health Visiting*. London: CETHV.

Scottish Home and Health Department (1973) *Towards an Integrated Child Health Service*. Chairman: Sir J Brotherston. Edinburgh: Her Majesty's Stationery Office.

Speakman J (1984) Measuring the immeasurable. *Nursing Times*, **80**(May 30): 56-58.

While A E (1980) *On Becoming a Health Visitor*. Unpublished MSc Thesis, Polytechnic of the South Bank, London.

While A E (1985) *Health Visiting and Health Experience of Infants in Three Areas*. Unpublished PhD Thesis, Chelsea College, University of London.

While A E (1986) To home visit or not to home visit? In: *Research in Preventive Community Nursing Care*, ed. While A E, pp. 165-176. Chichester: John Wiley.

While A E (1987a) Records as a data source: the case for health visitor records. *Journal of Advanced Nursing*, **12**: 757-763.

While A E (1987b) Health visitor contribution to pre-school child prophylaxis. *Public Health*, **101**: 229-232.

Wynn M and Wynn A (1974) *The Protection of Maternity and Infancy*. A study of the services for pregnant women and young children in Finland and some comparisons with Britain. London: Council for Children's Welfare.

Chapter 4

Observing Nurses' Talk in a Psychotherapeutic Community

Gillian Chapman

INTRODUCTION

The study described here was concerned with a group of nurses working in a psychotherapeutic community and with what they communicated to each other, to members of the multi-disciplinary team, to the hospital authorities and to the nursing profession about their work. In the community, neurotic, depressed and suicidal patients were treated without drugs. The therapeutic regime consisted of psychosocial nursing and psychoanalytically informed psychotherapy. The theoretical models that nurses used to understand patients, and the language they used to describe patients and events in the community, were key elements of the therapeutic programme. The term *nurses' discourse* is used in the study to describe this mix of theory, practice and language.

Two theoretical strands informed the research strategy and design. The first, concerned with professionalisation and status (Etzioni, 1969; Friedson, 1970, 1983) and its links with knowledge and power (Johnson, 1977; Foucault, 1961, 1973, 1981, 1982), led to an interest in nurses' access to knowledge, professional theoretical models and discourses. It was of interest to establish what, if any, therapeutic discourse informed nurses talk about their work in a therapeutic community, and to discover if this was reflected in the way they communicated with each other and members of the multidisciplinary team about their understanding of patients. The second theoretical strand was concerned with the epistemological debate about the relative merits of qualitative and quantitative methods when studying language in a natural setting (Hammersley and Atkinson, 1983). Both elements of the research, together with some of the main findings and their relevance to nursing, are discussed in this chapter.

BACKGROUND

With a few notable exceptions, nursing practice has rarely been examined in terms of its own intrinsic properties in the sociological and historical literature. Nursing has more often been viewed in terms of its secondary association with other professional interests (medicine) and social processes (deviance, professionalisation), or is seen as a special case of these processes. For example, recent feminist and Marxist analyses of the development of health-care systems mention nurses as a special case of class or gender subordination (Ehrenreich and Ehrenreich, 1975; Leeson and Gray, 1978; Doyal, 1979). Similarly, nurses have been viewed historically in terms of the professionalising activities of nursing's major figures (Abel Smith, 1979). Nurses' discourse in the early years is characterised as being essentially ideological and moral in nature (Maggs, 1983). The rhetoric of reform in nursing stressed prevailing nineteenth century values about what constituted a good woman/wife. Thus the personal attributes of the nurse became the hallmark of professional discourse about nursing at this time. Nurses' technical and theoretical expertise was not articulated. Apart from the studies mentioned earlier, and more recent anecdotal accounts provided by the Royal College of Nursing History of Nursing Group (Royal College of Nursing, 1984, 1985), the empirical reality of nurses' clinical practice and discourse in the formative years is largely lost to historical research.

In the sociological literature, on the other hand, there are two main areas in which nurses feature. First, in work associated with the profession and its organisation (Etzioni, 1969), and, second, in studies concerned with the experience of patients in organisations in which nurses work. In the one area nursing is portrayed as an unequal struggle with dominant medical and organisational forms, in the other as being organisationally passive with respect to superordinate processes of social and administrative control of different patient groups. Perhaps influenced by this assumption that nurses are closely bound and identified with the organisational procedures and regulations of the environment in which they work but do not control, other authors have concentrated on these aspects of nursing practice. In the substantive areas of mental and physical illness, writers like Glaser and Strauss (1965, 1968) on the social organisation of dying in hospital, Goffman (1970) on the underlife of the asylum, and Roth (1963) on the social processes of recovery from tuberculosis, refer to nurses through the organisational processes in which they work. Nurses, when identified, seem involved by virtue of the 'accident' of their participation in a particular organisational structure. In these and other studies, which focus on the experience of patients, nurses are portrayed either as cultural dupes facilitating oppressive organisational regimes or as culturally culpable for unreflexively acting as agents of those regimes that concentrate on the normalisation of social deviance (e.g. Holohan, 1977). Little attention seems to be paid to the meaning of nurses' clinical practices to the nurses themselves, or to the theories that underpin that practice, a notable exception being, perhaps, two studies of nurses in psychiatric settings (Clarke, 1978; Allen, 1981).

Research into clinical practice in nursing is in its infancy in Great Britain. Research in communications has tended to concentrate on nurse–patient interactions (Macleod Clark, 1984). Those studies that look at nurse-to-nurse reporting (Lelean, 1973; Shea, 1984) have been generated by pragmatic and normative concerns of what counts as good nursing practice. The view was taken in this research that nurses' utterances and talk and their written accounts formed part of a professional discourse – the set of meanings, beliefs and ideas that professionals bring to their everyday practices. It was, thus, treated neutrally with respect to 'good' practice, acting rather as a resource to discover what that practice was. This idea flows from Foucault and his critique of psychiatry and psychoanalytic discourse. Foucault (1982) argued that individuals are made subjects to psychiatric and psychoanalytic discourse and become tied to the identity it provides for them through their own self-knowledge. Like religion, psychiatric discourse requires that people expose their innermost secrets about fundamental experiences, and, far from liberation and self-actualisation, it makes them objects of their own knowing. Thus they become identities (say, a 'neurotic' mother) within a discourse they do not themselves produce and which predefines certain ideas, beliefs and behaviours as being normal or abnormal. The therapeutic community in which the research was undertaken was, on the one hand, part of a therapeutic movement that challenged the type of orthodox psychiatry Foucault criticised, while, on the other, was based on psychoanalytic and psychosocial principles of which he was equally critical. Therapeutic communities differ with client group and institutional setting (Clark, 1964) but they mostly attempt to work according to the following principles (Kennard and Roberts, 1983):

1. Respect for the individual client as a citizen with the capacity for autonomous action.
2. Shared decision-making with residents about day-to-day life in the community.
3. Use of the mechanism of meetings and groups to develop openness of communication about problems, feelings and conflicts.
4. Stressing an ordinary domestic environment in which clients can engage in meaningful, purposeful activity.

Clearly, talk, conversation and interactions with patients are the prime therapeutic tools. Recent research in other therapeutic communities suggested that it was also the means by which social reality was constructed, defined and reproduced (Bloor, 1980, 1981; Bloor and Fonkert, 1982; Baron, 1984). One purpose of the research was, therefore, to discover whether nurses' discourse reflected ideas of democracy, individuality and co-operation; another purpose was to discover the extent to which nurses' discourse defined patients in oppressive or pejorative ways.

STUDY DESIGN AND METHODS

The aims of the research were threefold:

1. To describe what nurses' discourse in the therapeutic community setting might be, and to establish the extent to which it reflected the principles noted above.
2. To test Foucault's ideas about the dominating elements of therapeutic discourse in a contemporary site of emergence.
3. To develop methods of data collection and analysis suitable for this purpose.

A range of methods of data collection and data analysis was used. Ethnographic techniques of observation and interview, together with representative sampling, were used to collect data. Examples of natural language (both verbal and written) were obtained without the imposition of the researcher's categories and constructs. This produced a wealth of material with associated problems of analysis (Atkinson, 1981). In order to surmount the problem of bias in the selection of data for analysis (Dingwall, 1981), and to avoid the irony of the researcher adjudicating between different accounts as if there were one truth (Garfinkel, 1967; Silverman, 1985), some quantitative techniques were used. Measures of statistical inference were used to strengthen, test and discover associations and conceptual relationships. The research was undertaken in three stages.

First stage

The hospital concerned was viewed as a case (Clyde Mitchell, 1983). It was one of the originators of the therapeutic community movement in Great Britain. Logical rather than statistical inference suggested that the central features of therapeutic community discourse would emerge in this setting. That is, while it was not claimed that the hospital and its therapeutic programme were representative of all therapeutic communities, the logic of discourse analysis is that elements of a particular therapeutic discourse will be revealed in any site of emergence. This is because language is a system of signs which derive their meaning only in relations to each other (Saussure, 1974; Hawkes, 1983). There is no necessary link between the sign (e.g. the word 'fire') and the event it symbolises. Each native language speaker, therefore, has a grasp of the abstract set of rules that govern the way these signs are structured in relation to each other, and he/she brings this competence in the language to each of his/her individual performances of that language. Each individual performance, however imperfect or complex, contains within it the structure of the language system from which it arose, in much the same way as the geneticist may identify the genetic structure of the body from the study of one cell. A more pertinent example might be concerned with how readily the rules governing surgical discourse (which might include references to swabs, incisions, forceps, scalpels, etc.) might be identified by observing the conversations in an operating theatre. Despite varied performances from surgeon or sister, certain features of the discourse would remain the same and could be identified at random sites of emergence.

A period of 9 months' participant observation helped to identify key sites of nurses' professional discourse, as well as to provide information about nursing practice. Given the range of sites in which nurses talked about their work, some sampling was required to ensure systematic and representative collection of data within the hospital. The criteria for selection of sites can be found in Chapman (1987). The sites included nurse-to-nurse accounts (nurse handover meetings), nurse-to-administration accounts (24-hour reports) and nurse-to-profession accounts (a published text).

Second stage

Nurses' 24-hour written reports were collected over a 4-month period prospectively, and a sample of 80 texts was obtained. A quantitative content analysis of topics of discourse, using the sentence as the unit of analysis, was undertaken. Criteria for coding and categorisation of material are to be found in Chapman (1988).

Third stage

Nurses' handover meetings were recorded with a tape-recorder over a period of 4 weeks, with the researcher present at the meeting observing and recording interactions. Four hours of material in total was transcribed. The methods of analysis were twofold: first, a thematic analysis in which unit ideas in sequences of conversation were identified, and, second, a structural analysis using techniques derived from literary criticism. Here the units of analysis were 'lexias'. [Barthes (1966) and Hawkes (1983) provide an explanation of these ideas.]

A key text selected by the senior nurse for distribution to nurse applicants was selected, and socio-linguistic techniques were used to identify underlying structures and relationships in the narrative. The unit of analysis was the phrase, and the results were tested for statistical significance. [Trew (1979) provides a detailed guide to the techniques used.]

FINDINGS

The data illustrated different aspects of nurses' use of language according to the site of discourse and method of analysis used.

24-hour reports

The majority of topics (86.1 per cent) recorded were associated with routine (mundane) domestic activity, and 23.3 per cent of topics were associated with patients' feelings about routines. A smaller percentage of topics was concerned with families (7.5), interpersonal relationships (2.9) and violence (2.8); non-routine resistance to the therapeutic programme, like smoking marijuana, was recorded on 0.4 per cent of occasions. The results were cross-tabulated to assess whether the variables of nurse seniority, report writing style or community size affected the topics recorded, but no relationship was found. New admission to the hospitals, however, was found to be statistically associated with the quantity and quality of topics recorded. In Figure 4.1, an increase in topics associated with violence and family, and a decrease in topics associated with interpersonal relationships, can be seen in February, when 57.8 per cent of all new admissions arrived. In a quite complex way it suggested that the 'life as usual' nature of the hospital was disrupted and that disturbance would increase at times of admission (see Figure 4.1).

Nurse handover meetings

The therapeutic community studied had a strong oral tradition. Talking about observations of self and others, the inner emotional states and outward social behaviour of staff and patient members of the community was a prime therapeutic activity in meetings. These meetings, like those observed by Turner (1972), demonstrated rule-governed, occasioned behaviour associated with assembling, beginning, handing over, moving on or ending, and turn-taking. It was found that nurses were theoretically eclectic, using psychosocial, psychoanalytic, psychopolitical and physiological models of human behaviour. Commonsense reasoning was a resource to which nurses returned in the light of puzzling events that were incompatible with the models in use. A striking aspect of nurses' talk was the frequency with which nurses used a psychosocial model. Nurses often made comments related to group cohesiveness or group cohesion, and contrasted it to either the social isolation of a patient or the disintegration

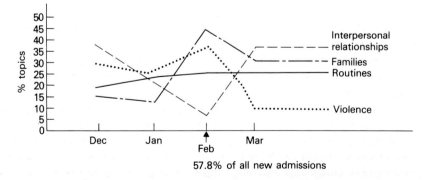

Fig. 4.1 Change of topics by month with admission rate

of the community. These approximated to Durkheim's notion of anomie and egoism (Durkheim, 1975).

The structural analysis of the handover meetings similarly emphasised the importance of the notion of the community as the subject of discourse. The disruptive nature of pairing and exclusive relationships was identified.

Published text

Domestic activity proved the essential backdrop against which the drama of patients' problems was enacted and revealed. Nurses and patients were portrayed as sharing similar characteristics, as human beings, but were sharply differentiated in terms of their response to events in the community. Nurses' feelings, thoughts and actions were seen in terms of the professional discourse; that is, when patients evoked feelings in the nurses, this was explained in terms of patients' individual psychopathology. On the other hand, patients' feelings, thoughts and actions for nurses or others were explained in terms of the patients' biography and early experiences of parenting – not the nurses' actions. Nurses were, then, dependent on differentiating themselves from patients on concepts derived from psychoanalytic theory, which they neither produced nor controlled.

DISCUSSION

There are three main areas in which the research described above is of relevance to nursing. These are the management of clinical practice, professional politics and nursing research.

Management of clinical practice

The 24-hour reports and nurse handover meetings illustrated the importance of observing mundane domestic events as a means of evaluating community cohesion or integration. Indeed, the research demonstrated that when the community was disrupted at times of admission, more untoward events were likely to be recorded. Patients were perceived, therefore, as having an effect on each other. In the context of a profession moving more firmly towards individualised care and the nursing process, it is perhaps useful to remind ourselves not to lose touch with the group dynamics of the ward or department, nor with the positive (and negative) effects that patients have on each other. In this hospital, individualised nursing care (each nurse had a caseload of patients from admission to discharge) was transformed into group/community nursing in the evening and at night. It is suggested here that in every specialty careful attention should be paid to identifying successful group nursing skills during these periods.

A further aspect of group dynamics identified in this research suggested that the rule-governed nature of nurse handovers inhibited supervision, by senior nurses, of the quality of care. Further research in other settings might help to identify the extent to which this occurs in handovers in other clinical areas and whether, for example, they are an appropriate vehicle for teaching student nurses or the supervision of clinical practitioners.

Professional politics

A question implicit in this research was concerned with whether nurses owned a theoretical framework and body of knowledge from which they worked, and the extent to which this was reflected in their communications. From the evidence in this study, it seemed that nurses in a therapeutic community did not own a unitary theory. They used a range of models drawn from the human sciences, but stressed a socio-community approach; this was reflected in their communication. However, while social status and prestige may not accrue to nurses because they lack a unitary theory, it does not follow that they were without authority or power. Their flexible discursive practices, informed by commonsense reasoning, located their power and body of knowledge in the taken-for-granted world of mundane domestic activity. This is in contrast to medical power, which is legitimised by claims that medical knowledge is based on objective methods, which in turn is presented as a mode of enquiry with privileged access to truth. As such, nurses' experience reflects women's experience generally, a point not lost to other analysts of nursing (Muff, 1982). It is difficult to establish, therefore, how nurses' domestic power could be transformed into 'scientific knowledge' based power, from which social prestige, status and rewards flow, without sacrificing that element of their discourse, domesticity and commonsense reasoning that provides patients with space to express and define their own subjectivity. In short, the development of a unitary nursing theory may replace a partnered patient with one subject to nurses' discourse.

Nursing research

Language, conversation and talk is not only the primary tool of nursing; it also forms the primary data upon which much social science and nursing research rests. Whether conversations and interactions are recorded as they arise in their natural setting, or are collected via people's responses to questionnaires and interviews, language and its analysis is the key to knowledge and understanding in nursing. Generally a variety of methods of data collection is well understood in nursing research - from participant observation to the construction of rating scales. Less well understood and discussed, perhaps, are the problems of analysing talk and language. In the research described here, an attempt to use methods of analysis underpinned by linguistic and social-linguistic theory (Cameron, 1985; Coulthard, 1985) was made, with varying degrees of success. It is hoped that nurse researchers will draw on the ideas to be found in this field of study when faced with the wealth of conversational and written data their field studies produce.

REFERENCES

Abel Smith B (1979) *A History of the Nursing Profession*. London: Heinemann.
Allen H (1981) Voices of concern - a study of verbal communication about patients in a psychiatric day unit. *Journal of Advanced Nursing*, **6**: 355-362.
Atkinson P (1981) Inspecting classroom talk. In: *Uttering Muttering*, ed. Adelman C, pp. 99-113. London: Grant McIntyre.
Baron C (1984) The Paddington Day Hospital: crises and control in a therapeutic institution. *International Journal of Therapeutic Communities*, **5**(3): 157-171.
Barthes R (1966) Introduction to the structural analysis of narratives. In: *Barthes: Selected Writings*, ed. Sontag S, pp. 251-296. London: Fontana.
Bloor M J (1980) The nature of therapeutic work in a Therapeutic Community: some preliminary findings. *International Journal of Therapeutic Communities*, **2**: 80-90.

Bloor M J (1981) Therapeutic paradox: the patient culture and the formal teaching programme in a Therapeutic Community. *British Journal of Medical Sociology*, **54**: 359-369.

Bloor M J and Fonkert J (1982) Reality construction, reality exploration and treatment in two Therapeutic Communities. *Sociology of Health & Illness*, **4**(2): 125-140.

Cameron D (1985) *Feminism & Linguistic Theory*. London: Macmillan.

Chapman G E (1987) *Text Talk and Discourse; A Study of Nurses' Use of Language in a Therapeutic Community*. Unpublished PhD thesis, London University.

Chapman G E (1988) Reporting therapeutic discourse in a therapeutic community. *Journal of Advanced Nursing*, **13**: 255-264.

Clark D H (1964) *Administrative Therapy*. London: Tavistock.

Clarke M (1978) Getting through the work. In: *Readings in the Sociology of Nursing*, eds. Dingwall R and McIntosh J, pp. 67-87. Edinburgh: Churchill Livingstone.

Clyde Mitchell J (1983) Case and situation analysis. *Sociological Review*, new series, May 1983, pp. 187-211.

Coulthard M (1985) *An Introduction to Discourse Analysis*. London: Longman.

Dingwall R (1981) Practical ethnography. In: *Sociology and Social Research*, eds. Payne G, Dingwall R, Payne J and Carter M. London: Routledge & Kegan Paul.

Doyal L (1979) *The Political Economy of Health*. London: Pluto Press.

Durkheim E (1975) *Suicide: A Study in Sociology*. London: Routledge & Kegan Paul.

Ehrenreich B and Ehrenreich J (1975) Hospital workers: class conflicts in the making. *International Journal of Health Services*, **5**(1): 43-51.

Ehrenreich B and English D (1973) *Witches, Midwives and Nurses: A History of Women Healers*. London: Writers and Readers Publishing Co-operative.

Etzioni E (1969) *The Semi-professions and their Organization*. London: (Free Press) Collier Macmillan.

Foucault M (1961) *Madness & Civilization*. London: Fontana.

Foucault M (1973) *The Birth of the Clinic*. London: Tavistock Publications.

Foucault M (1981) *The History of Sexuality*. London: Penguin.

Foucault M (1982) The subject and power. *Critical Enquiry*, **8**: 778-795 (University of Chicago Press).

Friedson E (1970) *Profession of Medicine. A Study of the Sociology of Applied Knowledge*. Chicago: Dodd, Mead and Company.

Friedson E (1983) The theory of professions - state of the art. In: *The Sociology of the Professions: Lawyers, Doctors and Others*, eds. Dingwall R and Lewis P. SSRC: Macmillan Press.

Garfinkel H (1967) *Studies in Ethnomethodology*. Englewood Cliffs, New Jersey: Prentice Hall.

Glaser B and Strauss A (1965) *Awareness of Dying*. Chicago: Aldine.

Glaser B and Strauss A (1968) *Time for Dying*. Chicago: Aldine.

Goffman E (1970) *Asylums*. London: Penguin Books.

Hammersley M and Atkinson P (1983) *Ethnography: Principles in Practice*. London: Tavistock Publications.

Hawkes T (1983) *Structuralism and Semiotics*. London: Methuen.

Holohan A (1977) Diagnosis is the end of transition. In: *Medical Encounters*, eds. Horobin G and Davis A. London: Croom Helm.

Johnson T (1977) *Professions and Power*. London: Macmillan.

Kennard D and Roberts J (1983) *An Introduction to Therapeutic Communities*. London: Routledge & Kegan Paul.

Leeson J and Gray J (1978) *Women and Medicine*. London: Tavistock Publications.

Lelean S R (1973) *Ready for Report, Nurse?* London: Royal College of Nursing.

Macleod Clark J (1984) Verbal communication in nursing. In: *Recent Advances in Nursing. 'Communication'*, ed. Faulkner A, pp. 52-74. London: Churchill Livingstone.

Maggs C J (1983) *The Origins of General Nursing*. London: Croom Helm.

Muff J (1982) (ed.) *Socialization, Sexism and Stereotyping - Women's Issues in Nursing*. St. Louis: C V Mosby.

Royal College of Nursing (1984) *The History of Nursing Group Bulletins 4, 5, 6*. London: Royal College of Nursing.

Royal College of Nursing (1985) *The History of Nursing Group Bulletins 6, 7, 8*. London: Royal College of Nursing.

Roth J (1963) *Time Tables*. Indianapolis: Bobbs-Merril.

Saussure E (1974) *Course in General Linguistics*. London: Fontana.

Shea H L (1984) Communication among nurses: The Nursing Care Plan. In: *Recent Advances in Nursing Communication*, ed. Faulkner A, pp. 145-166. London: Churchill Livingstone.

Silverman D (1985) *Qualitative Methodology & Sociology*. London: Gower.

Trew T (1979) What the papers say: linguistic variation and ideological difference. In: *Language & Control*, eds. Fowler et al., pp. 117-157. London: Routledge & Kegan Paul.

Turner R (1972) Some formal properties of therapy talk. In: *Studies in Social Interaction*, ed. Sudnow D, pp. 367-397. New York: The Free Press; London: Collier Macmillan.

Chapter 5

Evaluation of a Drug Guide for Old People in Primary Health Care: the Case for Information Sharing

Fiona Ross

INTRODUCTION

It is well known that many old people do not understand why they are taking certain drugs, and make errors of dosage and frequency (Knox, 1980; World Health Organisation, 1981; Royal College of Physicians, 1984). There is evidence that the proportion of the population receiving medication rises with age, that multiple drug therapy is age related (Skegg et al, 1977), and that 10 per cent of hospital admissions are due to drug-induced disease (Williamson, 1978). Thus as Shaw and Opit (1976) suggest, there is a case for providing old people with supervision and help with their drugs. The potential contribution of nurses in this respect has been recognised in respect of problem-solving (Crooks and Shepherd, 1975), supervision and monitoring (Neely and Patrick, 1968; Linn and Taylor, 1979; Wade and Finlayson, 1983; Royal College of Physicians, 1984). Linn and Taylor, for example, found that monthly supervisory visits from a nurse to old people was beneficial, in that the number of drugs was reduced, instructions and labelling were improved, and regular drug reviews were initiated.

In contrast to the general consensus that nursing has skills and expertise to tackle this problem, there is some evidence that district nurses do not regard it as a priority (Phillipson and Strang, 1984). That there is potential for district nurses to work in this area is undoubted; furthermore, there is tremendous scope for the nurse's partnership with the general practitioner to work towards an integrated and flexible policy for the prescribing and supervision of drugs for old people at home. To achieve this in an area where general practitioners have a legitimate primary role presupposes effective teamwork.

Effective teamwork makes the assumption that professionals share a core of knowledge, which matches that of the patient. Most studies on teamwork have focused on the nature of the collaboration and communication between health professionals, rather than on patient outcomes (Gilmore et al, 1974; Bond et al, 1985). There are some exceptions to this, which have discussed a professional team in a relationship of open access with the consumer (Anderson, 1969; Ross, 1980).

37

Webb and Hobdell (1980) take up this point and contend that some of the problems of teamwork are due to a failure to recognise two legitimating principles – *consumer sovereignty* and the *authority of relevance*. The first describes the patient as an active rather than a passive recipient of care. The second principle – the 'authority of relevance' – refers to the importance of valuing information equally from different team members, whatever their position in the hierarchy. Thus, for a team to function effectively the patient and all the team members must share in the common concern.

The evidence suggests that teamwork is not only a problematic theoretical concept, inadequately defined, but that there are many difficulties experienced by professionals in practice. A major gap in this literature is information on the extent to which professionals share the same knowledge about, and with, their patients.

The compliance debate

Patient knowledge and compliance are closely linked in the literature. Compliance is the extent to which a person's behaviour (in terms of taking medication, following diets or executing life-style changes) coincides with medical or health advice (Haynes, 1979, p. 2). Non-compliance is, therefore, a lack of adherence, even when the correct regime is known (Parkin et al, 1976, p. 688). Non-comprehension is deviation from prescribed drug treatment due to a failure to understand the nature of the regime (Parkin et al, 1976, p. 688); it is thus one aspect of non-compliance, and one of the concerns of this study.

One of the key issues in information sharing and patient knowledge is professional non-compliance, or the failure to follow recognised practice. Ley (1981) provides us with some explanations for professional non-compliance, including inadequacies in the organisation of care and discrepancies of professional knowledge. Ley gives a number of examples, but the most relevant in this context is the failure to maintain accurate records. There is growing research evidence that points to discrepancies between the patient's report (1981) and information contained in the record (Zander et al, 1978; Leinster et al, 1981). Clearly, this has implications for district nursing, because if the records are inaccurate, district nurses have no reliable database for reference. In this sense, district nurses are denied access to important information and cannot confidently monitor medication or deal confidently with queries.

The confusion may be as much the professionals' as it is the clients'. (Stimson and Webb, 1975)

Recently there has been a spate of published findings on discrepancies in general practice between doctors' and patients' knowledge of prescribed medication (Arcand and Williamson, 1981; Bowling and Cartwright, 1982). In separate studies, Price et al (1986) and Claoue and Elkington (1986) reported the identical figure of 46 per cent of patients taking drugs not reported by general practitioners. These findings suggest that theories of non-compliance are over-simplified, and that other factors such as inadequate communication and professional lack of knowledge must also be taken into account. This raises the question of how far drug information is shared between members of the primary health-care team, in particular the district nurse. In this study the congruence of information was one measure of teamwork.

Information sharing, self-care and the case for a personal drug record

If clients and professionals are to work together effectively to promote self-care, then it follows that as well as directing health promotion strategies at the patient, the weaknesses of professional care should be addressed. This point has been made by Tones (1977), who argues that behavioural change is as important for the service providers as for the consumers. This was the rationale for the nurse and doctor peer review of prescribing, which in this study meant that the general practitioners and district nurses compared their information on drugs with the patient.

There is considerable evidence that records present problems in general practice. Problems leading to discrepancies in knowledge have been referred to earlier; others include keeping information up to date (Stuart, 1972), repeat prescribing that takes place without a consultation (Drury, 1982) and lost or mislaid records (Metcalfe, 1980).

Little systematic research has been done in the area of district nursing records. However, McIntosh (1978) and Poulton (1981) note that district nursing records are often incomplete, reporting treatment given, and not problem orientated. Reasons for this include the difficulty of obtaining information and the problem of leaving the information accessible in the patient's home. The district nurse's record (as that of the general practitioner) may be criticised for contributing to poorly co-ordinated information and control of knowledge by health professionals.

Partly as a consequence of these problems, and partly due to the growing consumer lobby, there is pressure for patients to have access to information in their medical record. Such innovations in sharing information have been evaluated for general health records (Michael and Boardley, 1982), obstetric records (Lovell et al, 1987) and personal medication records (Erskine et al, 1978; Jackson and Edwards, 1981). The medication record is designed to record all medicines, whether advised by general practitioners, hospital doctors or another agency. Many also include self-medication. Only in some of these studies are the records retained by the patient.

INFORMATION GIVING AND THE DRUG RECORD

Information giving includes a number of different approaches: teaching individually and in groups, structured educational packages and written advice. There are a growing number of studies evaluating written instructions for medication. There is some evidence that drug information leaflets are read and used by the elderly (Morris and Olins, 1984) and are related to patient satisfaction with treatment (George et al, 1983). These studies fall into two groups: those that evaluate written instructions on single or selected drugs (Ley et al, 1976; George et al, 1983), and, second, those evaluating the complete range of medication (Wandless and Davie, 1977). As an example of the second group, Ellis et al (1979) found that patients receiving written instructions on all their drugs were significantly better informed on diagnosis, general advice and drug treatment than were a control group. They acknowledge that an inevitable difficulty of an out-patient record is the drug omissions due to self-medication or deficiencies in the doctor's recording practice. It is for these very reasons that the patient should be given responsibility for the record.

Although comparison of these studies is difficult, because of different methods used and populations studied, there is some evidence that written information for the patient can be an effective way of improving knowledge of drugs. Health promotion strategies that seek to improve patient knowledge must also be aimed at co-ordinating professional knowledge. This implies a multidisciplinary approach. Thus the main focus here is the meaningfulness, accessibility and reliability of information to both patient and professional. I contend that a shared interdisciplinary record, held by the patient, would overcome the problems of separate professional records as well as providing reliable information to patients of their current medication.

STUDY DESIGN AND METHODS

The objectives of the study were:

1. To compare the patient's, district nurse's and general practitioner's knowledge of prescribed medication.
2. To measure the effect of a patient-held drug guide.

The context: a joint appointment in district nursing and research

This study was carried out by a practising district nurse with a half-time commitment to research. As a working member of the team, the district nurse researcher was in regular contact with the problems, conflicts and demands of primary health care. Therefore, the key partnership between these two roles was an inevitable and powerful influence on the identification of the research question and subsequent design. The joint appointment had important implications for the methodological approach – a key issue here is subjectivity. Subjectivity is an inevitable component of evaluative research, and may reflect the perspective of the organisation, funding agency or individual researcher. Hockey (1977) contends that researchers should acknowledge their personal values and state clearly the extent to which their frame of reference influenced the research design. I would go further and suggest that in some contexts the value of research is heightened when the researcher writes herself into the study (James, 1984). In this way she brings to the research something of the urgency of patients' needs, as well as the uncertainty of working outside a narrowly defined role.

Procedure

The study took place in an inner London group practice of 8500 patients with 5 general practitioners, 2 trainee general practitioners and 4 attached district nurses, including myself. It was designed as a 'before and after' study using the patients as their own controls.

The drug guide (Figure 5.1) was developed after discussion with the primary health-care team, the local pharmacist and a pensioner's health group, and was introduced to patients as a 'tablet and medicine guide'. It was important to avoid technical language and jargon, which may have resulted in misunderstandings. The aim was to develop a simple, problem-orientated chart, incorporating the patient's description of her problems.

The sample studied included all patients in the practice aged 60 years and over who were receiving district nursing care. Each patient was visited at home by a fieldworker who recorded details of the patient's description of her current medication. The patient's doctor was then presented with the medical records, and from this and his knowledge of the patient, he completed a record of medication. The district nurse, who had access to both medical and nursing records, was also asked to provide details of the patient's current medication. The information collected included prescribed drugs, dosage, reason for prescribing and frequency of administration. The information from these three sources was then compared.

DATE	NAME AND PURPOSE OF TABLET OR MEDICINE	COMMENTS

1   Write down any changes in your tablets or medicines, or ask the doctor or nurse.

2   Write down any problems with your medicines or tablets in the column marked 'Comments'.

3   Please take this guide when you (or a relative) visit the doctor in the surgery.

Name

Address

GP   Nurse

Allergies

Fig. 5.1   Tablet and medicine guide

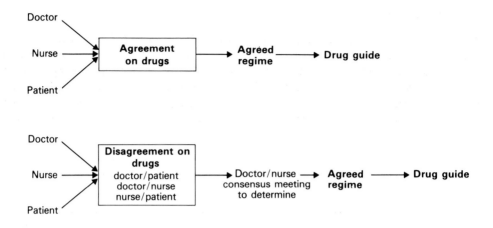

Fig. 5.2 Procedure to determine the agreed regime

An agreed regime of treatment

Where drugs recorded by doctor, nurse and patient were identical, this was defined as the 'agreed regime'. Where there was any discrepancy the doctor and nurse consulted together to decide on the agreed regime, i.e. medication the patient was supposed to be taking. The method of agreeing the regime is outlined in Figure 5.2. At these meetings, the doctor and nurse had access to the information supplied by the patient, as well as their own previously completed questionnaires, and the medical record. The current consultation sheet in the medical record was checked to ensure that a complete record of medication was entered. If not, the appropriate changes were made.

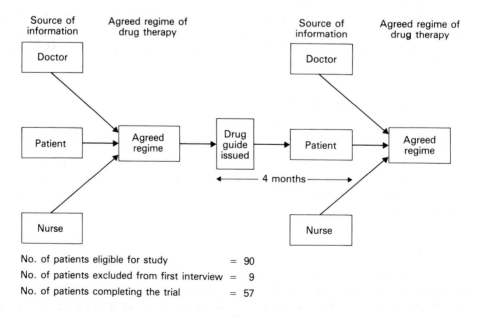

No. of patients eligible for study   = 90
No. of patients excluded from first interview = 9
No. of patients completing the trial   = 57

Fig. 5.3 The study design

The drug guide

This was completed on the basis of the drugs, dosage and frequency of administration included in the agreed regime and was delivered personally to the patient. The drug guide was retained by the patient. At the end of 4 months, patient, doctor and nurse were again asked independently to complete a record of medication that they believed the patient to be taking. It was then possible to compare the knowledge of the patient, nurse and doctor about medication before and after the drug guide was used. The study design is summarised in Figure 5.3.

FINDINGS

This chapter focuses on the 57 patients who were interviewed both at the start and at the end of the study. In particular, it sets out to assess the effectiveness of the drug guide on information sharing in terms of four measures of outcome: the number of prescribed drugs for the majority of patients in the study, patient and professional reported discrepancies on medication, doctor and nurse consensus on individual patients' medication, and the organisation of drug information in the medical record.

Characteristics of the study population

Eighty-one patients were included in the original sample, of whom 40 (49.3 per cent) were aged over 80 years, and 56 (69.1 per cent) were women. Many suffered from physical disabilities that could have caused difficulties with their medication. For example, 52 (64.2 per cent) were not able to open a child-proof drug container, and 18 (22.2 per cent) could not read the typed print of a drug label.

Twenty-four patients were not included in the second-stage interviews, either because they had recovered and needed no further district nursing care (5) or because they were admitted to hospital, had died or had left the district (13). Six patients in the original sample were receiving no drugs.

The number of prescribed drugs

The 57 patients followed up reported themselves to be taking 3.5 drugs on average (a total of 201) before, and 3.7 drugs on average (209 in total) after, using the drug guide. One patient reported taking as many as 10 drugs. Both before and after patients reported taking a higher total number of drugs than had been recorded by either the doctor or the nurse. Furthermore, there was a consistent pattern in that the number of drugs in the agreed regime was higher than that reported by any single source.

Agreement

Patient and professional knowledge must first be analysed in terms of the proportion of cases, for which there was complete agreement. Out of 57 patients there were only 3 (5.3 per cent) cases at the first interview for whom there was complete patient, nurse and doctor agreement. This number was doubled at the follow-up. There was complete doctor and nurse agreement for 20 patients at the end of the study, that is twice as many as previously. However, this only accounted for just over a third (35.1 per cent) of the study group. Discrepancies in knowledge must be interpreted in this context.

Discrepancies in patient and professional knowledge of prescribed drugs

Discrepancies are discussed in terms of three outcome measures: drugs reported by the patient only, drugs reported by the doctor and nurse only, and discrepancies of the patient's knowledge of drugs (appearance, function, dose and frequency).

Drugs reported by the patient only

Of the total of 57 patients, 25 (44 per cent) reported taking drugs that were recorded by neither the doctor nor the nurse (Table 5.1). The initial meeting between the doctor and the nurse led to the majority of these drugs being included in the agreed regime of treatment. Many of these were minor drugs, such as prescribed skin ointments and iron supplements.

Table 5.1 Numbers of patients reporting drugs not mentioned by either the doctor or the nurse before and after introduction of the drug guide

	Patients completing the study	
	Before (n=57)	After (n=57)
Number of patients reporting drugs independently of doctor and nurse	25	25
Number of drugs involved		
Subsequently included in agreed regime	32	28
Subsequently excluded from agreed regime	8	6
Total	40	34

Table 5.2 Numbers of patients not mentioning drugs reported by doctor and/or nurse before and after introduction of the drug guide

	Patients completing the study	
	Before (n=57)	After (n=57)
Number of patients in disagreement with doctor and/or nurse	15	9
Drugs involved		
Digoxin	1	0
Diuretic	1	0
Analgesic	3	4
Hypnotic/tranquilliser	4	0
Other	7	6
Total	16	10

There were, however, some important drugs that neither the doctor nor the nurse had reported, such as glyceryl trinitrate, digoxin (one case) and anti-inflammatory drugs (four cases). At the end of the study there was a reduction in the total number of these drugs, but there were still 25 patients who reported prescribed medication not mentioned by either the doctor or the nurse.

Drugs reported only by the doctor and/or the nurse

At the beginning of the study there were 15 patients for whom either the doctor or the nurse reported drugs that had not been reported by the patient (Table 5.2). These included important drugs such as digoxin, diuretics and hypnotics. At the end of the study there were only nine patients for whom the doctor and/or the nurse reported drugs not mentioned by the patient. Just one of these 10 drugs was of major consequence. The remainder included simple analgesics, aperients and topical agents.

Patient knowledge of drugs

Patients were asked to describe the appearance, function, dose and frequency of the drugs they were taking. Fewer errors were recorded at the end of the study period than at the beginning (Table 5.3). There was a significant improvement in patient knowledge of drug function, the number of errors falling from 56 to 35, significant at the 0.05 level.

Discrepancies in knowledge between doctors and nurses on individual patients' medication

The information obtained from the doctors and nurses at the beginning of the study showed some disagreement for 38.0 per cent of drugs. At the end, this disagreement had fallen

Table 5.3 Numbers of errors made by patients in knowledge of drug appearance, action, dose and frequency before and after introduction of the drug guide

	Number of errors in follow-up group	
	Before	After
Appearance	21	21
Action	56	35
Dose	33	27
Frequency	34	28
Total number of drugs	201	209

Table 5.4 Number of patients involved in doctor and nurse disagreement on drugs, before and after introduction of the drug guide

Disagreement on drugs	Number of patients (n = 57)	
	Before	After
Doctor not nurse	24 (42.1%)	14 (24.6%)
Nurse not doctor	25 (43.9%)	15 (26.3%)

to 19.6 per cent of drugs. The number of patients involved in these doctor and nurse dis-agreements was reduced by 17 per cent at the end of the study (Table 5.4). However, important drugs were not mentioned by either the doctor or the nurse both before and after the introduction of the drug guide. Those not reported by the nurse included digoxin, diuretics and analgesics. Those not reported by the doctor included digoxin, diuretics and anti-inflammatory agents.

The organisation of drug information in the medical record

In completing the medication questionnaire the doctors and nurses used the medical record as a source of information. Since district nurses use their own notes as well as the medical record, they were asked about other sources of information. The main focus of the analysis was to assess the extent to which information was clearly presented on the consultation sheet compared with 'scattered elsewhere', for example in letters and discharge summaries. A comparison of before and after was undertaken to assess the impact of the drug guide and the interdisciplinary review on the organisation of the medication record.

At the beginning of the study the drug information was found on the current consultation sheet by the nurses in 27 (47.4 per cent) records, and by doctors in 39 (68.4 per cent). At the end the information was found on the consultation sheet by the nurses in 40 (70.2 per cent) records and by doctors in 47 (82.5 per cent). At both times nurses were more likely than doctors to refer to other parts of the record. Explanations given included 'no information anywhere' and 'slightly confusing as to what she is presently taking'. Similar comments were made by doctors: 'it wasn't clear from the consultation sheet which drugs she is still taking'.

For each patient, nurses were asked whether they felt they had access to complete information about that individual's drugs. At the beginning of the study district nurses felt confident about drug information in the records for only 26 (45.6 per cent) patients, and at the end this had risen to 41 (71.9 per cent) patients.

DISCUSSION

The discussion of the findings draws attention to the mismatch of patient and professional knowledge of drugs and the effect of the drug guide on information sharing. The major contribution of these findings is in terms of the lack of knowledge doctors and nurses have of a key and substantive area of practice, namely what drugs their elderly patients are taking. The second new perspective offered by this study is the use of a drug guide to provide access to health information, opportunities for participation and a bridge between the health-care system and the patient. There are clear links here between ideas of self-care, information sharing and the professional response in terms of teamwork and prevention.

The patients in the sample studied were found to be reasonably typical of a district nurse's caseload in terms of age (Hockey, 1972), living alone (Wade et al, 1983), clinical problems and prescribed drugs (Moir and Dingwall-Fordyce, 1980). There was evidence that the drug guide contributed to patients' knowledge; for example, at the end of the study patients were better informed about the dose, frequency and purpose of their drugs.

There was a disturbingly high rate of disagreement between professionals and the patient, given that both doctor and nurse had access to the patient's record in completing their questionnaires. A remarkably similar pattern of findings emerged both at the beginning and at the end of the study. Over a third of patients on both occasions (25, 44 per cent) reported drugs that were unknown to the doctor and the nurse. This is in line with the recent findings of Price et al (1986) and Claoue and Elkington (1986).

There are a number of probable reasons for this, which include self-medication, lay advice, the dual system of prescribing and the frequent failure of communication between hospital and community (Bliss, 1981). This important last point is illustrated by a patient who, at the second interview, reported taking a laxative, an antibiotic and an anti-inflammatory agent, none of which had been reported by the doctor or the nurse. The doctor commented: 'it is impossible to tell what she is taking, because the hospital consultant's last letter says he has taken her off all her old drugs. I don't know what he has restarted'. In addition, agencies in the community, such as day hospitals, and terminal care support teams, may initiate or change treatment. Another factor contributing to poor communication is that treatment decisions for the elderly are often made in the home, when the record may be unavailable, or in discussion with a third person such as a relative, warden or other carer. It is sometimes difficult to ensure that some of these decisions are entered in the medical record.

There were also discrepancies in terms of the drugs reported by the doctor or nurse only and not the patient. This finding confirms the work of others that between 3 per cent (Bowling and Cartwright, 1982) and 25 per cent of old people (Das et al, 1977) fail to report drugs prescribed by their general practitioner.

Finally there were serious differences in knowledge between general practitioners and district nurses about the drugs each believed the patient was taking. Clearly these findings have implications for information sharing, teamwork and district nursing practice. Although the role of teams in patient teaching is relatively unstudied, there is a consensus that the multidisciplinary approach is the way forward (Tones, 1977). The doctor and nurse consensus on medication, resulting from the meeting and recorded on the drug guide, provided unambiguous information on drugs, which it was hoped would produce a positive outcome in terms of patient knowledge and comprehension. It was found that poor agreement on drugs between doctors and nurses was associated with a lack of patient knowledge and that both improved as a result of the intervention. The doctor and nurse meeting to discuss the drugs of these patients with disagreements was a positive indicator of collaboration as well as being methodologically innovative. Thus, it would be reasonable to propose that effective information sharing within the team would lead to enhanced patient awareness. This has important implications for developing strategies to promote information sharing with patients and for an open access model of care.

In summary, the drug guide was associated with an improvement in patient knowledge of drugs, a reduction in disagreements between doctors and nurses and between professionals and patients, and an improvement in the organisation of information in the medical records. In addition, the district nurses were more confident in their use of the record. There was, however, a slight increase in the total number of prescribed drugs at the end of the 4 months. It is likely that considerable benefits resulted from the interdisciplinary review and discussion of medication required to determine the agreed regime of treatment, which was in itself a necessary consequence of using the guide. Thus the drug guide was only one factor that probably influenced the outcome measure.

IMPLICATIONS OF THE RESEARCH

Since this study is rooted in the practice setting in which the researcher was also a district nurse, it has a number of implications for both future practice and research. Bearing in mind the dangers of generalising from one academic practice, a number of points can be made.

First, the problem of drugs and the elderly needs to be tackled on more than one front. It is not sufficient merely to focus narrowly on the patient's role in compliance. Rather it is important to look at other aspects of care delivery, for example the professionals' knowledge, and the effects of other agencies on prescribing. This study showed that even in a motivated and committed primary health-care team, there was a lack of consensus about drugs. The methods used here could be usefully replicated in other practices to provide further descriptive information. Future work in this area, however, would need to take into account the influence of the restricted drugs list (introduced after this study) on patient knowledge and professional consensus.

Secondly, although numerous recommendations have been made to develop medication records, there have been few attempts at systematic evaluation. These findings suggest that there is scope not only for development, but also for careful evaluation of similar records. The third area for which this study has implications is in the context of interdisciplinary collaboration. The method developed for this study, using an interdisciplinary review as a key part, could be replicated to investigate other issues of common concern. Further work needs to be done on records in general practice and their potential for planning co-ordinated care.

Finally, implications can be drawn for district nursing. Although only a small group of district nurses participated in this study, their lack of confidence reflected deficits in knowledge of drugs. This opens up numerous research possibilities to explore the learning experience of district nurses in the post-registration courses and in-service development, particularly important in the light of the Cumberlege recommendations for district nurses to prescribe. There are also implications for the future development of joint appointments in district nursing. It has been acknowledged frequently that district nurses are key members of the primary health-care team and central to community care policies for the elderly. However, developments in district nursing have been limited, and more work is urgently needed to define and evaluate the district nurse's role and contribution to care in a challenging and changing primary health-care system.

REFERENCES

Anderson J A D (1969) The health team in the community. *Lancet*, **20**: 679-681.

Arcand R and Williamson J (1981) An evaluation of home visiting of patients by physicians in geriatric medicine. *British Medical Journal*, **283**: 718-720.

Bliss M R (1981) Prescribing for the elderly. *British Medical Journal*, **283**: 203-206.

Bond J, Cartlidge A, Gregson B, Phillips P, Bolam F and Gill K (1985) *A Study of Interprofessional Collaboration in Primary Health Care Organisations*. University of Newcastle upon Tyne: Health Care Research Unit.

Bowling A and Cartwright A (1982) *Life after Death. A Study of the Elderly Widowed*. London: Tavistock.

Claoue C and Elkington A (1986) Informing the hospital of patient's drug regimes. *British Medical Journal*, **292**: 101.

Crooks J and Shepherd A (1975) Drugs and the elderly – the nature of the problem. *Health Bulletin*, **33**: 222-227.

Das B, Maddock S and Whittingham E (1977) Special problems of medication in a survey of 114 elderly people at home, in welfare homes and in hospital. *Modern Geriatrics*, **7**(1): 22-23.

Department of Health and Social Security (1982) *Nurses Working in the Community*. London: OPCS.

Drury V W M (1982) Repeat prescribing – a review. *British Medical Journal*, **2**(6090): 799-802.

Ellis D, Hopkkin J, Leitch H and Crofton J (1979) 'Doctors Orders' controlled trial of supplementary, written information for patients. *British Medical Journal*, **1**: 456.

Erskine Z, Moir D, Jeffers T and Petrie J (1978) An outpatient medication record. *British Medical Record*, **2**: 1606-1607.

George C, Waters W and Nicholas J (1983) Prescription information leaflets: a pilot study in general practice. *British Medical Journal*, **287**: 1193-1196.

Gilmore M, Bruce N and Hunt M (1974) *The Work of the Nursing Team in General Practice*. London: Council for the Education and Training of Health Visitors.

Haynes R B (1979) Introduction. In: *Compliance in Health Care*, eds. Haynes R B, Wayne Taylor D and Sackett D L. Baltimore: The Johns Hopkins University Press.

Hockey L (1972) *Use or Abuse? A Study of the State Enrolled Nurse in the Local Authority Nursing Service*. London: Queen's Nursing Institute of District Nursing.

Hockey L (1977) Indicators in nursing research with emphasis on social indicators. *Journal of Advanced Nursing*, **2**: 239-250.

Jackson R and Edwards N (1981) A self medication aid for patients on multiple drug therapy. *Pharmaceutical Journal*, **226**: 401-403.

James N (1984) A postscript to nursing. In: *Social Researching. Politics, Problems and Practice*, eds. Bell C and Roberts H. London: Routledge and Kegan Paul.

Knox J (1980) Prescribing for the elderly in general practice. *Journal of the Royal College of General Practitioners*, suppl. **30**(1).

Leinster K, Edwards W, Christensen D and Clark H (1981) A comparison of patient drug regimes as viewed by the physician, pharmacist and patient. *Medical Care*, **12**(6): 658-664.

Ley P (1981) Professional noncompliance - a neglected problem. *British Journal of Clinical Psychology*, **20**: 720-724.

Ley P, Jain V and Skilbeck C (1976) A method for decreasing patient medication errors. *Psychological Medicine*, **6**: 599-601.

Linn J and Taylor W (1979) Medications for the elderly. *Medical Journal of Australia*, **1**(8): 315-316.

Lovell A, Zander L, James C, Foot S, Swan A and Reynolds A (1987) The St Thomas's Hospital maternity case notes study. *Paediatric and Perinatal Epidemiology*, **1**: 57-66.

McIntosh J (1978) Record keeping - a boon or a bind. *Nursing Mirror*, **147**(1): 43-44.

Metcalfe D (1980) Why not let patients keep their own records? *Journal of the Royal College of General Practitioners*, **30**: 420.

Michael M and Boardley C (1982) Do patients want access to their medical records? *Medical Care*, **20**(4): 432-435.

Moir D and Dingwall-Fordyce I (1980) Drug taking by the elderly at home. *Journal of Clinical and Experimental Gerontology*, **2**(4): 329-332.

Morris L and Olins N (1984) The utility of drug leaflets for elderly consumers. *American Journal of Public Health*, **74**(2): 157-158.

Neely E and Patrick M (1968) The problems of aged persons taking medication at home. *Nursing Research*, **72**: 52-55.

Parkin D, Henney C, Quirk J and Crooks J (1976) Deviation from prescribed drug treatment after discharge from hospital. *British Medical Journal*, **2**: 686-688.

Phillipson C and Strang P (1984) *Health Education and Older People - the Role of Paid Carers*. The Health Education Council with the University of Keele.

Poulton K (1981) *Perceptions of Needs and Wants by Nurses and their Patients*. Unpublished PhD thesis, University of Surrey.

Price D, Cooke J, Singleton S and Feely M (1986) Doctors' unawareness of the drugs their patients are taking - a major cause of over prescribing? *British Medical Journal*, **292**: 99-100.

Ross F M (1980) Primary health care in Thamesmead. *Nursing Times*, Occasional Paper, **76**(18 and 19): 81-88.

Royal College of Physicians (1984) Medication for the elderly. *Journal of the Royal College of Physicians*, **18**(1): 3-10.

Shaw S and Opit L (1976) Need for supervision in the elderly receiving long term prescribed medication. *British Medical Journal*, **1**: 505-507.

Skegg D, Doll R and Perry J (1977) Use of medicines in general practice. *British Medical Journal*, **1**: 1561-1563.

Stimson G and Webb B (1975) *Going to See the Doctor*. London: Routledge and Kegan Paul.

Stuart J (1972) The use of a home record for permanently housebound patients. *Journal of the Royal College of General Practitioners*, **22**: 63-64.

Tones B (1977) *Effectiveness and Efficiency in Health Education: a Review of Theory and Practice*, Occasional Paper. Edinburgh: Scottish Health Education Unit.

Wade B and Finlayson J (1983) Drugs and the elderly. *Nursing Mirror*, **156**(18): 17-21.

Wade B, Sawyer L and Bell J (1983) *Dependency with Dignity*, Occasional Papers in social administration. London: Bedford Square Press.

Wandless I and Davie J (1977) Can drug compliance in the elderly be improved? *British Medical Journal*, **1**: 359-361.

Webb A and Hobdell M (1980) Coordination and teamwork in the health and social services. In: *Teamwork in the Personal Social Services and Health Care*, ed. Lonsdale A. London: Croom Helm.

Williamson J (1978) Prescribing problems in the elderly. *The Practitioner*, **220**(5): 749-755.

World Health Organisation (1981) Health care of the elderly: report of the technical group on use of medicaments by the elderly. *Drugs*, **22**: 279-294. Geneva: WHO.

Zander L, Beresford S A and Thomas P (1978) Medical records in general practice. *Journal of the Royal College of General Practitioners*, Occasional Paper 5.

Chapter 6

The Treatment of Leg Ulcers with Occlusive Hydrocolloid Dressings: a Microbiological Study

Brian Gilchrist

INTRODUCTION

Although no accurate figures exist, it is estimated that there are about 100 000 patients in the UK with active leg ulceration (Callam et al, 1985). The choice of treatment remains controversial; while some doctors advocate surgery (Negus, 1985) and others argue that it is a condition to be managed medically (Allen, 1985), at least one group argues that, once established, there is 'no cure' (Browse, 1983).

One fact, however, is in no doubt – leg ulcers are a condition that is managed mainly by nurses, especially those in the community. A recent survey (*Journal of District Nursing*, 1987) reported that venous leg ulcer treatment was more than double that of any other ailment encountered, and 98 per cent of the respondents reported that they had patients with ulcers. Forty-five per cent said that they dressed ulcers every other day, and the Lothian Study (Callan et al, 1985) confirmed that 87 per cent of all the leg ulcers that they found were cared for by the primary health team.

Despite the considerable size of the problem, there is surprisingly little evidence to guide the nurse towards an appropriate treatment for the often painful, open, granulating wound that she is regularly asked to dress. Stewart et al (1985) found that 28 different dressing agents were being used in their district, and a recent review of the wide variety of products available (*Drug and Therapeutic Bulletin*, 1986) concluded that: 'claims of efficiency in ulcer healing are rarely supported by well designed clinical trials'. A recent handbook (Morgan, 1987) listed 57 wound management products currently available for the treatment of leg ulcers; clearly, there is a need for much further study in this area if nurses are to be reassured that the dressing they are using is both safe and effective. This chapter describes one such study, and looks briefly at the problems of such research.

OCCLUSION AND WOUND HEALING

The observation that wounds covered with polythene healed twice as fast as those left exposed to the air was first reported over 20 years ago (Winter, 1962). This effect, it was argued, results from the prevention of dehydration of the serous exudate, thus preventing the formation of a scab. The epidermal cells are thus free to migrate unhindered across the moist wound surface, rather than having to burrow beneath the scab. Although this effect was confirmed by others (Hinman and Maibach, 1963), serious doubts were expressed that the accumulation of diluted serous exudate beneath the dressing would promote bacterial growth, an effect that could be demonstrated even on intact skin (Marples and Kligman, 1969; Aly et al, 1978). The introduction of a semi-permeable film dressing ('OpSite', Smith and Nephew), which allowed some of the water vapour to escape, and the demonstration that the exudate under the dressing was actively bacteriocidal (Buchan et al, 1980), did, however, allow this concept to be utilised clinically.

In 1983, a new type of occlusive dressing, called an *occlusive hydrocolloid* (HCD), was introduced, and because the dressing absorbed exudate to form a moist swollen gel that expanded to fill the wound cavity, it, too, seemed suitable for granulating wounds.

Although the dressing was shown in clinical trials to be an effective treatment for leg ulcers (Cherry et al, 1984; van Rijswijk et al, 1985), nurses using the product ('Granuflex', Squibb Surgicare, also known as 'DuoDerm' outside the UK) continued to be worried by the offensive smell of the pus-like exudate, and as the dressing is impermeable to oxygen (Lawrence, 1985) and to bacteria (Mertz and Eaglstein, 1984), questions were raised concerning the effect of the dressing on bacteria, especially anaerobes.

The aims of this study, therefore, were:

1. To assess whether there are any changes in the bacterial flora of a venous ulcer that is being treated with the HCD.
2. To attempt to assess the growth of anaerobic bacteria under the HCD.
3. To determine whether the bacterial flora has any effect on the healing rates of the ulcers.

METHOD OF STUDY

The general design of the study is shown in Figure 6.1. Patients with established ulceration were first screened by a specialist nurse to ensure that any with a predominantly arterial aetiology were excluded. The subjects were then asked to attend a special out-patient clinic at the local hospital, where the purpose of the study was explained to them and their written consent was obtained. They were required to attend the clinic each week for at least 8 weeks, and on each occasion the ulcer area would be traced onto clear acetate in order to monitor healing, and the specimens would be collected. Each week a routine wound swab was taken and placed in Stuart's medium and a measured amount of exudate was collected using a sterile plastic pipette. The exudate was placed into a specially prepared bottle of transport media, which had been treated so that there was minimal oxygen present and so that maximal growth would take place.

The specimens were taken immediately to the laboratory, where they were processed, using conventional techniques, in an attempt to grow any bacteria that might be present. Special efforts were taken to culture any anaerobic bacteria, and serial dilutions were made so that quantitative counts could also be made.

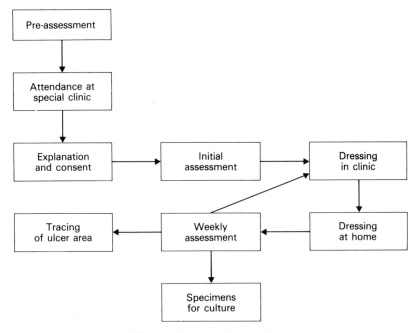

Fig. 6.1 Design of the study

The dressing was changed once during the week by a district nurse, who had been provided with the dressings and a written instruction sheet explaining the purposes of the trial and giving a contact telephone number to call should she experience any difficulties. Throughout the trial, standard compression was applied using either double-layer shaped 'Tubigrip' or 'Venosan 2000' elastic stockings.

FINDINGS

Ulcer healing

Twenty chronic venous ulcers were studied for 8 weeks. All the ulcers were resistant to at least two previous conventional treatments, and all the subjects were screened using Doppler ultrasound to exclude significant arterial disease. The average ulcer size was 994 mm² and the average time present was 6.6 months.

Nine out of 20 ulcers studied healed completely in an average of 11 weeks, while the average healing over the 8-week period was 58.3 per cent. With the totally healed ulcers excluded, the non-healing ulcers decreased in area by 44.4 per cent in the same period.

Aerobic bacteria

The findings of the initial pretreatment swab are shown in Table 6.1. This revealed a wide variety of common skin organisms with *Staph. aureus* predominating, as would be expected. Most of the ulcers had at least two species present; the most in any one ulcer was, however, five species. Overall, there was very little change in the aerobic flora in the 8-week period,

Table 6.1   Findings of pretreatment swab

Staph. aureus	12	Strep. Group B	2
Proteus mirabilis	7	Strep. Group G	2
Ps. aeruginosa	5	Ps. stutzeri	2
Staph. albus	3	E. coli	1
Strep. faecalis	3	Strep. Group A	1
Ent. cloahae	2	Anaerobes	1
Kleb. oxytoca	2	No growth	1

n=25; this number includes five ulcers that were not studied for the full 8 weeks

in that, once an organism was present, it became a permanent feature of the flora. Seventeen ulcers gained at least one further species, usually within the first 4 weeks.

The most striking feature was the acquisition of *Strep. faecalis*, which appeared in eight ulcers in the week following the commencement of the treatment, and in two others in weeks 2 and 3 respectively. Overall, 13 out of 20 ulcers contained this organism at some point in the trial. Only nine ulcers lost any species during the trial, in each case one species only. The main feature of this loss was the complete disappearance of the *Pseudomonas* species from all except one ulcer within 4 weeks. In the one remaining case, *Pseudomonas* was still present after 16 weeks, when it was established by close questioning that the subject had been lifting the dressing each morning to squeeze out the exudate in order to prevent accidental leakage. This practice was discontinued, and the *Pseudomonas* was absent 7 days later.

Anaerobic bacteria

Anaerobic bacteria were cultured from 12 out of 20 ulcers, but there was no consistent pattern to the week of first appearance, which ranged from week 1 to week 8. Anaerobes were present at some time in six of the nine ulcers that healed completely, and the predominant species cultured was *Petococcus magnus*, although *Bacteroides* was cultured on three occasions. Serial dilutions did not show any significant increase in numbers over time.

Healing rates

The healing rates were calculated from the slope of the log(area) *vs* time graph, using the method described by Ryan (1985). No significant difference in healing rates could be demonstrated between those ulcers that contained anaerobes and those that did not ($p=0.26$).

DISCUSSION

The main finding of this study – that there is very little change in the bacterial flora of an ulcer treated with HCD, and that the flora appears to have little influence on the healing of the ulcer – will help to relieve some of the very real worries that nurses may have had about this product. It is generally agreed that any such ulcer is likely to be contaminated with bacteria; the difficulty facing the nurse is the question of whether or not particular bacteria are pathogenic or not, as this will depend on a number of factors, and opportunistic infections can also occur as the result of bacteria that are normally harmless commensals.

Despite this, there is increasing evidence that the presence of bacteria does not necessarily adversely affect wound healing (Leaper, 1986), and one study even suggests that, as the presence of bacteria does not seem to influence diagnosis, treatment or prognosis, the practice of sending routine swabs to the laboratory is both unnecessary and wasteful (Eriksson et al, 1984).

What, then, should the nurse look for? Observations from this study and from previous reports (Allen, 1985) suggest that the best indicators of bacterial invasion are the classic symptoms of cellulitis, i.e. redness, increased swelling, heat and, most especially, a sudden increase in pain, which is of a different nature to that associated with the ulcer itself. It is agreed that, at this point, the most appropriate treatment is systemic antibiotics (Allen, 1985). Although a swab might be indicated at this time, it should be remembered that the result may be misleading and should be interpreted with caution as either: (i) the organism cultured might not be the one causing the cellulitis, or, (ii) the organism causing the cellulitis might not be cultured at all. Nevertheless, there is now general agreement that topical antibiotics must never be used in the routine treatment of venous ulceration.

The rapid colonisation by *Strep. faecalis* is unexplained. Although the intact skin around the ulcer is the obvious potential source, control swabs from the intact skin did not indicate that this was the case. It is tempting to argue that the organism was introduced via the hands of the district nurses, but this would require a further study to examine this question. The apparent anti-Pseudomonal effect of the dressing is consistent with previously published papers (Katz et al, 1986; Varghese et al, 1986) and although a number of mechanisms have been suggested, the evidence of the subject who lifted the dressing appears to support the theory that eradication of oxygen is fatal to this obligate aerobe.

The incidence of anaerobic bacteria is greater than that previously reported in another study using the same dressing (Eriksson, 1985). This is thought to be due to the special specimen collection technique that was developed for this study, as anaerobic bacteria are very difficult to isolate normally. Nevertheless, in this study the presence of anaerobic bacteria could not be shown to adversely affect wound healing.

This study showed, therefore, that hydrocolloid dressings are a safe, effective treatment for out-patient use, and that they do not appear to promote harmful bacterial growth. The study did, however, raise some interesting and important issues with respect to nurses carrying out clinical research.

Access to patients

Clinical trials depend for their success on an adequate number of suitable patients. There are now a number of nurses in the UK who have been able successfully to combine their daily work with such trials (see, for example, Millward, 1986), but in many cases nurses wishing to conduct such trials will first have to obtain the 'consent' of a consultant before being allowed access to patients, and such permission may be one of the conditions laid down by the ethical committee. This will mean, therefore, the nurse gaining the support of an appropriate medical colleague. While there are some outstanding examples of such support in the field of leg ulcer treatment, this is not always the case.

Such trials can also be difficult to conduct on an in-patient basis because of the length of time to the end of the trial and the necessity to discharge patients as soon as possible. Once in the community it may be much more difficult to control all the variables and ensure a standard treatment.

Ethical issues

There is as yet no standard policy on nursing and clinical research, and the attitude will vary from area to area. The protocol for this study, for example, was submitted simultaneously to two different ethical committees in two London teaching hospitals; approval for the study was granted within a week by one committee, while the other would not approve the study at all. Another interesting ethical problem arose in the course of this study: despite the approved protocol stating that 'No systemic therapy will be given unless there is concurrent evidence of cellulitis, and deterioration of the surrounding tissue', the appearance of Group A *Streptococcus* in one ulcer prompted the medical staff to insist that antibiotics must be given. Although it is accepted that a risk might be present (Schraibman, 1987), this was a clear breach of the protocol, and there was no clinical indication that therapy should be started. Indeed, had the patient not been taking part in a trial, there is little doubt that a swab would not even have been taken. Nevertheless, once the result was known, an ethical problem arose which was resolved by the attending medical staff taking unilateral action.

Time

Studies such as this require a great deal of time. Even if the trial is conducted as part of a normal daily routine, time over and above this must be devoted to analysis of the results, the performing of calculations, etc., and in writing up the results. The setting up of a special clinic also necessitated a time commitment of one half-day every week for nearly a year – a difficult problem for the charge nurse of an acute ward, and one that requires much co-operation from other staff.

Co-operation of others

This trial depended very much for its success on the willingness of the district nurses to provide back-up and to follow the trial protocol. Although they may well have been attracted by the fact that the protocol actually reduced their workload, it could not have proceeded without them. During the trial two nurses phoned for advice, and such availability is critical for good co-operation.

Clearly, this trial also required considerable assistance in the culture and identification of microorganisms, and the invaluable help of Dr Caroline Reed is acknowledged. In the current climate, however, such help may be limited simply by lack of time and space in an otherwise busy laboratory.

Availability of products

When this study was conducted hydrocolloid dressings were not available on FP10 prescription. This meant that the researcher had to provide all the necessary materials for the nurses if the trial was to proceed at all, and in this instance the manufacturers agreed to provide an adequate supply for research purposes. Nevertheless, if the treatment is shown to be successful (as was the case in this instance), the nurse has the problem of not being able to use a treatment that she believes is going to benefit the patient.

This does not mean, however, that such trials should not be conducted. Rather, it is only with evidence such as this that the nurse can successfully argue that new products should be approved. This problem was recently highlighted by Dale (1986), and there is now increasing awareness that nurses are ideally placed to conduct such trials and that they have the expertise.

Such trials must, however, be well planned, contain sufficient numbers and be meticulously carried out. Perhaps it is time for nurses to carry out 'multi-centre trials' too. Such exercises will be costly and time consuming, but they are, I believe, essential if nurses are to identify those treatments that will best meet the needs of this difficult patient group.

ACKNOWLEDGEMENT

This study was financed by a grant from Squibb Surgicare, and their support and encouragement is gratefully acknowledged.

N.B. Since this study was undertaken, 'Granuflex' dressings have been made available on FP10 prescription, but only in one size.

REFERENCES

Allen S (1985) Leg ulcers and their management. *Nursing Times*, **81**(25): 49-56.

Aly R, Shirley C, Cunico B and Maibach H (1978) Effect of prolonged occlusion on the microbial flora, pH, carbon dioxide and transepidermal water loss on human skin. *Journal of Investigative Dermatology*, **71**(6): 378-381.

Browse N (1983) Venous ulceration. *British Medical Journal*, **286**: 1920-1921.

Buchan I A, Andrews J K, Lang S M et al (1980) Clinical and laboratory investigation of the composition and properties of human skin wound exudate under semipermeable dressings. *Burns*, **7**: 326-334.

Callam M J, Ruckley C V, Harper D P and Dale J J (1985) Chronic venous ulceration of the leg: extent of the problem and provision of care. *British Medical Journal*, **298**: 1855-1856.

Cherry G W, Ryan T and McGibbon D (1984) Trial of a new dressing in venous leg ulcers. *Practitioner*, **228**: 1175-1178.

Dale J (1986) Treatments on trial. *Community Outlook*, October, pp. 32-37.

Drug and Therapeutic Bulletin (1986) Dressings for leg ulcers. *Drug and Therapeutic Bulletin*, **24**(3): 1-4.

Eriksson E (1985) Comparative study of hydrocolloid dressing and double layer bandage in the treatment of venous stasis ulceration. In: *An Environment for Healing: the Role of Occlusion*, ed. Ryan T J, pp. 45-49. London: Royal Society of Medicine.

Eriksson E, Eklund A-E and Kallings L O (1984) The clinical significance of bacterial growth in leg ulcers. *Scandinavian Journal of Infectious Disease*, **16**(2): 175-180.

Hinman C D and Maibach H (1963) The effect of air exposure and occlusion on experimental human skin wounds. *Nature*, **200**(4904): 377-378.

Journal of District Nursing (1987) Your data on leg ulcers. *Journal of District Nursing*, **5**(9): 4-6.

Katz S, McGinley K and Leyden J J (1986) Semipermeable occlusive dressings. *Archives of Dermatology*, **122**: 58-62.

Lawrence J C (1985) The physical properties of a new hydrocolloid dressing. In: *An Environment for Healing: the Role of Occlusion*, ed. Ryan T J, pp. 69-76. London: Royal Society of Medicine.

Leaper D (1986) Antiseptics and their effect on healing tissues. *Nursing Times*, **82**(23): 45-47.

Marples R R and Kligman A M (1969) Growth of bacteria under adhesive tapes. *Archives of Dermatology*, **99**: 107-110.

Mertz P M and Eaglstein W H (1984) The effect of a semi-occlusive dressing on the microbial population in superficial wounds. *Archives of Surgery*, **119**(3): 287-289.

Millward P (1986) The use of hydrocolloid dressings. *Care Science and Practice*, **4**(3): 24-25.

Morgan D (1987) *The Management of Leg Ulcers*, 2nd edn. Cardiff, Whitchurch Hospital.

Negus D (1985) Prevention and treatment of venous ulceration. *Annals of the Royal College of Surgeons of England*, **67**: 144-148.

Ryan T J (1985) Current management of leg ulcers. *Drugs*, **30**: 461-468.

Schraibman I G (1987) The bacteriology of leg ulcers. *Phlebology*, **2**(4): 265-270.

Stewart A, Foster M and Leaper D (1985) Treating ulcers. *Nursing Mirror*, **161**(12): suppl. 56-58.

van Rijswijk L, Brown D, Friedman S et al (1985) Multicentre clinical evaluation of a hydrocolloid dressing for leg ulcers. *Cutis*, **35**: 173-176.

Varghese M, Balin A K, Carter D M and Caldwell D (1986) Local environment of chronic wounds under synthetic dressings. *Archives of Dermatology*, **122**: 52-57.

Winter G D (1962) Formation of the scab and the rate of epithelialisation of superficial wounds in the skin of the young domestic pig. *Nature*, **193**: 293-294.

Chapter 7

Nursing Process Evaluation Working Group

Jack Hayward

The reader may find it a little strange that here, nestled in a book on 10 years of nursing research at King's College, is an account of the activities and findings of a working party. 'Surely', some may exclaim, 'a working party cannot and does not employ methods as rigorous and controlled as even the more qualitative aspects of research reported elsewhere in this volume. What place can it justifiably occupy?'

There are two answers. First, the main task of the working party was to identify research priorities in relation to the nursing process, as seen by carefully selected members of the nursing profession, a review of the literature and the views of numerous organisations and interested parties. Second, the working party is an established method of seeking and ordering perceptions, beliefs and opinions that prevail at a certain time about a given issue. Provided that the membership is chosen carefully and the evidence is drawn from the widest possible range of sources, such evidence possesses a 'collective validity', a fact recognised by the wide use of working parties as a basis for policy formation in governmental and other circles. Indeed, for the task in hand, it was difficult to envisage a viable alternative.

BACKGROUND

What, then, are the circumstances that favour the working party approach? Perhaps the most obvious concern size and complexity of the topic: any new aspect of social, economic or professional policy aimed at bringing about changes nationwide is bound to have local variations in interpretation and implementation. For instance, some schemes will be considered 'better' than others, hence there is a value component; some may claim to be 'more efficient in the use of resources', an economic slant; yet others may argue that important aspects of professional practice and development are at stake. The nursing process has advocates who claim that its adoption will improve the quality of nursing care and sceptics who complain that time spent on laborious documentation could be better spent on direct patient care.

So, where the focus of interest has great size and complexity, together with substantial regional or local variations, problems are created for orthodox research approaches. Additionally, to gain insight into a phenomenon that is developing and changing at a rapid pace, even a sizeable research project taking, say, 5 years or more may not only be horrendously complex to initiate and manage, but may, after much endeavour, end up having dubious validity because of the rate of change. If other ingredients, such as cost, appropriate personnel and the necessity of obtaining both quantitative and qualitative data, are added, any idea of a national survey becomes daunting; however, if more discreet targets for research are first identified by a specially convened working party, there is a fair chance that selection of priorities will be relevant to broad as well as specific aspects.

From a number of articles and reports it was clear that although the advent of the nursing process was a key discussion point during any debate on nursing, ambiguities existed about its precise nature, for instance an agreed definition, the meaning of full or part implementation and the degree to which this has taken place in British nursing. In other words, by 1985 a great deal was known about these matters but, equally, a great deal was not known. Unknowns often indicate the need for research, but before the Nursing Research Liaison Group (NRLG) of the Department of Health and Social Security could pin-point specific priorities much exploratory work was needed.

METHODS OF WORKING

It was for this reason that the Nursing Process Evaluation Working Group (NPEWG) was appointed in April 1985 'to tease apart the various issues involved in evaluating the effectiveness of the Nursing Process as a guide to both teaching and practice and then make recommendations to the NRLG on priorities for future research'. Chaired by Dame Phyllis Friend, formerly Chief Nursing Officer at the DHSS, the membership was drawn from National Health Service nursing services and academic institutions. To ensure a range of views, National Health Service members were selected from over 150 nominations submitted by regional nursing officers, and represented management, practice, education and nursing process co-ordination.

The terms of reference required the group to 'consider the present position relating to preparation for and implementation of the Nursing Process in the provision of . . . acute care; care of the elderly . . .; to identify problems and issues arising in implementation of the Nursing Process in these sectors', also in midwifery and health visiting, and to 'report to DHSS by Spring 1986 incorporating outline protocols/problems statements (including suggested research methods) for each priority area amenable to research'.

The working party held 11 formal meetings and numerous ad hoc discussions as specific aspects were organised by small groups of members, all of which fed material into the main proceedings.

After consideration of background papers the group drew heavily on a number of sources of information. Paramount among these was published material, literature reviews prepared for the DHSS and information based upon local knowledge, including visits to see the nursing process in action. These activities were supplemented by evidence submitted by a wide spread of organisations, groups and individuals.

Inevitably, although the working group remained resolutely focused on the nursing process, from time to time almost the whole of nursing was mentioned. Sticking to the job in hand often necessitated much discipline. Early on, considerable discussion took place as to the eventual style and nature of the report. It needed to be clear, distinctive and unmistakable in its intention; in no way was it to be seen as a text on 'how to implement the Nursing Process'. Rather, it was to be descriptive of the current situation, not only its introduction, but ways by which the nursing process might be viewed as a basis for practice and education. Above all, the working group aimed to identify areas of the nursing process amenable to research and to rank these in order of priority.

PROBLEMS OF DEFINITION

First, however, the group had to clarify what it meant by the nursing process. Mindful of the fact that a plethora of definitions exist – including some that appear to confuse rather than clarify – the group took the view that, for an adequate understanding, two important aspects need to be grasped. First, that the nursing process has been one of the greatest self-generated processes of change the nursing profession has ever witnessed; developed entirely from within rather than as a reaction to external events, it has been an internal revaluation in the way nurses view the delivery of care. This fact alone makes the nursing process a fascinating area of study for anyone interested in self-generated change within professional groups. Second, the nursing process has both ideological and procedural components – the former largely because of its relationship with certain schemata or models of care (the nursing process may have its theoretical underpinnings here), and the latter because the oft-quoted four-stage process of assessment of need, the setting of objectives that form part of a care plan, implementation of this plan and, finally, evaluation of the outcome provides system and structure to what the nurse does. In view of this orientation the group agreed that, for its purpose, the nursing process is:

'. . . a planned systematic approach to the care of the individual patient'.

Ideally, then, the nursing process is the practical realisation of ideas about care that have their roots in one or more models of care.

For research purposes, however, a deeper consideration of the problems of definition was undertaken, because precision and clarity of definition is often the first stage in a process characterised by rigour in thought and action; in other words, if the group's eventual recommendations were to be soundly based, they should, so to speak, incorporate certain theoretical and conceptual ideas.

RESEARCH AND THE NURSING PROCESS

An example of such consideration would be the choice of appropriate research methods. For instance, it would be convenient if the effectiveness of implementation of the nursing process could be measured by means of a controlled trial – nursing process versus non-nursing process wards or districts. But, even if this rather simple-minded empiricism would have been at any time valid, it would certainly have faced serious problems at the time of the working group's study (1986). For one thing, recent developments then meant that it was virtually impossible to find a hospital or district that remained immune to recent influences, and for another, the range and subtlety of data would require a variety of research methods if the total exercise was to have any degree of credibility. For instance, the semantic properties of the term 'nursing process' and of its conceptual underpinnings assume considerable importance because many of these ideas may, on the face of it, be unresearchable in any empirical sense. 'But', the reader may exclaim, 'surely certain aspects of the four stages described above contain processes and procedures that may be examined within a broadly empirical framework?'. This may be so, but, equally, there are other important constituents of a metaphysical or ethical nature not amenable to an empirical approach; the study of one aspect is of little use without the other. By widening the range of possible research approaches there is little of the nursing process that does not become open to some sort of investigation in three broad areas: semantic analysis to clarify meanings, ethical analysis to examine value systems and empirical research into the effects of practice.

WIDER EFFECTS OF THE NURSING PROCESS

It has for some time been abundantly clear that the nursing process has had far-reaching effects on nursing. Perhaps not always manifestly, but by 1985 it would have been rare to find a trained nurse who was not in some way conversant with its principles. The nursing process has affected all sections of the profession, even though large numbers of more senior nurses have not themselves practised it. Most notably, however, it has affected the way in which nurses think about the care of patients, many would claim for the better. It is here that the nub of the debate emerges: many of those who use the nursing process believe it has not only improved their practice but has brought increased job satisfaction in its train. The part research can play is to investigate and, if possible, illuminate, substantiate or refute such claims. In 1985, although a sizeable literature existed, only a lamentably small proportion of this could be described as research.

Because of this, the group felt it important to gather the greatest possible amount of information – factual, anecdotal and impressionistic – in order to paint a reasonable picture of the way in which the nursing process had affected nursing and the scale of its take-up, and, from this information, to pin-point research priorities.

The first and most obvious ploy was to examine the literature, which falls into fairly distinct groups: advocatory, prescriptive, descriptive and, rarely, evaluative. The shortcomings of experiential accounts are well documented, but it can be argued that if similar perceptions are reported by a wide spread of people, or if reported experiences are backed by evidence from a variety of sources, individuals or groups, then a certain weight or validity can be accorded them. The collecting of evidence was, therefore, the logical next step.

Not all of the evidence received or heard raised issues that were in any way researchable but, after a while, certain threads or strands began to emerge – a discernible similarity between evidence in specific areas, a growing consensus as to what were the strengths and weaknesses of developments to date. This is not to exaggerate the level of agreement achieved or to deny that on some issues conflicting evidence was received, but without doubt broad agreement emerged, for example on the belief that, where practised well, the nursing process aids morale and provides increased job satisfaction among nurses, or that, in some cases, insufficient discussions with professional colleagues are held before changes in practice occur. This latter problem of poor interprofessional communication was highlighted on numerous occasions.

IMPLEMENTATION

In spite of all the evidence taken from individuals and organisations, the literature reviews and the sifting and sorting, it remained difficult to identify to any degree of precision the extent to which the nursing process had been implemented nationally. It seemed likely that, by 1986, attempts had been made in the majority of health districts but, in itself, this remains only a rough guide to the extent and effectiveness of implementation. One thing that became very clear, however, was the great disparity between health districts in the style and manner of their attempted introduction. Some districts tried very hard to bring it in with tact and in a planned manner. However, evidence from a number of other health districts as well as numerous articles and letters told a different and rather sad story, often where senior nurses appear to have pushed their staff into using the nursing process without adequate preparation of either the staff themselves or of others in the workplace. Predictably, this often produced resentment and a tendency for the nurses concerned to reject the whole idea: the nursing process simply became yet another task! Alternatively, the group heard of instances where one group of nurses were keen to try out the nursing process, only to be met with hostility from other nurses opposed to the idea.

Overall, the impression received from widely ranging sources was that in the years following the General Nursing Council policy document (1977), some authorities tried to implement the nursing process with the misguided zeal and untimely haste of a shot-gun marriage. Sometimes a date was set and only token recognition given to the essential preparation required if service and educational personnel were to undergo the change in a knowledgeable and confident manner. The group was careful to emphasise that this criticism in no way detracts from those who put a great deal into preparation; it merely highlights the fact that these instances were all too few.

IDENTIFYING RESEARCH PRIORITIES

After all the evidence was collected and collated, the group set about looking for trends and directions, for out of this great mass of information the aim was to identify research priorities. In addition to general nursing, specialised areas of midwifery, psychiatric nursing, health visiting and mental handicap all come under scrutiny, so the task was formidable.

Finally, however, the need for some degree of classification became apparent. The research issues, themselves, seemed to fall into nine areas, which could then be put into two categories as in Figure 7.1. Substantial overlap will occur between areas, and between issues contained

Category	Area
Scope of research	Management and organisation
	The change process
	Education
	Practice
	Quality of care
Scale of research	National
	Local
	Ward level
	Individual

Fig. 7.1 Classification of the research issues

Table 7.1 Research classification grid

Scope	Scale			
	National	Local	Ward/care setting	Individual
Management and organisation	1	2	3	4
Change process	5	6	7	8
Education	9	10	11	12
Practice	13	14	15	16
Quality of care	17	18	19	20

within areas, but when the two categories of Figure 7.1 are transferred to a grid format or matrix, a useful framework emerges (Table 7.1).

Chapter 6 of the report discussed these topics in detail, together with possible research approaches under the headings of:

1. extent of implementation;
2. quality of care;
3. perceptions, beliefs and expectations;
4. professional competencies;
5. the learning environment;
6. accountability;
7. effects on staff, patients and relatives; and
8. historical background;
   together with some of the main research questions.

After a year's work, the group succeeded in identifying a number of areas in which research might be useful. The list is not exhaustive or definitive, but was felt to be a useful addition to the DHSS research commissioning process whereby decisions about priorities for funding are made. The group took the view 'that there should be a systematic and coordinated programme of research relating to the Nursing Process. Individual and small-scale projects and dissertations on their own are of limited value, but if their findings corroborate the findings of others, their reliability and hence their usefulness assume greater importance. We recommend that the feasibility of setting up such a group be explored with professional and education bodies, the NHS and higher education sector'.

This short chapter has merely highlighted some of the background and procedural aspects of what in the end became a sizeable endeavour. Obviously, the full report (Hayward, 1986) contains very much more detail, and is required reading for any researcher intending to work on the nursing process, those nurses closely involved with decisions about implementation or, in fact, anyone with more than a passing interest in the subject.

ACKNOWLEDGEMENT

The working group was exceedingly fortunate to have Frances Cooper as Research Officer, whose reviews of relevant publications and theses were especially helpful.

REFERENCES

General Nursing Council for England and Wales (1977) *A Statement of Educational Policy*, Circular 77/19A.

Hayward J (ed.) (1986) *The Nursing Process Evaluation Working Group*, NERU Report No. 5. King's College, University of London: Nursing Research Unit.

Chapter 8

Midwives' Responsibilities for Decision-making

Sarah Robinson

BACKGROUND TO THE STUDY

Midwives trained in Britain are qualified to provide care throughout pregnancy, labour and the puerperium on their own responsibility, to recognise those signs of abnormality that require referral to medical staff, and to provide advice, information and emotional support to women from early pregnancy to the end of the postnatal period. During the late 1970s, however, much concern was expressed that a number of factors were preventing midwives from fulfilling this role: these included increased medical involvement in normal maternity care, fragmentation of care between an increasing number of health professionals and staff shortages (e.g. Royal College of Midwives, 1977; Barnett, 1979; Brain, 1979).

This chapter describes a study of midwives' responsibilities, undertaken in 1979, when concern about their role was at its height. It was commissioned and funded by the Department of Health and Social Security and supported from the outset by the Royal College of Midwives and the then Central Midwives Board.

Prior to this time, little research had in fact focused on the responsibilities of midwives. One of the earliest examples of research that did exist was a national survey of the views and work experience of midwives, carried out by a Ministry of Health Working Party in 1947 (Ministry of Health et al, 1949). They concluded that the role of the midwife, with its focus on the normality of childbirth, had been overshadowed by the 1920s' and 1930s' campaign to reduce maternal mortality. This had emphasised the potential abnormalities of childbirth and focused on the role of medical staff at the expense of the role of midwives.

Subseqent research included a study of midwives' work conditions and reasons for entering and leaving the profession (Ramsden and Radwanski, 1963) and a study of the perceptions held by midwives and medical staff of the midwife's responsibilities (Walker, 1976). The latter study demonstrated a diversity of views in that doctors regarded themselves as responsible for decision-making in all aspects of normal and abnormal maternity cases and were willing to delegate some of this responsibility to midwives, whereas midwives regarded themselves as independent practitioners, taking responsibility for normal cases and providing assistance to medical staff in abnormal cases (Walker, 1976). Most of the other studies undertaken in this period were concerned with determining how many midwives were required to staff the maternity services adequately (Sheffield Regional Hospital Board, 1972; Auld, 1974; Croydon Area Health Authority, 1976; Papakyriakou, 1977).

In view of the concern about restrictions on opportunities for midwives to fulfil the role for which they were trained, this study aimed to document the activities and procedures they were undertaking and the degree of responsibility they were able to exercise for decision-making in antepartum, intrapartum and postpartum care. Views on respective responsibilities for maternity care were also sought from midwives and other health professionals with whom they worked. Related topics such as views on adequacy of staffing levels, opportunities to provide continuity of care and views on extending the role of the midwife into areas such as family planning were also explored in the course of the study. All these data are available in Robinson et al (1983), and publications focusing on specific aspects of the study include Robinson (1980 and 1985a, b, c). This chapter focuses on midwives' responsibilities for decision-making.

METHODS

Exploratory interviews with midwives and other personnel involved in maternity care revealed considerable diversity in the level of responsibility exercised by midwives and in opinions concerning the role that they should fulfil in maternity care. In view of this diversity and the paucity of earlier work in the field, a national survey by questionnaire of midwives, health visitors, obstetricians and general practitioners was chosen as the most appropriate method for achieving the aims of the study. This strategy provided information on the diversity of practice and on overall trends, as well as providing sufficient numbers for statistical analysis within sub-groups.

The survey design was a two-stage random sample, stratified by region. One in four of the health districts was selected randomly from each of the 14 regional health authorities and from Wales, providing a total of 60 districts in all. The sample sizes required were provided by including all the midwives and medical staff in obstetrics in post in each district, a one-in-two sample of the health visitors and a one-in-three sample of general practitioners on the obstetric list in each district.

Attempts to ensure validity of the questionnaires were of two kinds: first, extensive piloting of the questionnaires, and, second, by interviewing and observing sub-samples of respondents who had completed pilot questionnaires. The latter procedure, described as *between-method triangulation* (Denzin, 1978), indicated whether data obtained by different methods produced the same findings. Data obtained from questionnaires, interviews and observations revealed a high degree of concordance, indicating that the questionnaire satisfied the criteria of validity as well as those of representativeness and reliability. Seventy-eight per cent (4128) of the midwives returned their questionnaires, and this represented one-fifth of those in practice in 1979. Response rates for health visitors, obstetric staff and general practitioners were 87 per cent (1177), 56 per cent (333) and 67 per cent (1122) respectively. In this chapter data from midwives only are presented.

FINDINGS

Antenatal care

The data showed that a substantial majority of both hospital and community midwives performed the various tasks involved in normal antenatal care – interviewing the woman and

Table 8.1 Hospital and community midwives' responsibilities for abdominal examination

Responsibility for abdominal examination	Percentage of respondents	
	Midwives in consultant units %	Community midwives %
Usually carried out by midwife only	4.3	13.9
Usually carried out by doctor only	33.4	16.7
Carried out by midwife, but usually repeated by doctor	57.3	48.7
Carried out by midwife at one visit and by doctor at next visit	—	6.8
Situation varies from one clinic to another	—	8.6
No answer	5.0	5.3
Total	100% (634)	100% (1159)

recording her history, and carrying out procedures to assess the clinical condition of the woman and foetus. Even though a midwife carries out these procedures, she may not *necessarily* be required to take responsibility for the overall decision that pregnancy is progressing normally, as in many clinics this is regarded as the doctor's responsibility. If so, the doctor will carry out the abdominal examination, even if it has already been carried out by a midwife, as it is when this examination is performed and the results of the other routine investigations are available that the overall assessment of pregnancy is made.

Consequently, the hospital and the community midwives were asked who usually carried out the abdominal examination in the clinic in which they worked; their answers are shown in Table 8.1. The data in column 1 of the table show that the great majority of hospital midwives worked in clinics in which medical staff were responsible for the assessment of pregnancy, in that 33.4 per cent said the examination was carried out by a doctor only and 57.3 per cent said it was carried out by a midwife but then repeated by a doctor.

It can, of course, be argued that one of the reasons why many women attending hospital antenatal clinics are always examined by a doctor is that, with the advent of 'shared antenatal care' with the general practitioner, visits to the hospital clinic are regarded as for the specific purpose of assessment by the obstetrician. However, figures in the second data column of the table show that when women visit community antenatal clinics, they are also likely to be assessed by medical staff, in that 16.7 per cent of the community midwives said the abdominal examination was usually carried out by the doctor only and 48.7 per cent said it was carried out by the midwife but usually repeated by the doctor. Just under a third of the community midwives were responsible for the abdominal examination in some or in all of the clinics in which they worked, but this was the case for less than 5 per cent of the hospital midwives.

The survey data also indicated that few other opportunities existed for midwives to make antenatal assessments on their own responsibility. Although midwives' clinics were held in 26 of the 71 consultant units included in the survey, in 19 of these units medical staff referred only a very small proportion of women to the midwives' clinic. Community midwives do have the opportunity to make antenatal assessments when they visit women at home during the antenatal period, but the majority of those who participated in this study made few home visits for this purpose.

Intrapartum care

Investigating the division of responsibility between midwives and medical staff for the care of women during labour and delivery was more complex than the corresponding division of responsibility for antepartum care. Although there was an increase in the 1970s in the proportion of operative and instrumental deliveries, the majority of deliveries in the UK, as in previous decades, continued to be undertaken or supervised by a midwife (Chamberlain et al, 1978; Cartwright, 1979; Department of Health and Social Security, 1978). Changes were, however, taking place in the extent to which the midwife was responsible for determining the pattern of care during labour and delivery. This was due both to an increase in the involvement of medical staff in the assessment of women in the labour ward, and to the introduction of policies specifying the procedures to be followed in the management of labour and delivery, such as the frequency of vaginal examinations, the length of time allowed for the second stage of labour and whether or not to use routine continuous foetal heart rate monitoring.

Midwives in this study were asked which of the situations described in Table 8.2 usually applied in the labour ward in which they worked. A substantial majority said that women in normal labour are cared for by a midwife and only examined by a doctor at a midwife's request.

Midwives may be exercising their clinical judgment when making decisions concerning the care of women in normal labour, or they may be required to follow a unit policy or a decision made by a doctor with regard to some aspect of this care. The figures in Table 8.2 show that a total of 91.5% (1445) of the midwives said they worked in units in which normal labours were managed by the midwife. In order to ascertain the proportion of these midwives who, nonetheless, worked in units in which aspects of this management were determined by unit policy or medical decisions, they were asked who was responsible for the decisions listed in Table 8.3.

The data on decision-making show that by 1979 the midwife's freedom to make decisions, basic to the care of women in normal labour, had to some extent been curtailed. The proportion of respondents who said that the midwife made the decision varied from one procedure to another – from 36.9 per cent for using continuous foetal heart rate monitoring machines to 94.3 per cent for carrying out an episiotomy. Just under half of the respondents said that

Table 8.2 Midwives in consultant units: management of normal labour

Management of normal labour	Percentage of respondents
Patients in normal labour are cared for by a midwife and only examined by a doctor if this is requested by a midwife	79.8
All patients are examined by a doctor on admission and then normal labours are managed entirely by a midwife, unless a problem arises	11.7
All patients are examined by a doctor on admission, and visited at regular intervals throughout labour, and the decisions as to management of labour are made by a doctor	4.6
No answer	3.9
Total	100.0 (1579)

Table 8.3 Midwives in consultant units: responsibility for decision-making in normal labour

Responsibility for decision-making	Decisions made in the management of normal labour				
	When to carry out vaginal examinations	At what point during labour to rupture membranes	Whether to give intra-muscular analgesics	Whether to carry out an episiotomy	Whether to use a continuous monitoring machine
	%	%	%	%	%
Decision is usually made by a midwife	47.4	56.3	79.4	94.3	36.9
Decision is usually made by a member of the medical staff	0.3	10.2	2.0	0.3	30.2
There is a unit policy which specifies the usual procedure to be followed	49.3	29.7	19.6	4.0	28.2
No answer	2.9	3.8	3.0	2.1	4.6
Total	100 (1445)	100 (1445)	100 (1445)	100 (1445)	100 (1445)

the frequency with which vaginal examinations were carried out was determined by unit policy, and a substantial minority said that this was the case for rupturing membranes, using continuous foetal heart rate monitoring machines and giving intramuscular analgesics.

As expected, the data showed that most community midwives had little involvement in the care of women during labour and delivery. The number of home deliveries has declined steadily with the move to hospital confinements and 45 per cent of the respondents had not undertaken any home confinements in the year prior to the survey. Of those who had done so, most had carried out five or fewer. Seventy-six per cent had not undertaken any domino deliveries in that year, and of those who had, the majority had undertaken fewer than 10.

Postpartum care

Medical involvement in normal postnatal care is not usually an issue for community midwives as they provide this on their own responsibility in the woman's home, calling in medical staff if necessary. It is an issue, however, in the hospital context, and data from this study demonstrated a duplication of midwifery and medical roles similar to that found in assessment during pregnancy.

Midwives are qualified to assess the condition of the normal postpartum woman, and make daily examinations to do so. The majority participating in this study, however, worked in consultant units in which medical staff also examined normal postnatal women, either once or twice during their stay (55 per cent) or daily (26 per cent). Just 17 per cent of respondents said that medical staff examined normal postnatal women only if asked to do so by a midwife. Additionally, over 80 per cent of midwives worked in units in which medical staff always made the decisions as to whether the woman and her baby were fit to go home – decisions that midwives are also qualified to make.

IMPLICATIONS OF THE FINDINGS

The research demonstrated that although midwives carried out a major part of the care provided for childbearing women, a substantial proportion were not required to exercise fully the degree of clinical responsibility for which they were trained and qualified, as they worked in situations in which medical staff had assumed this responsibility. These constraints on the midwife's role raise a number of important implications for the maternity services.

First, resources are wasted. Midwives are trained at some considerable cost, but, once qualified, those parts of their training that concern decision-making, particularly in the assessment of pregnancy, are likely to be underused or duplicated. Second, the medical take-over of decision-making for normal pregnancy, labour and the puerperium limits opportunities for students to develop confidence in their skills and decision-making ability and for qualified midwives to maintain their confidence in this respect. Unit policies, whether formulated by medical staff alone or by medical staff in consultation with senior midwives, require midwives to follow predetermined courses of action, whether or not they regard it as appropriate in particular cases; as Chalmers et al (1989) have argued, many of these policies insist on practices of unproven benefit. Insistence on their implementation restricts the development and maintenance of clinical judgment by midwives. This in turn may lead to problems when policies change, as the necessary skills may have been lost with the retirement of experienced midwives and not developed in more recently trained practitioners. Third, the research demonstrated wide variation in the degree of responsibility midwives were able to exercise, and this in turn creates difficulties in the development of appropriate curricula for midwifery training. If training is designed to enable midwives to assume a particular level of responsibility, many are likely to experience the frustration and lack of job satisfaction that results from unfulfilled expectations.

Finally, and most importantly, the data from this study have a number of implications for the quality of care available to women. Failure to make full use of the clinical skills and judgment of the midwife also affects the kind of support they are able to provide. Thus, when medical staff undertake the assessment of normal pregnancy, care is likely to be fragmented into a number of tasks undertaken by different personnel – by doctors and midwives and in some clinics by nursing and auxiliary staff as well. This fragmentation reduces opportunities for midwives to develop the kind of supportive and continuous relationships within which women feel encouraged to discuss their pregnancy and voice their problems or concerns. Medical involvement in the care of all pregnant women also contributes to long waiting times, and means that medical staff have less time to spend with those women who do require their specialist medical and obstetric expertise.

It can be argued that if midwives are not entrusted with the care of normal pregnant women, then they may lose confidence in their own skills and abilities and become less able to increase the confidence of women who look to them for support. Cartwright's 1979 study demonstrated that many women felt they were given insufficient information during the course of labour. This point has been further explored by Kirkham (1983), who concluded that one of the reasons why midwives fail to provide women with information during labour is that they themselves are unhappy with the policies they are required to implement in the management of their care.

SUBSEQUENT DEVELOPMENTS AND DIRECTIONS
FOR FUTURE RESEARCH

Since this research was completed, subsequent studies have substantiated many of the findings (DHSS, 1984; Garcia et al, 1985), and concern about the underuse of the midwife's skills has been voiced continually by individual midwives, by their professional and statutory bodies and by parliamentary and government committees (see, for example, Social Services Committee, 1980; Maclean, 1980; Fisher, 1981; Morrin, 1982; Towler, 1982; Roch, 1983; Central Midwives Board for Scotland et al, 1983; Ashton, 1987).

The main question to be addressed in considering the future of maternity care provision is whether it matters, in terms of neonatal and perinatal outcomes and satisfaction with the experience of childbirth, that midwifery skills and knowledge are underutilised. Very few valid studies exist that have attempted to answer this question. Randomised controlled trials to compare the effectiveness of midwifery with medical care have been undertaken by Runnerstrom (1969), Slome et al (1976) and Flint and Poulengeris (1987), and these studies are the only three listed in the Oxford Database of Perinatal Trials (Chalmers, 1988). Retrospective studies to compare these two types of care, and studies that have examined the effect of introducing midwives into areas where access to such care was not previously available include Dillon et al (1978) and Levy et al (1971) respectively. Reviews of these studies have concluded that, although not all are perfect methodologically, they provide no indication that midwives achieve worse neonatal and perinatal outcomes than medical staff (Thompson, 1986; Robinson, 1989). Studies that have explored satisfaction with care in pregnancy and childbirth demonstrate high levels of satisfaction with care provided by midwives (e.g. Humphrey, 1985; Williams et al, 1985; Flint and Poulengeris, 1987). There appears to be no evidence to justify restricting the midwife's role in the care of normal pregnant women; to do so deprives women of the midwife's clinical skills and hinders midwives in the provision of information, advice and support.

Two trends in particular, however, militate against midwives having more responsibility for the care of women who experience a normal pregnancy, labour and puerperium. First, the continuing emphasis on the potential abnormalities of childbirth inevitably diminishes the role of the midwife in favour of the obstetric specialist; as noted, this trend was identified in the 1940s by the 1947 Midwives' Working Party (Ministry of Health et al, 1949). While there is no dispute that the specialist should have responsibility for the clinical management of women with medical or obstetric complications, there is a lack of clarity as to how much responsibility they should have for the care of women who experience normal childbirth and how much of this care should be provided by midwives acting on their own responsibility. Second, responsibilities for maternity care are increasingly seen in terms of the relative roles of the consultant on the one hand and the general practitioner on the other. Under the system of 'shared' antenatal care, for example, the care of high risk women is assigned to the obstetrician and that of low risk women to the general practitioner with intermittent assessment by the obstetrician. Care of the latter group is thus divided between two groups of medical staff, yet it is precisely this group of women for whom the midwife is specifically trained to care. Suggestions that general practitioners should care for a greater proportion of low risk women in labour (Royal College of Obstetricians and Gynaecologists, Royal College of General Practitioners, 1981) will lead to a duplication of resources in the intrapartum period similar to that which already characterises antenatal care.

In the 1980s, a number of government and professional reports have recommended that the midwife's skills be used more fully (Social Services Committee, 1980; Royal College of Obstetricians and Gynaecologists, 1982; Maternity Services Advisory Committee, 1982; Central Midwives Board et al, 1983; Royal College of Midwives, 1987), and midwives themselves have sought to restore their role by devising and in many cases implementing schemes that use their skills to the full. Midwives' clinics and delivery suites where midwives provide care for low risk women have been established in many areas (Towler, 1981; Morrin, 1982; Flint, 1982; Stuart and Judge, 1984; Curran, 1986; Flint and Poulengeris, 1987). Schemes whereby small teams of midwives provide continuity of care for women from early pregnancy to the end of the postnatal period have been implemented (Curran, 1986; Flint and Poulengeris, 1987) and in the latter case evaluated by means of a randomised controlled trial. Studies to assess the effect of midwifery support in pregnancy for women designated as high risk are in progress (Davies and Evans, 1986; Oakley and Elbourne, 1989). A wide range of aspects of care provided by midwives has now been the subject of evaluation; reports of many of these studies are available in 'Research and the Midwife Conference Proceedings' (Thomson and Robinson, 1982, 1983, 1984, 1985, 1986). If childbearing women are to be provided with effective and satisfying care, commitment is required not only to full use of midwifery skills and knowledge but also to the continuing evaluation of the way in which these are deployed.

REFERENCES

Ashton R (1987) Interview with Ruth Ashton, General Secretary, Royal College of Midwives. *Midwife, Health Visitor and Community Nurse,* **23**(7): 292-300.

Auld M (1974) *How Many Nurses?* London: Royal College of Nursing.

Barnett Z (1979) The changing pattern of maternity care and the future role of the midwife. *Midwives' Chronicle and Nursing Notes,* **92**(1102): 381-384.

Brain M (1979) Observations by a midwife. In *Report of a Day Conference on the Reduction of Perinatal Mortality and Morbidity.* London: Children's Committee and Department of Health and Social Security, HMSO.

Cartwright A (1979) *The Dignity of Labour.* London: Tavistock.

Central Midwives Board for Scotland, Northern Ireland Council for Nurses and Midwives, An Bord Altranais, Central Midwives Board (1983) *The Role of the Midwife.* Suffolk: Hymns Ancient and Modern Ltd.

Chalmers I (ed.) (1988) *The Oxford Database of Perinatal Trials.* Oxford: Oxford University Press.

Chalmers I, Enkin M and Keirse M (1989) Evaluation of care during pregnancy and childbirth. In: *Effective Care in Pregnancy and Childbirth,* eds. Enkin M, Keirse M and Chalmers I. Oxford: Oxford University Press.

Chamberlain G, Phillip E, Howlett B and Master K (1978) *British Births 1970, Vol. 2, Obstetric Care.* London: Heinemann Medical.

Croydon Area Health Authority (1976) *The Use of the Qualified Midwife.* Surrey: Croydon Area Health Authority.

Curran V (1986) Taking midwifery off the conveyor belt. *Nursing Times,* **82**(34): 42-43.

Davies J and Evans F (1986) Evaluating an inner city community care project. In: *Research and the Midwife Conference Proceedings 1986,* eds, Robinson S and Thomson A. London: King's College, London University, Nursing Research Unit.

Denzin N K (1978) *The Research Act: a Theoretical Introduction to Sociological Methods.* New York: McGraw-Hill.

Department of Health and Social Security (1984) *Study of Hospital Based Midwives - a Report by Central Management Services.* London: Department of Health and Social Security.

Dillon T, Brennan B, Dwyer J, Risk A, Sear A, Dawson L and Wiele R (1978) Midwifery 1977. *American Journal of Obstetrics and Gynecology*, **130**(8): 917-926.

Fisher C (1981) Community midwife: the gentle approach (comments made in interview). *Nursing Focus*, **3**(4): 562.

Flint C (1982) Antenatal clinics. *Nursing Mirror*, 24 Nov; 1, 8, 15 & 22 Dec; 5, 12, 19, & 26 Jan; **155**(21-24), **186**(1-4).

Flint C and Poulengeris P (1987) *The 'Know Your Midwife' Report*. Published by C Flint, 49 Peckarmans Wood, Sydenham Hill, London SE26.

Garcia J, Garforth S and Ayers S (1985) Midwives confined? Labour ward policies and routines. In: *Research and the Midwife Conference Proceedings 1985*, eds. Thomson A and Robinson S. London: Nursing Research Unit, King's College, London University.

Humphrey C (1985) The community midwife in maternity care. *Midwife, Health Visitor and Community Nurse*, **21**(10): 349-355.

Kirkham M (1989) Midwives and information-giving during labour. In: *Midwives, Research and Childbirth*, Vol. 1, eds. Robinson S and Thomson A. London: Chapman and Hall.

Levy B, Wilkinson F and Marine W (1971) Reducing neonatal mortality rate with nurse-midwives. *American Journal of Obstetrics and Gynecology*, **109**(1): 50-58.

Maclean D G (1980) Where have all the midwives gone? *Midwives' Chronicle and Nursing Notes*, **93**(1108): 158.

Maternity Services Advisory Committee (1982) *Maternity Care in Action. Part 1 - Antenatal Care*. London: HMSO.

Ministry of Health, Department of Health for Scotland, Ministry of Labour and National Service (1949) *Report of the Working Party on Midwives* (Chairman: Mrs M Stocks). London: HMSO.

Morrin H (1982) Are we in danger of extinction? *Midwives' Chronicle*, **95**(1128): 17.

Oakley A and Elbourne D (1989) Interventions to alleviate stress in pregnancy. In: *Effective Care in Pregnancy and Childbirth*, eds. Enkin M, Keirse M and Chalmers I. Oxford: Oxford University Press.

Papakyriakou J K (1977) *A Qualitative Examination of Some of the Factors Relevant to the Determination of a Manpower Planning Policy for Midwives at a Health District Level*. MSc Thesis, Department of Management Studies, University of Manchester, Institute for Science and Technology.

Ramsden P and Radwanski P (1963) *Some Aspects of the Work of the Midwife*. London: The Dan Mason Nursing Research Committee of the National Florence Nightingale Memorial Committee.

Robinson S (1980) *Midwifery Manpower*, NERU Occasional Paper No. 4. Chelsea College, London University: Nursing Research Unit.

Robinson S (1985a) Normal maternity care: whose responsibility? *British Journal of Obstetrics and Gynaecology*, **92**(1): 1-3.

Robinson S (1985b) Responsibilities of midwives and medical staff: findings from a national survey. *Midwives' Chronicle*, **98**(1166): 64-71.

Robinson S (1985c) Midwives, obstetricians and general practitioners: the need for role clarification. *Midwifery*, **1**(2): 102-113.

Robinson S (1989) The role of the midwife: opportunities and constraints. In: *Effective Care in Pregnancy and Childbirth*, eds. Enkin M, Keirse M and Chalmers I. Oxford: Oxford University Press.

Robinson S, Golden J and Bradley S (1983) *A study of the role and responsibilities of the midwife. NERU Report No. 1*. London: Chelsea College, London University: Nursing Research Unit.

Roch S (1983) Is the midwife accountable? *Nursing Times*, **79**(39): 38-39.

Royal College of Midwives (1977) *Evidence to the Royal Commission on the National Health Service*. London: Royal College of Midwives.

Royal College of Midwives (1987) *The Role and Education of the Future Midwife in the United Kingdom*. London: Royal College of Midwives.

Royal College of Obstetricians and Gynaecologists, Royal College of General Practitioners (1981) *Report on Training for Obstetrics and Gynaecology for General Practitioners by a Joint Working Party of the RCOG and RCPG*. London: RCOG/RCPG.

Royal College of Obstetricians and Gynaecologists (1982) *Report of the RCOG Working Party on Antenatal and Intrapartum Care*. London: Royal College of Obstetricians and Gynaecologists.

Runnerstrom L (1969) The effectiveness of nurse-midwifery in a supervised hospital environment. *Bulletin of the American College of Nurse Midwives*, **14**(2): 40-52.

Sheffield Regional Hospital Board (1972) *Report of the Working Party to Study the Hospital Midwife.* Sheffield: Sheffield Regional Hospital Board.

Slome C, Wetherbee H, Daly M, Christensen K, Maglen H and Thiede H (1976) Effectiveness of certified nurse-midwives: a prospective evaluation study. *American Journal of Obstetrics and Gynecology,* **124**(2): 177–182.

Social Services Committee, House of Commons (1980) *Report on Perinatal and Neonatal Mortality* (Chairman: R Short). London: HMSO.

Stuart B and Judge E (1984) The return of the midwife? *Midwives' Chronicle,* **97**(1152): 8–9.

Thompson J B (1986) Safety and effectiveness of nurse midwifery care: research review. In: *Nurse Midwifery in America,* eds. Rooks H P and Haas J E. A report of the American Nurse Midwives Foundation, Washington.

Thomson A and Robinson S (1982, 1983, 1984, 1985, 1986) *Research and the Midwife Conference Proceedings.* King's College, London University, Nursing Research Unit; University of Manchester, Department of Nursing Studies.

Towler J (1981) Out of the ordinary. Park Hospital Maternity Unit. *Nursing Mirror,* **152**: 32–33.

Towler J (1982) A dying species: survival and revival are up to us. *Midwives' Chronicle,* **95**(1136): 324–328.

Walker J (1976) Midwife or obstetric nurse? Some perceptions of midwives and obstetricians of the role of the midwife. *Journal of Advanced Nursing,* **1**: 129–138.

Williams S, Hepburn M and McIlwaine G (1985) Consumer view of epidural analgesia. *Midwifery,* **1**(1): 32–36.

Chapter 9

Defining a Role for Nurse Practitioners in British General Practice

Barbara Stilwell

THE PROBLEM

In 1986 the government-initiated Community Nursing Review (DHSS, 1986) recommended that: 'The principle should be adopted of introducing the nurse practitioner into primary health care'. The role that the review team envisaged was wide-ranging and encompassed the diagnosis and treatment of specific diseases, counselling, screening and care of the chronic sick. This recommendation is supported by the Royal College of Nursing, who see the key to the nurse practitioner role as the autonomy to admit and discharge patients from the primary health-care system (Royal College of Nursing, 1986).

The Social Services Committee of the House of Commons examined and reported on the Community Nursing Review team's findings and also recommended that the role of the nurse practitioner should be developed. They say: 'Properly trained practitioners, working closely with general practitioners, could perform a valuable complementary service for elderly patients' (Social Services Committee, 1987).

These attempts at a definition of a role for nurse practitioners have led to confusion, particularly among nurses who are employed by general practitioners to work in treatment rooms; such nurses are known as practice nurses. Practice nurses have jobs that vary considerably and their work has been the subject of many studies since the mid-sixties, when general practitioners were offered a 70 per cent subsidy of a nurse's salary.

Most studies that have described the roles of practice nurses have been undertaken by doctors and have concerned various aspects of delegation of tasks (Bowling, 1985). Some delegation has been extensive, one practice studying the effects of a nurse undertaking first home visits (Weston-Smith and Mottram, 1967; Weston-Smith and O'Donovan, 1970), while Reedy (1972) noted that some practice nurses performed venepunctures, sutured wounds, gave simple physiotherapy and assessed patients attending surgery without an appointment. It may be the extension of the nursing role into these traditionally medical areas that has led some authors to compare the role of the practice nurse with that of the American nurse practitioner (Harris, 1970; Devlin, 1985; Cater and Hawthorn, 1987). In some practices nurses are now employed with the title of nurse practitioner (Fawcett-Henesy, 1987; Restall, 1987).

The problem, then, is one of definition. Is a practice nurse role the same as that of a nurse practitioner, or is it more akin to a physician's assistant, as Reedy (1980) suggested in his analysis of practice nurses' work?

PREVIOUS RESEARCH

As stated earlier, most research into the work of nurses in general practice has been undertaken by doctors and has tended to focus on tasks rather than on an analysis of total nursing care (Rea, 1962; March, 1967; Hasler et al, 1968; Kuenssberg, 1971; Bowling, 1981). Some writers have alluded to the nurse's role as listener or counsellor (Cartwright and Scott, 1961; Weston-Smith and Mottram, 1967; Kuenssberg, 1969; Reedy, 1972), although no attempt has been made to assess the importance of these functions to patients.

A recent study by Stilwell et al (1987) describes what happened when a specially trained nurse practitioner was introduced into an inner city general practice. The nurse practitioner (a woman) worked with one female and two male doctors, and patients had free access to nurse practitioner care.

The study was planned to demonstrate that:

1. a nurse practitioner offered a safe alternative for patients to seeing a doctor;
2. this expanded and extended role was acceptable to patients; and
3. the role was acceptable to colleagues.

The nurse worked in a consulting room similar to that of the doctors. Clients were offered 20-minute appointments, and were advised of the nurse practitioner's presence by a large notice in the waiting room that described the nurse as having further training in the management of the common family health problems. Consultations were informal, people being encouraged to talk about themselves and their life-style. Health teaching was held to be an important component of nursing practice (Stilwell, 1985). The aim of each consultation was to deal with the presenting problem, taking into account factors other than physical symptoms, and focusing on long-term health education.

Analysis of the work of the nurse practitioner over a 6-month period showed that the majority of people consulting her were women. Most people were under 40 years of age, and over half had chosen to consult her. The majority of problems presented to the nurse practitioner (60 per cent) concerned social or emotional problems, or health education.

An analysis of the public's attitudes to nurse practitioner care in the British study (Stilwell, 1988) showed that most people who had consulted the nurse practitioner would do so again. Although this sample of patients was small (126 respondents from a random sample of 140), their views are reflected in a large study by Levine and colleagues (1978) in which 700 patients expressed views about care from a total of 58 nurse practitioners working in a variety of settings.

It has been mentioned earlier that some authors have likened the practice nurses to the American nurse practitioner. Interestingly, Reedy (1980, p. 489), in a study of 153 practice nurses' activities and opinions, had said:

'There is . . . a close analogy between the role and organisational position of the employed nurse in Great Britain and the physician's assistant in America . . . It remains to be seen if [the nurses'] apparent acceptance of technical activities becomes associated with the dependence on doctors which characterizes the physician's assistant role . . .'

Greenfield et al (1987) reported that most nurses currently performed conventional nursing tasks such as giving injections and applying dressings, but that many had an extended role. Over 70 per cent took cervical smears, 62 per cent examined breasts and 69 per cent undertook auroscopic examination of the ears, nose and throat. Only a few had roles extended into conventional medical areas: 8 per cent of nurses used a stethoscope to examine the heart and chest and 4 per cent carried out abdominal palpation, for example. Eighty-two per cent of nurses felt that practical tasks were the most important aspect of their work, and that preventive and screening procedures came second. Sixty per cent of nurses thought that counselling and advising patients about coping with illness was of only moderate importance in their work; 69 per cent of nurses thought that their role extended beyond that of basic training. There were enormous variations in the patterns of work of this sample of practice nurses, highlighting a lack of role definition. Others have expressed concern at the practice nurses' role perhaps deserting the caring ethic of nursing in favour of delegated medical tasks (Skeet, 1978; Hockey, 1984). Certainly, in this sample of nurses, practical tasks, some of them taken over from doctors, were the most important aspect of their work.

If the role of nurse practitioner is to be developed in the British health care system, as has been advocated, then certain issues need clarification. These issues include the difference between what practice nurses do now and what nurse practitioners could do, the style of nursing care that is most helpful to patients, the attitudes of doctors to professional autonomy for nurses, and the attitudes of nurses to role expansion for themselves.

THE PRESENT STUDY

Aims

This study has been designed to provide a functional definition of the term 'nurse practitioner' by observation of nurses working in general practice, and by interviews with patients who have consulted these nurses to ascertain their expectations of satisfaction with the nursing care they have experienced. Nurses and doctors have also been interviewed for their views on the extended and expanded nursing role in general practice.

Sample

A sample of 13 nurses in general practices was chosen from the large sample of nurses responding to Greenfield et al's study of practice nurses both in the West Midlands (1987) and nationally (not yet reported). Criteria for choosing this sample were:

1. The nurse's name had to be given on the questionnaire as willing to help further with the study.
2. Patients had open access to the nurse.
3. The nurse claimed to have an extended role.
4. The nurse had expressed an interest in the development of a nurse practitioner role.

Two of the sample chosen had a title of 'nurse practitioner'. Of the 13 practices approached to take part in the study, eight agreed to do so. So far, six practices have been studied;

some employed more than one practice nurse, so a total of 11 nurses were observed in consultation with patients. Practices were located in urban, rural and inner city areas.

Methods of research

The following methods were used to study each nurse's role:

1. There was continuous observation of 339 consultations carried out by 11 nurses. Three to five days were spent with each nurse, though the days were not always consecutive. The observer was non-participant in the consultation, sitting in an unobtrusive position. Everyone consulting the nurse was asked before the start of their consultation for permission for an observer to be present while they were with the nurse.

   The observer noted verbal and non-verbal aspects of communication used by the nurses, as well as any remarks made by the clients that were particularly relevant to their choice of nursing rather than medical care, or in any way related to their appreciation of nursing care.

   The reasons given initially for consulting the nurse were noted. Matters other than the presenting concern, discussed during the consultation, were also noted.

2. A sample of 37 consultations (10.9 per cent of all consultations) was audio-recorded. No recordings were attempted until the observer had sat in on a nurse's consultation for at least one whole day, and until the observer felt the nurse had relaxed while being watched.

3. Interviews were conducted with patients, nurses and doctors in each practice to ascertain their views on the usefulness of an expanded role for nurses in general practice and satisfaction with the nurse's current role in their practice.

   Semi-structured interviewing schedules were used, and closed questions supplemented by open-ended questions. Ample time was given for free responses. Thirty patients, eight doctors and seven nurses were interviewed, and all these interviews were audio-recorded.

FINDINGS

Nurse consultation

What the nurses did

The average length of time each nurse spent with patients was calculated; this ranged from 6.7 minutes for one nurse to 18.1 minutes for another. Nurses spending the least time with patients did not have seating for them and the patients in their room; instead the patient sat or lay on a couch. In one practice there were two couches side by side, separated by a curtain; in the mornings a nurse worked in each cubicle. For these nurses the average consultation time was 7.7 minutes. One of the nurses, who had the title 'nurse practitioner', worked in a consulting room that could also be used by a doctor; her consultations were the longest, lasting 18.1 minutes on average. Neither she nor the other nurse practitioner wore a uniform; the remainder of the sample, who called themselves practice nurses, did.

Nurses with longer consultation times tended to ask more questions and to engage in more social conversation with clients. In all the practices patients had open access to nursing care, and 48 consultations were observed in which the nurse was chosen as the first point of contact. Fifty-two of all the consultations observed were for immunisation procedures, and 47 were for injections, dressings or suture removal. Twenty-three patients came for blood tests, referred by the general practitioners.

Blood pressure checks and screening patients for other risk factors were the reasons for 30 consultations. Twenty-one consultations were for cervical smears, and seven for some form of contraception (including oral contraception). Some of this sample of nurses shared with the doctor the care of patients with asthma or diabetes, and 27 patients consulted about these conditions. Eighty-four consultations were for a range of other reasons.

It is clear that nurses are consulted for a large number of reasons. It was observed that the nurses who considered themselves to have the most extended roles and who consulted with patients seated at a desk, rather than a couch, had the most complex presentations and were more likely to be consulted by patients coming to surgery without appointments.

At five out of six practices the nurses had an appointment system for patients. At the sixth practice, where the nurse had an extended role, she saw whoever came in to see her during surgery hours, including emergency presentations.

Styles of nurse consultation

All the nurses observed were friendly in their approaches to clients, remembering details of previous conversations and consultations. They gave the impression of being genuinely interested in the clients' stories.

It was common for nurses to ask general questions such as: 'How are you feeling now?', which allowed patients to give subjective views of the ways in which illness or treatment affected them. Side-effects and management of drugs were also a common nursing concern, again usually introduced by questions. Explanation and teaching about diseases or health promotion usually came later in the consultation. Four nurses were observed on more than one occasion drawing explanatory diagrams. Books and leaflets were commonly given by all nurses.

Perhaps not surprisingly, nurses who spent more time with clients were likely to give fuller explanations and answer more questions than nurses whose consultation times were short. Permission was often asked of patients before procedures were carried out:

> 'While you're here, would you like me to check your blood pressure?
> I'll check your breast, if that's OK with you.'

This sample of nurses (11) commonly thanked people for coming.

Questions regarding follow-up were also common, and included this example:

> 'N: Would you like to come back and see me in 1 month?
> P: No
> N: When would you like to come back?
> P: About 3 months
> N: OK then, that's fine, we'll make the appointment for then.'

Clients were often asked if there was anything else they wished to talk about or if they had questions. All the nurses were 'good listeners' and maintained eye contact with their patients. All had a relaxed manner, displayed by an open posture (Fast, 1978).

Although this sample of nurses did not acknowledge that they used any particular model of nursing care, their observed styles of care were consistently those of mutual participation, exhibiting empathy and friendship and eliciting patients' preferences (Szasz and Hollander, 1956). All the nurses observed during this study were skilled at making people feel at ease. They did so by the use of time, so clients felt they were not hurried, by their non-verbal behaviour, which displayed an open posture, and by interest in their clients' stories. The nurses displayed warmth towards their clients and often talked for a while about the clients' personal lives and concerns before dealing with the presenting 'problem'.

The following patients' comments reflect the nurses' skills in communication.

What the patients said

A small sample of patients (30) was interviewed regarding their views about the nursing care they had experienced in their practice. The majority of them (21) had consulted a nurse before when attending their general practice. The most typical comments were related to the accessibility and approachability of the nurse:

> If I have any worries, no matter how trivial, I can pop in and talk them over with Sister. I don't feel I'm taking up a busy doctor's time' (man, retired, aged 66 years).

The time that the nurse spent with patients was seen by them as an important characteristic of nursing consultations.

Spending time with the nurse was associated by many people with receiving fuller explanations of their illness and treatment. This was, in fact, observed to be the case, nurses commonly using consultation time for detailed explanations of patients' conditions or medication. People were not actually aware of the time available to them in consultations with the nurse, or, indeed, with the doctor. It seems that they gained the impression that the nurse had more time because they felt relaxed.

All patients felt that consulting a nurse was helpful. They were asked to explain why. A typical response was:

> 'Well, I suppose she (nurse) talks more in layman's terms, draws little diagrams, explains it simply, whereas with the doctor I always have to ask questions . . .' (woman aged 40 years).

Many people said that they thought the nurses were 'caring' or 'nice'. This was usually difficult for patients to define exactly, but was often associated with voice tone or explanation; for example:

> 'Interviewer: What made you think she (the nurse) cared?
> Patient: Well the way she was talking, explaining everything while she was taking the blood, and what it was going to be tested for. You don't always know that (woman aged 43 years).'

The attitude of patients to nursing care, revealed in this study, are similar to those found by Stilwell (1987) in the study of nurse practitioner care, in that time given and approachability were considered to be important components of care.

The doctors' opinions

Eight doctors (six men, two women) were interviewed regarding their attitudes to their nurse colleagues' role in particular and their views about some more general aspects of nursing. All doctors talked of benefits to their practice and patients.

All the doctors felt that the nurses with whom they worked were approachable and accessible for patients. One young female doctor said:

'People find nurses more approachable, appreciate the time and consideration that nurses will offer them.'

All the doctors except two commented on the nurses' ability to follow protocols methodically. The two doctors who did not comment on this aspect of nurses' care both employed nurses called 'nurse practitioners'. Although most doctors held this view, paradoxically most of them felt that their nurses were adaptable to changing practice needs.

Two doctors said that they had employed nurses who could develop their own role. One of these was called a nurse practitioner. The doctor who worked with the nurse practitioner said that her main contribution to care was to 'develop areas which are no-one's job to do well now, e.g. asthma care'.

It seems, then, that doctors think of nurses as methodical and thorough, which, for some, may imply a lack of imagination or an inability to make decisions. However, doctors also wanted adaptable nurses who could develop their roles.

In all cases, except one, doctors and nurses called each other by first names; the one exceptional dyad called each other by title and surnames at all times. This more formal pair talked to each other only about work; the other nurse–doctor pairs conversed on more general and social topics.

All the doctors perceived role overlap between themselves and the nurses but did not find this a threat. The greater the nurse's role extension in a practice, the more likely the doctors were to be in some way unconventional. In one where a nurse practitioner worked, for example, two doctors had not started to read medicine until they were in their thirties. The practice in which nurses had the least extended role was one in which the doctors had been through conventional career pathways and now did nothing but general practice.

The nurses' opinions

Seven nurses of the 11 observed were interviewed regarding their extended nursing role. All acknowledged a role extension, although on observing them, one nurse was noted not to have as extended a role as she thought she had.

None of the nurses had done similar work before becoming practice nurses. Most of them had received training from their predecessors in the practice, but all said that their role had changed in response to client demand. When asked why they thought people occasionally chose to consult them rather than a doctor, all the nurses thought it was because they were more accessible than the doctors.

All the nurses aimed to incorporate health education into their consultations and stated this as a major aim of each consultation. Other aims included discovering the real reason why the patient had come, and for one nurse:

'To encourage the patients with whatever is wrong with them to ordinary, normal life. That's probably always been my aim during my nursing career.'

All the nurses saw their roles as continually developing and changing. They felt that, with suitable training, nurses could prescribe safely. They were all enthusiastic about further training as nurse practitioners, though most of them already had extended roles in that they carried out tasks or gave care previously undertaken by doctors.

CONCLUSIONS FROM RESEARCH

How has this study of nurses' consultations and clients', doctors' and nurses' attitudes to them helped to define a nurse practitioner role?

First, important functions of nurses in British general practice have been expressed. These have included communication skills, client teaching and an ability to be methodical in planning and implementing care. Clients have particularly valued nurses' skills, especially their ability to empathise. Second, it has been possible to identify key principles of nursing practice in this particular field, which are sensitive to clients' needs as well as acceptable to nurses and doctors. Third, it has been possible to compare different styles of nursing practice and to differentiate between conventional practice nursing and a more autonomous nursing role which involves case management and time organisation. A nurse practitioner is concerned with the past, present and future care of all aspects of a person's health, and takes responsibility for the care given and its outcome.

Data from the consultations between nurses and their clients will be further analysed. However, preliminary results indicate the kind of educational preparation that should benefit nurse practitioners and increase their confidence as decision-makers.

It is, therefore, intended to plan a course for nurse practitioners in British general practice based on the results of this study.

REFERENCES

Bowling A (1981) *Delegation in General Practice. A Study of Doctors and Nurses*. London: Tavistock Publications.

Bowling A (1985) Delegation and substitution. In: *Health Care U.K.*, eds. Hamson A and Gretton J. London: Chartered Institute of Public Finance and Accountancy.

Cartwright A and Scott R (1961) The work of a nurse employed in general practice. *British Medical Journal*, 1: 807–813.

Cater M L and Hawthorn P J (1987) *Survey of Practice Nurses in the U.K. - their Extended Roles*. Paper given at a conference on Nurse Practitioners and Practice Nurses. St Bartholomew's Hospital, London, 31 Jan 1987.

Department of Health and Social Security (1986) *Neighbourhood Nursing: a Focus for Care*. Report of the Community Nursing Review. London: HMSO.

Devlin R (1985) Training the 5000. *Community Outlook*, Jan 7, p. 9.

Fast J (1978) *Body Language*. London: Pan Books.

Fawcett-Henesy A (1987) Chairman of the Royal College of Nursing Working Party on Nurse Practitioners, personal communication.

Greenfield S, Stilwell B and Drury M (1987) Practice nurses: social and occupational characteristics. *Journal of the Royal College of General Practitioners*, 37: 341–345.

Harris M (1970) The work of a nurse practitioner. *Nursing Times*, 66: 1402–1403.

Hasler J C, Hemphill P M R, Stewart T I, Boyle N, Harris A and Palmer E (1968) Development of the nursing section of the community health team. *British Medical Journal*, 3: 734–736.

Hockey L (1984) Is the practice nurse a good idea? *Journal of the Royal College of General Practitioners*, 34: 102–103.

Kuenssberg E V (1969) The nurse - a luxury or a necessity in general practice? *Journal of the Royal College of General Practitioners*, 19 (supp. 3): 34–39.

Kuenssberg E V (1971) General practice through the looking glass. *Practitioner*, 206: 129–145.

Levine J I, Orr S T, Sheatsley D W, Lohr J A and Brodie B M (1978) The nurse practitioner: role, physician utilization, patient acceptance. *Nursing Research*, 27: 245–253.

Marsh G N (1967) Group practice nurse: an analysis and comment on six months' work. *British Medical Journal*, **1**: 489–491.

Rea J N (1962) The nurse as an ancillary medical worker *Medical World*, **97**: 291–293

Reedy B L E C (1972) Organisation & management: the general practice nurse. Update, **5**: 75–78.

Reedy B L E C (1980) A comparison of the activities and opinions of attached and employed nurses in general practice. *Journal of the Royal College of General Practitioners*, **30**: 483–489.

Restall D (1987) Nurse practitioner, Scotland, personal communication.

Royal College of Nursing (1986) *Response to the Consultation on Primary Health Care*. London: Royal College of Nursing.

Skeet M (1978) Health auxiliaries: decision makers and implementers. In: *Health Auxiliaries and the Health Team*, eds. Skeet M and Elliot R. London: Croom Helm.

Social Services Committee on Primary Health Care (1987) First report. House of Commons Paper 37–41. London: HMSO.

Stilwell B (1985) Prevention and health: the concern of nursing. *Journal of the Royal Society of Health*, **105**: 60–62.

Stilwell B (1988) Patients' attitudes to the availability of a nurse practitioner to general practice. In: *The Nurse in Family Practice*, Bowling A and Stilwell B. London: Scutari Press.

Szasz T and Hollender M H (1956) A contribution to the philosophy of medicine, the basic models of the doctor–patient relationship. *Archives of Internal Medicine*, **97**: 585–592.

Weston-Smith J and Mottram E M (1967) Extended use of nursing service in general practice. *British Medical Journal*, **4**: 672–672.

Weston-Smith J and O'Donovan J B (1970) The practice nurse – a new look. *British Medical Journal*, **4**: 673–677.

Chapter 10

The Role of the Nurse in the Management of Parasuicide in the Community

Edana Minghella

INTRODUCTION

The Parasuicide research project was set up in Camberwell Health Authority in South London to encompass both research and clinical development. The overall aim was to develop and evaluate a service using specially trained community psychiatric nurses (CPNs) in the assessment and management of patients attending the district general hospital Accident and Emergency Department after deliberate self-harm (parasuicide).

For the purposes of this research, *parasuicide* is defined as:

Any non fatal act of of deliberate self-injury or taking of a substance (excluding alcohol) in excess of the generally recognised or prescribed dose. (Kreitman and Kennedy, 1980)

The project is concerned only with patients aged 16 years and over and not in school.

PARASUICIDE AND PSYCHIATRIC NURSING

Parasuicide presents as a relevant problem to psychiatric nurses for several reasons. First, the sheer number of patients demonstrates the importance of parasuicide as a major problem for the health services in general. At least 100 000 people attend hospital following an overdose or deliberate self-harm each year (Office of Health Economics, 1981). This is undoubtedly an underestimation of the total number of parasuicides; for example, Kennedy and Kreitman (1973) suggested that GPs might be seeing as many as 30 per cent more cases than those referred to hospital. Moreover, the Samaritans are reported to estimate a number as high as 210 000 annually (*The Observer*, 21 September 1986).

Second, research in Oxford, Cambridge and elsewhere has suggested that specially trained professionals other than psychiatrists could carry out assessments of parasuicide patients. Although the research has major implications for psychiatric nurses, most of it has been instigated by doctors. However, in Oxford, psychiatric nurses have been actively involved (Catalan et al, 1980).

85

The DHSS responded to the research with a circular advising that there should be a multidisciplinary team approach to the management of patients who have deliberately harmed themselves, and confirming that professionals other than psychiatrists could be used in the assessment and management of this patient group (Department of Health and Social Security, 1984). Until recently, most hospital policies have conformed with earlier recommendations, which advised that all parasuicide patients should be admitted to the general hospital and assessed by a psychiatrist (Ministry of Health, 1968).

Finally, only about a quarter to a third of patients are given a formal psychiatric diagnosis. The majority have relationship and family difficulties, chronic social problems and/or alcohol problems. At the same time, patients remain vulnerable to psychiatric illness and are at a higher risk of suicide than the general population; consequently, psychiatric knowledge and skills are crucial requirements for patient assessment.

Given these factors, CPNs are ideally equipped to work with this group of patients. They have a broad range of physical and psychosocial skills and knowledge and an eclectic approach, and work within hospital, community and clinic settings. However, basic psychiatric nurse training does not usually provide nurses with the special expertise required for the safe assessment and management of parasuicide patients.

THE LOCATION OF THE RESEARCH PROJECT

Approximately 800 patients a year attend the Accident & Emergency Department at King's College Hospital following deliberate self-harm. The health authority – Camberwell – covers a socially deprived, inner-city area that includes Brixton. Jarman indicators rank it as the sixth most deprived health district in the country (Jarman, 1983). Characteristics include poor housing, overcrowding, high unemployment, violence, a high crime rate, a prevalence of one-parent families and a racially mixed population of around 200 000.

METHODS

Three main studies were undertaken as the research element of the project, and a number of assessment instruments, listed in Table 10.1, were used.

Table 10.1 Summary of research instruments

Aim of assessment	Instrument
Psychiatric assessment	General health questionnaire* (Goldberg and Hillier, 1979) Standardised psychiatric interview** (Goldberg et al, 1970)
Suicidal risk	Suicidal Intent Scale (Pierce, 1981)
Psychosocial assessment	Semi-structured interview schedule
Alcohol use	CAGE questionnaire (Mayfield et al, 1974)

*GHQ not used after Study 1
**SPI not used in Study 1

First, there was an initial pilot study to examine the existing service, pilot research instruments, and to provide an epidemiological profile of our parasuicide patients (Study 1).

Next, there was a second pilot study to explore safe threshold scores in the assessment of suicidal risk and psychiatric 'caseness' (Study 2).

Finally, there was an intervention/follow-up study, and this will be described more fully (Study 3).

Intervention study

There were three main stages in this study:

1. a nurses' training programme;
2. an experimental study comparing a specially designed CPN service with the existing traditional psychiatric service;
3. a follow-up study (in progress) to compare the outcomes of the patients allocated to the experimental service with those allocated to the existing service.

Patients were allocated alternately to the two different services and were to be followed up 8–12 months later to compare outcomes.

The main hypotheses were as follows:

Hypothesis 1. The experimental CPN parasuicide service will be more efficient than the present service, by reaching a higher proportion of patients, with more appropriate use of hospital, community and manpower resources and skills.

Hypothesis 2. This new service will be as safe as the present service, in that suicidal and/or mentally ill patients requiring a psychiatrist's intervention will be screened out by the nurses and appropriately referred before leaving the hospital.

Hypothesis 3. The new service will be more effective than the present service, with lower rates of repeated parasuicide and a higher take-up of services offered.

Training programme

Two experienced nurses, one male and one female, were specially appointed to the posts of CPNs (parasuicide) in order to take part in the experimental service. A training programme was devised, with the overall aim of ensuring that the nurses would be well-informed, competent and confident to work in the new service, and would be able to use the research instruments. The list of topics covered in the programme is shown in Table 10.2, and included sessions on assessment skills, counselling and attitudes to parasuicide, as well as on the use of the research instruments and general information about suicide and parasuicide. A variety of different teaching methods and teachers was used, including experiential learning, the use of video, didactic lectures and general discussion. A period of intensive supervised practice was an essential part of the package.

Intervention study: selection of patients

Adult patients were selected from all the parasuicide patients attending the Accident & Emergency Department over a specified period of 14 weeks. Patients who required an emergency psychiatric assessment (normally outside the working hours of the services to be compared) were excluded from the study (Group E). All remaining patients were allocated

Table 10.2 Training programme: summary of topics

Knowledge
Social/psychological/psychiatric aspects of
  suicide and parasuicide
Nursing depressed and suicidal patients
Hospital and community resources
Crisis intervention theory
The nursing process
Research methods
The parasuicide research project
Child protection and social services
The Samaritans
Welfare rights

Process
Assessment skills
Counselling skills
Use of research instruments
Recording skills
Teaching skills
Supervised practice

Values
Recognising own fears
Labelling/prejudice
Hostility
Nurses' limitations
Ethics of the research project

'blindly' by alternating between two groups: P and N. Patients allocated to Group P were subject to the existing hospital-based psychiatric service, while patients in Group N were offered the new CPN experimental service described below. The selection process is shown in Figure 10.1.

Description of the CPN parasuicide service

During the research period, only Group N patients were offered the CPN service. (Following the end of the research period, the service has continued to run in collaboration with the psychiatrists.)

   The service operates from Monday to Friday, 9 a.m.–5 p.m. Referrals are picked up from the Accident & Emergency Department first thing every morning. Patients admitted to a

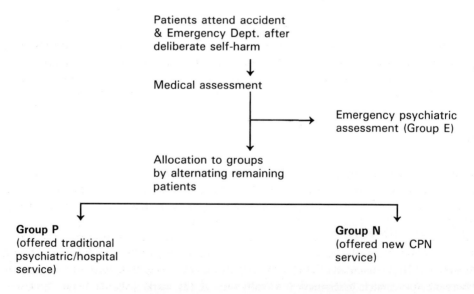

Fig. 10.1 Intervention study (Study 3) flowchart

medical bed are seen on the ward. If a patient has been discharged, one of the CPNs writes to offer an appointment in one of the health centres or at home.

The CPNs carry out an extensive assessment interview, lasting 2–3 hours. This includes a screen for mental illness (the standardised psychiatric interview or SPI) and Pierce's Suicidal Intent Scale to assess the patient's suicidal risk. The rest of the assessment includes the patient's psychosocial circumstances, alcohol and drug use, physical health, relationships and reason(s) for the act.

If there is evidence of formal mental illness and/or suicidal risk, the CPN refers the patient for a psychiatrist's opinion. The psychiatrist may then refer the patient back to the CPN if he/she considers that psychiatric intervention is not necessary.

If there is no formal mental illness or suicidal intent, the CPN may offer follow-up. This happens in about 50 per cent of cases. Otherwise, the CPN may refer or advise on other statutory and voluntary services. In all cases, the patient's GP is informed of the parasuicide.

Follow-up clinics are held in designated community health centres, and less often, in the patient's home. Follow-up consists of short-term, problem – focused counselling, with the general aim of avoiding further parasuicide by helping the patient to make more effective use of his or her own resources in coping with problems.

Nursing supervision is provided at all stages of assessment and management. Because of the vulnerable nature of this group of patients, and especially the increased risk of suicide, the availability of such supervision is essential. A senior psychiatric registrar provides medico-psychiatric advice and supervision.

Because of the very stressful nature of this work and the high level of responsibility assumed by the CPNs, the need for support is recognised and built into the service. There is a close relationship with the psychiatrists, psychotherapists, hospital social workers and the Accident & Emergency Department. A senior social worker is available to offer advice to the CPN parasuicide team, especially in cases where children may be at risk.

Follow-up

The research follow-up is in progress. The aim is to trace and interview as many patients as possible from Groups N and P, and to compare the outcomes. Follow-up indices include repeated parasuicide and suicide, changes in psychosocial circumstances and changes in mental state. Patients are also asked to complete a Consumer Satisfaction Schedule.

FINDINGS

Summary results from Study 1, which examined the existing service and provided baseline data for the project, are shown in Table 10.3. One of the most important findings was that the hospital policy for the existing service was not being implemented, and, consequently, many patients were not offered psychosocial assessment.

Study 2 aimed to pilot research instruments and explore safe threshold scores. It produced working cut-off scores for the research instruments measuring mental state (SPI) and suicidal intent (Pierce's Suicidal Intent Scale), which, when used by the research nurse with 31 patients, compared favourably with routine assessments of the same patients made by junior psychiatrists.

Table 10.3 Summary of findings of Study 1: parasuicide in the district

General description	
Numbers:	2–3 patients/day (over age 16 years)
	800–900 patients/year
Sex:	Females 55%, males 45%
Age:	75% under age 40 years
	Modal average age: 20 years
Method:	Overdose 90%
	Self-injury 12%
	Alcohol featured in 45% of cases
Interviewed patients (n=64)	
Socioeconomic status:	Married 28%
	Employed full-time 25%
	Jobless for >1 year 39%
	In debt 31%
Health:	Saw psychiatrist within last week 10%
	Psychiatric history 58%
	Saw GP within last week 17%
Common problems:	Relationship difficulties 36%
	Alcohol abuse 22%
	Unemployment 48%
	Physical problems 39%
Traditional parasuicide service	
POLICY	PRACTICE
Admit all parasuicide patients to a general medical bed	34% (62 patients) not admitted
All patients to be seen by a psychiatrist	32% (57 patients) not seen by a psychiatrist

Preliminary findings: Study 3

Findings from the final study are described in more detail.

Two hundred and twenty-four patients attended the hospital over the 14 weeks. The mean age was 31 years, with 60 per cent women and 40 per cent men. Forty-four patients were excluded (Group E), and the remaining 180 were evenly spread between groups N and P.

There are some data available for Group N, but not for Group P as yet. Of the 90 Group N patients, 48 (53 per cent) were female and 42 (47 per cent) male, and the mean age was 33 years. Sixty-five patients (72 per cent) were interviewed. The remaining 25 consisted of patients who had been discharged, or who had discharged themselves before assessment, except for one elderly patient whose care was taken over by the hospital's team for the elderly. In most of these cases there was no response to CPN letters offering out-patient assessment. The figure of 72 per cent pick-up rate compares favourably with the traditional service rate of 66 per cent found in Study 1 (see Table 10.3).

Follow-up data

As follow-up is still in progress, the only information available about the outcome of the patients from the two groups relates to the repeat rate. So far, 32 patients (around 18 per cent)

have attended the Accident & Emergency Department having repeated the parasuicide, although it is worth remembering that other repeaters may have attended different hospitals in surrounding areas. There is no difference in repeat rate so far between Groups N and P, implying that the CPN service is as safe and effective as the traditional psychiatric service. Interestingly, males have repeated more than females: 21 per cent of men compared with less than 10 per cent of women. It is known that three patients have died, one of whom committed suicide the day after discharging himself from the Accident & Emergency Department.

Establishing the new service

There were problems in setting up the service. Economic problems, such as arranging funding and trying to find clinic space within the hospital and the community, were perhaps the most predictable.

There were also socio-psychological problems. In particular, these were connected with the question of psychiatric nurses working within the general hospital and the effects of this on general nursing and medical staff. At first, the team encountered some hostility, with general nurses appearing to feel threatened and defensive; for example, they needed to emphasise that their busy-ness prevented them from spending time 'just talking' with patients.

Perhaps the most difficult problems to overcome were our own feelings of insecurity. We needed to acquire more confidence in the service and in the considerable skills developed by the CPNs. This lack of confidence was not related to the opinions of the psychiatrists who, rather than resisting the idea of the service, seemed to feel relieved that this difficult group of patients could be managed by CPNs. As the service has continued and become established, confidence in the service in all quarters has improved, and the link between the CPNs and the psychiatrists has strengthened, with more cross-fertilisation of ideas and cross-referrals.

DISCUSSION AND NEED FOR FURTHER INVESTIGATION

Although the research is not yet finished, early results suggest that the CPN service is at least as efficient and as safe and effective as the traditional psychiatric service for parasuicide patients. The CPNs reach more patients and the rate of repeated parasuicide is divided equally between the two services.

Furthermore, the project has some important implications. First, the project shows the expanded role of the psychiatric nurse in practice. In the parasuicide service, the CPNs are involved in primary psychiatric and psychosocial assessment, autonomous treatment and referral, and work as an independent service. There are links with, rather than responsibility to, psychiatrists and other disciplines. The CPNs are not working as substitute psychiatrists – for example, the CPN does not attempt to make a psychiatric diagnosis – but as specialist practitioners with particular objectives and modes of practice. In demonstrating one way in which an extended nurse's role may be evaluated, it is hoped that this project might stimulate further investigation and expansion within this and other specialist areas.

However, it was only after further post-registration training that the CPNs were able to function in this extended role. I have reported elsewhere that the nurses themselves perceived the need for further training (Brooking and Minghella, 1987). Their basic Registered Mental Nurse (RMN) course did not provide the necessary assessment, interviewing or counselling skills, or the considerable knowledge of suicide and parasuicide, required for the work.

Thus, a second implication of this research project is that, as psychiatric nursing becomes more community oriented, and if the professional role of the nurse is to develop and be accepted and respected by other professionals, these important, fundamental skills need to be included in the RMN syllabus. The knowledge base should address primary and secondary health care mental health problems, such as deliberate self-harm, sub-clinical depression and general anxiety, rather than emphasising the knowledge associated with hospitalised patients and psychiatric diagnoses. That is not to deny that specialist teams, such as the parasuicide team described here, would not continue to demand specialist knowledge, skills and experience, but rather to suggest that basic training should acknowledge the need for a broader skills and knowledge base in order to encompass the widening range of patient problems and disorders that, increasingly, psychiatric nurses can be expected to confront.

A third point is that, while the research did not set out to address the question of the efficacy of different kinds of nursing interventions, this would be the next logical step. The project concentrated on a particular kind of intervention involving short-term, problem-solving counselling; however, as the service has developed, it has become clear that a counselling relationship is not always appropriate or possible. Family and couples work may be considered, given that many of the patients present with relationship problems. Another suggestion would be group therapy, particularly with well-defined sub-groups, such as a young women's group. A cognitive–behavioural approach may also be worth investigating, perhaps based on the notion of attempting to change the patient's perception of the motivation behind his actions. Nursing interventions such as these need to be tested and evaluated to measure their effectiveness in reducing patient distress, minimising the risk of suicide or further parasuicide and enabling the patient to achieve some personal growth and development.

All of the points in this discussion suggest the need for further research. This project utilises a particular traditional experimental approach to nursing research, and we have been quite successful in confronting many of the practical, ethical and methodological difficulties that such an approach often presents. However, other methods could also be adopted to good effect. For example, in the evaluation of nursing interventions, the research design could range from the descriptive (e.g. reporting the outcome of patients involved in a specific, predetermined nursing intervention) to the more experimental, where different nursing practices could be compared with each other and with a control group.

In summary, this project indicates that there is a role for community psychiatric nurses as relatively autonomous, safe, efficient and effective practitioners in a field that is acknowledged as difficult, unpopular and precarious. It highlights the need for improved basic nursing education and post-registration training, and opens up the arena for further investigation into the extended role of the nurse, training requirements, and the use and efficacy of specific psychiatric nursing interventions.

ACKNOWLEDGEMENTS

Many thanks to Gill Turnbull, John Staines, Professor Robert Cawley, Dr Julia Brooking and Dr Stuart Turner, without whom this project would not have been possible.

REFERENCES

Brooking J I and Minghella E L (1987) Parasuicide. *Nursing Times,* **83**(21): 40–43.

Catalan J, Marsack P, Hawton K E, Whitwell D, Fagg J and Bancroft J (1980) Comparison of doctors and nurses in the assessment of deliberate self-poisoning patients. *Psychological Medicine,* **10**: 483–491.

Department of Health and Social Security Circular (1984) *The Management of Deliberate Self-Harm* CMHN(84)25/LASL(84)5. London: HMSO.

Goldberg D P and Hillier V (1979) A scaled version of the General Health Questionnaire. *Psychological Medicine,* **9**: 139–145.

Goldberg D P, Cooper B, Eastwood M R, Kedward H B and Shepherd M (1970) A standardised psychiatric interview for use in community surveys. *British Journal of Preventive and Social Medicine,* **24**(1): 18–23.

Jarman B (1983) Identification of under privileged areas. *British Medical Journal,* **286**: 1705–1709.

Kennedy P and Kreitman N (1973) Epidemiological survey of parasuicide in general practice. *British Journal of Psychiatry,* **123**: 23–24.

Kreitman N and Kennedy J A T (1980) Suicide in relation to parasuicide. *Medical Education,* **14**: 18–30.

Mayfield D, McLeod G and Hall P (1974) The CAGE questionnaire: validation of a new alcoholism screening instrument. *American Journal of Psychiatry,* **131**: 1121–1123.

Ministry of Health (1968) *Hospital Treatment of Acute Poisoning (Hill Report).* London: HMSO.

Office of Health Economics (1981) *Suicide and Deliberate Self-Harm.* London: HMSO.

Pierce D W (1981) Predictive validation of a suicide intent scale. *British Journal of Psychiatry,* **139**: 391–396.

Section 2

**The Consumer Perspective:
Patients' and Relatives'
Experiences and Opinions**

Chapter 11

A Survey of Current Practices and Opinions Concerning Patient and Family Participation in Hospital Care

Julia I Brooking

INTRODUCTION

This chapter describes a survey of patients, relatives and nurses that examined current practices, opinions and attitudes towards patient and family participation in nursing. The study originated from observations during clinical practice that patients and their families in general hospitals often adopted passive and dependent roles. This behaviour appeared to result from their expectations about appropriate behaviour, their uncertainty in a strange environment and the behaviour of hospital staff, which seemed to reinforce acquiescence. The researcher questioned whether passivity was widespread and whether it was in the best interests of patients and their families.

In recent years, it has been widely proposed that patients and their families should be more involved in decision-making about care and the delivery of care. This view also seemed to be an assumption of the nursing process, which is being developed in some British hospitals. The idea of giving patients control over their care has become fashionable and fits in with other social trends, such as the general upsurge of consumerism and interest in nursing ethics and patients' rights. The extent to which the notion of increasing patient and family participation has actually been incorporated into nursing practice is questionable. More importantly, the effects of these recommendations have never been systematically evaluated.

AN OVERVIEW OF THE LITERATURE

Psychological and sociological concepts

There is an impressive body of psychological research (reviewed by Langer, 1983) that shows that control over aversive events reduces stress, is preferred by subjects and has other beneficial effects. The different types of personal control, identified by Averill (1973) as behavioural, cognitive and decisional, are each related to stress in different and complex ways. It has been shown that choice, self-administration of aversive stimuli, information and prediction are all aspects of control.

Most of these studies were conducted in psychological laboratories, but this research is relevant to patient participation because there is much evidence (reviewed by Wilson-Barnett, 1979) that being ill and in hospital is seen by patients as stressful and unpleasant. In most experiments control was easy to exercise, and it is probable that control that is difficult to exercise may not reduce stress and may be relinquished by subjects (e.g. Solomon et al, 1980). Patient control over care in hospital may be seen by patients as difficult to exercise, but this has not been tested.

Personality variables and coping styles that are theoretically likely to interact with control include locus of control (Lefcourt, 1980), self-efficacy (Bandura, 1977), reactance (Brehm, 1966) and helplessness (Garber and Seligman, 1980). Relevant demographic variables may include age, sex, education and social class. Relationships between the exercise of control and these variables have not been elucidated, although predictions are possible.

The traditional sociological conception of the sick role sees the patient as passive (Parsons, 1951) and the carer as powerful and controlling (Greenwood, 1957). There is evidence that patients recognise that passivity is expected of them and are rewarded for conformity (Armitage, 1980). It seems that junior nurses prefer passive patients more than senior nurses do (Anderson, 1973). Patient satisfaction surveys (reviewed by Locker and Dunt, 1978) show that lack of information is patients' main complaint.

It is clear that families tend to be excluded from care-giving in hospital (Rosenthal et al, 1980). Families of hospital patients experience much distress (Stember, 1977), but nurses have minimal contact with them (Bond, 1982). It is possible that family stress may be reduced by increased participation in care.

Consumerism in health care

Traditional medical practice appears to be based on a deterministic, mechanistic view of the nature of humans. The moves towards patient participation, control and self-care have their philosophical antecedents in the opposing view that humans have free will and self-determination.

The widespread national and international commitment to democracy, personal autonomy and human rights justifies taking these notions seriously in health care. This is supported by various nursing codes of ethics and patients' bills of rights (e.g. American Hospital Association, 1972). Nevertheless, much medical and nursing practice is based on 'benevolent paternalism', which may be incompatible with personal autonomy (Bassford, 1982). The increasing influence of the health-care professions over every aspect of life has become recognised as a potentially dangerous form of social control (Zola, 1971; McKeown, 1976; Kennedy, 1980) and is one of the many factors that has contributed to the development of consumerism in health care.

Consumer participation in many areas of life has become increasingly influential since the 1960s (see Richardson, 1983). Consumerism in health care exists at various levels: individual and community, in sickness and in health, and as both a radical alternative and an adjunct to professional care. Reasons for the recent interest in self-care include changes in society and in the health-care professions (Levin et al, 1977).

Many examples of lay participation in community care exist. These include the community health councils (Levitt, 1980), patient participation groups in general practice (Pritchard, 1981), and self-help groups (Robinson and Henry, 1977). Few of these developments have been systematically evaluated.

Some studies of patient participation in hospital care have been carried out. Relevant studies with psychiatric patients include work on institutionalisation. Wing and Brown (1970) have shown that increasing patient choice, autonomy and responsibility is important to reverse institutionalisation. Therapeutic communities (see Hinshelwood and Manning, 1979) are an example of a development in psychiatry that operates on democratic principles and promotes patient autonomy. One general hospital study with myocardial infarction patients (Cromwell et al, 1977) indicated the importance of congruent combinations of participation, information and personality, but the relationships among them remain unclear.

American experiments with elderly nursing home residents, which have manipulated responsibility and choice (Langer and Rodin, 1976) and control and predictability (Schulz, 1976), have found significant improvements in physical and psychological well-being in the experimental group patients. At 18-month follow-up, Rodin and Langer (1977) found a significant difference in death rates between their experimental and control groups, in the predicted direction.

There is convincing evidence that giving surgical patients various types of preparatory information results in better postoperative recovery on a variety of physical and psychosocial measures (Kendall and Watson, 1981). Several writers have argued that information provides patients with increased control (e.g. Auerbach, 1979). The few studies that have directly examined the relationship between active patient involvement and the outcomes of surgery or aversive medical procedures have found that involvement enhanced recovery and the effectiveness of procedures (e.g. Tryon and Leonard, 1965; Greer et al, 1979; Taylor and Levin, 1977).

Descriptive studies have demonstrated the ability of patients to carry out procedures usually performed by professionals. For example, self-monitoring of blood pressure by hypertensives resulted in reduced blood pressure and improved drug compliance (Carnahan, 1973; Wilkinson and Raftery, 1978).

From these and other studies it can be seen that beneficial effects have resulted from giving patients more control over their care. Appropriate information and education seem to be essential prerequisites. The relationship between appropriate amounts of participation and individual difference variables requires further study. Most of the work reviewed is American, so should not be generalised to British patients.

Very little research or other literature was found on family participation in care. There is a little evidence that family involvement and positive family attitudes can have beneficial effects on patient outcomes (Brownell, 1978). Several writers have argued that families should participate in practical care during hospitalisation (e.g. Castledine, 1978), but there is little research on the extent of family participation, their attitudes to participation or its effects on patient and family well-being.

Professional attitudes to patient and family participation in care are important because of the power of doctors and nurses to support or prevent these developments. There is much descriptive and prescriptive nursing literature extolling the advantages of patient and family participation in care (e.g. Williamson, 1981), and this is supported by the World Health Organisation (Mahler, 1982). Nevertheless, some hostility from professionals is inevitable, given the assumptions on which self-care is based (Levin et al, 1977). Studies of doctors' and nurses' attitudes (Pankratz and Pankratz, 1974; Citron, 1978; Linn and Lewis, 1979) revealed that high levels of education and senior appointment were generally associated with more positive attitudes to patient self-determination. The attitudes of patients and relatives towards these issues have been little investigated and show no consistent patterns (Chang, 1978; Krantz et al, 1980).

Nursing process and nursing theory

Patient and family participation in nursing process is advocated in the British (Ashworth, 1982; McFarlane and Castledine, 1982) and American (Yura and Walsh, 1967) literature. Various writers have discussed patient participation in assessment (Crow, 1979), planning (Jasmin and Trygstad, 1979), implementation (Tiffany, 1979) and evaluation (Royal College of Nursing, 1979). Marriner (1980) pointed out the importance of educating patients to supply them with a foundation upon which to base rational and informed decisions.

Patient participation is the central proposition in the work of several nursing theorists, such as Hall (1966) and Orem (1980). Orem argues that all humans possess self-care capability, which is influenced by health status, age and knowledge. Inadequate self-care is, according to Orem, the main justification for nursing intervention, which is designed primarily to compensate for lack of self-care capacity and to restore the patient to independent self-care capacity as soon as possible.

DESIGN AND METHOD

In view of the paucity of empirical work in this area, it was decided to assess current practices, opinions and attitudes concerning patient and family participation in nursing.

The aims of the study

These were to provide further information on the following questions:

1. To what extent do patients and their relatives participate in the assessment, planning and implementation of nursing?
2. What are the attitudes of nurses, patients and relatives towards patient and family participation in nursing?
3. Do wards and units have policies about patient and family participation in care?
4. What are nurses taught about this topic?
5. What is the relationship between the use of nursing process and patient and family participation in care?

The research instruments

Three separate but closely related self-completion questionnaires were designed for nurses, patients and relatives. These eight-page questionnaires took about 20 minutes to complete and contained:

1. questions about demographic and other factual information;
2. a 24-item Likaert scale to measure attitudes towards patient and family participation in nursing;

3. a scale to measure the extent to which the nurse encouraged patient and family participation or the extent to which the patient or relative perceived they had participated in care during the stay in hospital;
4. a scale assessing the extent to which the patient or relative would ideally like to participate in care;
5. a scale assessing actual participation in 20 common nursing procedures;
6. questions for nurses about ward policies and what they had been taught about these issues;
7. a scale to measure nurses' attitudes towards nursing process.

After comprehensive pre-testing the questionnaires were pilot tested on 28 subjects in a different hospital from the main study.

The main study

Data were collected from 18 general medical and surgical wards in two London hospitals. Half the wards were using nursing process to some extent and half not at all. The use of nursing process was quantified using a scale designed by Brooking (1986). Questionnaires were completed by 107 nurses, 114 patients and 72 relatives, an overall response rate of 82 per cent. All the patients were adults who had been in-patients for at least 4 days and who were judged to be physically and mentally capable of completing the questionnaires. As far as possible, relatives were linked to patients in the study. Nurses had worked on the ward or unit for at least a week and ranged in seniority from managers to students.

The data were analysed using the Statistical Package for the Social Sciences (Nie et al, 1975). Data from the three subject groups were examined separately and then compared using a range of descriptive and inferential parametric and non-parametric statistics. Qualitative data were content analysed. In designing the scales, attention was given to all aspects of their validity and reliability. Using the main study data the questionnaires were tested for internal consistency, and most of the scales achieved reasonable levels of reliability, which are reported fully in Brooking (1986).

SUMMARY OF THE MAIN FINDINGS

1. The nurses were mainly young, unmarried women who had more qualifications than the patients or relatives. The patients and relatives were mostly married and more than half were employed, with social classes II and III predominating. Most patients and relatives had some knowledge of the patient's illness, tests and treatment; high levels of knowledge were associated with previous admissions, higher social class and more qualifications. More than half the patients and relatives had been hospital patients at least twice. More than half the relatives were the spouses of a patient, and relatives tended to be more worried about this admission than the patients themselves.

2. The use or lack of use of nursing process had negligible effects on practices and attitudes in relation to patient and family participation. None of the wards was using nursing process fully. In most wards highest scores were obtained for patient assessment, then problem identification and planning nursing actions, suggesting that these aspects of nursing process were developed first and/or were easiest to implement and sustain. Most wards obtained lowest scores for goal setting and evaluation.

3. Nurses expressed generally positive attitudes towards nursing process, except for complaints about the quantity of paperwork associated with it.

4. Nurses expressed generally positive attitudes towards patient and family participation in care and obtained higher attitude scores than patients or relatives.

5. Nurses who held most positive attitudes towards nursing process and towards patient and family participation in care tended to be older, in more senior positions and had more qualifications.

6. Many nurses claimed to organise care to facilitate patient and family participation, but there was little actual evidence of this. Patients and relatives claimed to have much less participation in care than nurses indicated they provided.

7. None of the wards had formal or informal policies about patient and family participation. Within wards there was little consensus about practice, which seemed to vary according to nurses' personal opinions and often conflicted with the views of the sister. Senior nurses described practices more idealistically than did juniors. There was little indication that patients were encouraged to participate in care planning, and the notion of relative participation in planning received even less support. There was agreement that patients were encouraged to be as independent as possible, but that patient choice about self-care was limited. Relative participation in care giving seemed confined to simple tasks.

8. Nurses reported that little was taught during training about patient and family participation, either in the wards or the school of nursing.

9. Patients and relatives reported little participation in planning and giving care and generally wanted increased participation.

10. Patients and relatives who held most positive attitudes and reported the highest levels of participation tended to be knowledgeable about the patient's condition and treatment and familiar with hospitals. They were of higher social class, had more qualifications and were more worried about this admission.

11. Patients and relatives who most wanted increased participation were those who already had the greatest participation.

12. Relatives expressed more positive attitudes towards patient and family participation in care than patients, and expressed a stronger desire than patients for increased participation.

DISCUSSION

The findings

The importance of demographic and personality variables in response to patient and relative control are revealed in the findings of this study. Unlike most of the psychological experiments on control, this study differentiates the characteristics of subjects who do and do not want control and identifies circumstances in which control may not be preferred, i.e. in highly complex tasks and at times of stress. The survey confirms the findings from medical sociology that the traditionally passive, acquiescent patient role is still accepted by some patients and still expected and preferred by many nurses. However, this study shows that patients' and relatives' roles are modified by factors such as social class, education, knowledge of the condition, age, anxiety, and familiarity with the hospital environment. The widely discussed consumer movement had limited impact on these patients and relatives, some of whom appeared willing to accept the subservient role that they believed was required of them. The study confirms the importance of patient education as the basis for informed participation in decision-making and self-care. Attitudes of staff were found to be similar to those found in previous American work. Family participation in care was found to be minimal. The difficulties in obtaining data from relatives help to explain the general lack of research on patients' relatives. The findings provide indirect support for Orem's notion that nurses compensate for self-care deficits. The findings add to Orem's theory in elucidating the causes of self-care deficits, which are associated with psychological and organisational factors rather than the patients' pathology only.

Practical implications of the research

The survey was carried out in only two hospitals, both in London, and had a small sample. Therefore, the results have limited generalisability, and recommendations for practice are made with caution.

It is possible to recommend that nurses need more knowledge about the nature and potential psychological and practical benefits of patient and family participation in care. More attention should be given to these topics in pre- and post-registration nursing education. Sisters, charge nurses and nurse managers should consider whether to formulate ward or unit policies in relation to these issues, which would be preferable to practice based on nurses' personal views.

Not all patients and relatives want to share in decision-making or engage in self-care, and a passive role may be preferred by some. Nevertheless, many patients and relatives are dissatisfied with the amount of involvement in care currently permitted and would welcome an increase. Patients should be allowed to choose the extent to which they wish to share in decision-making and participate in care giving. They should also be given a choice about the extent to which they wish their relatives to be involved. Patients' preferences may change during their admission as they become familiar with the environment and learn more about their condition. Consequently, patients' wishes concerning participation should be reviewed every few days. In the case of helpless patients, their relatives should be offered the same choices, but, whenever possible, the wishes of patients should be of paramount importance.

Familiarity with the hospital environment and knowledge about the condition were found to be important determinants of patient and family participation. Familarity with the environment could be enhanced by making hospitals more accessible to the public, with pre-admission visits, open days, organised tours, etc. Patient education and information giving should be seen as an important part of the nurse's role, to provide the basis for informed decision-making. Information booklets should be available to supplement verbal information. Teaching should include practical care skills, particularly for patients with chronic disorders who require continuing care after discharge.

Evaluation of the methods used

Due to the paucity of empirical work in this area, it was essential to obtain data on current practices and attitudes among relevant subject groups. This provides a baseline upon which further studies of patient and family participation in nursing may be developed.

During the course of the study the limitations of survey methods and these questionnaires in particular became very apparent. Self-completion questionnaires may not be the best way of obtaining data about the complex, abstract and controversial subject of patient and family participation in care. Had time permitted, observation and semi-structured interviews would have increased confidence in the findings.

Nevertheless, this method still achieved the overall aims of the study and provided some evidence in relation to the hypotheses. The scales developed for the study achieved moderate levels of validity and reliability and, with modifications, could be used in further research.

REFERENCES

American Hospital Association (1972) Statement on a patient's bill of rights. Chicago: The Association. Cited in Bandman E and Bandman B (1977) There is nothing automatic about rights. *American Journal of Nursing*, **77**(5): 867–872.

Anderson E (1973) *The Role of the Nurse*. London: Royal College of Nursing.

Armitage S K (1980) Non compliant recipients of health care. *Nursing Times* Occasional Paper, **76**(1): 1–3.

Ashworth P M (1982) Change from what? In: *Proceedings of the Royal College of Nursing Research Society XXIII Annual Conference*, eds. Harrisson S P, Hockey L, Keighley T C and Sisson A R, University of Durham. London: Royal College of Nursing.

Auerbach S M (1979) Preoperative preparation for surgery: a review of recent research and future prospects. In: *Research in Psychology and Medicine*, eds. Osborne D J, Gruneberg M M and Eiser J R. London: Academic Press.

Averill J R (1973) Personal control over aversive stimuli and its relationship to stress. *Psychological Bulletin*, **80**: 286–303.

Bandura A (1977) Self-efficacy: towards a unifying theory of behavioural change. *Psychological Review*, **84**: 191–215.

Bassford H A (1982) The justification of medical paternalism. *Social Science and Medicine*, **16**: 731–739.

Bond S (1982) Communicating with families of cancer patients. 1. The relatives and doctors. 2. The nurses. *Nursing Times*, **78**: 962–965 and 1027–1029.

Brehm J W (1966) *A Theory of Psychological Reactance*. London: Academic Press.

Brooking J I (1986) *Patient and Family Participation in Nursing Care: the Development of a Nursing Process Measuring Scale*. Unpublished PhD thesis, University of London, King's College.

Brownell K D (1978) The effect of spouse training and partner cooperativeness in the behavioural treatment of obesity. *Dissertation Abstracts International*, **38**: 11–18, 5559.

Carnahan J E (1973) The effects of self-monitoring by patients on the control of hypertension. *Dissertation Abstracts International*, **34**(68): 2922.

Castledine G (1978) Involving the family in patient care. *Nursing Mirror*, **147**: 14.

Chang B L (1978) Perceived situational control of daily activities: a new tool. *Research in Nursing and Health*, **1**(4): 181–188.

Citron M J (1978) Attitudes of nurses regarding the patients' role in the decision-making process and their implications for nursing education. *Dissertation Abstracts International*, **38**(128): 584.

Cromwell R L et al (1977) *Acute Myocardial Infarction: Reaction and Recovery*. St Louis: C V Mosby.

Crow J (1979) Assessment. In: *The Nursing Process*, ed. C R Kratz. London: Baillière Tindall.

Garber J and Seligman M E P (1980) *Human Helplessness: Theory and Applications*. New York: Academic Press.

Greenwood E (1957) Attributes of a profession. *Social Work*, **11**: 45.

Greer S et al (1979) Psychological response to breast cancer: effect on outcome. *The Lancet*, **ii**: 785–787.

Hall L E (1966) Another view of nursing care and quality. In: *Continuity of Patient Care: the Role of Nursing*, eds. Straub K M and Parker K S. Washington, DC: Catholic University Press.

Hinshelwood R D and Manning N (eds.) (1979) *Therapeutic Communities – Reflections and Progress*. London: Routledge & Kegan Paul.

Jasmin S and Trygstad L N (1979) *Behavioural Concepts and the Nursing Process*. St Louis: C V Mosby.

Kendall P C and Watson D (1981) Psychological preparation for stressful medical procedures. In: *Medical Psychology: Contributions to Medical Psychology*, eds. Prokopc and Bradley L. London: Academic Press.

Kennedy I (1980) *Unmasking Medicine. The Reith Lectures, 1980*. Published in six parts in *The Listener*, 6 November–11 December.

Krantz D S, Baum A and Wideman M V (1980) Assessment of preferences for self-treatment and information in health care. *Journal of Personality and Social Psychology*, **39**(5): 977–990.

Langer E J (1983) *The Psychology of Control*. California: Sage.

Langer E J and Rodin J (1976) The effects of choice and enhanced personal responsibility for the aged: a field experiment in an institutional setting. *Journal of Personality and Social Psychology*, **34**(2): 191–198.

Lefcourt H M (1980) Locus of control and coping with life's events. In: *Personality: Basic Issues and Current Research*, ed. Staub E. New Jersey: Prentice-Hall.

Levin L S, Katz A H and Holst E (1977) *Self-Care: Lay Initiatives in Health*. London: Croom Helm.

Levitt R (1980) *The People's Voice in the NHS: Community Health Councils after Five Years*. London: King Edward's Hospital Fund for London.

Linn L S and Lewis C E (1979) Attitudes toward self-care among practising physicians. *Medical Care*, **17**(2): 183–190.

Locker D and Dunt D (1978) Theoretical and methodological issues in sociological studies of consumer satisfaction with medical care. *Social Science and Medicine – Medical Psychology and Sociology*, **12**: 283–292.

Mahler H (1982) Paper given by the Director General of WHO at the 11th International Conference on Health Education, Hobart, Tasmania.

Marriner A (1980) *Guide to Nursing Management*. St Louis: C V Mosby.

McFarlane J and Castledine G (1982) *A Guide to the Practice of Nursing using the Nursing Process*. London: C V Mosby.

McKeown T (1976) *The Role of Medicine*. Nuffield Provincial Hospital Trust. Oxford: Oxford University Press.

Nie N H, Hadlai Hull C, Jenkins J G, Steinbrenner K and Bent D H (1975) *Statistical Package for the Social Sciences*, 2nd edn. New York: McGraw-Hill.

Orem D E (1980) *Nursing: Concepts of practice*, 2nd edn. New York: McGraw-Hill.

Pankratz L and Pankratz D (1974) Nursing autonomy and patients' rights: development of a nursing attitude scale. *Journal of Health and Social Behaviour*, **15**(3): 211–216.

Parsons T (1951) *The Social System*. New York: Free Press.

Pritchard P (1981) *Patient Participation in General Practice*, Occasional Paper 17. London: Royal College of General Practitioners.

Richardson A (1983) *Participation: Concepts in Social Policy, I*. London: Routledge & Kegan Paul.

Robinson D and Henry S (1977) Self-help and health: mutual aid for modern problems. London: Martin Robertson.

Rodin J and Langer E J (1977) Long-term effects of a control-relevant intervention with the institutionalised aged. *Journal of Personality and Social Psychology*, **35**: 897–902.

Rosenthal C J, Marshall V W, Macpherson A S and French S E (1980) *Nurses, Patients and Families*. London: Croom Helm.

Royal College of Nursing (1979) *Implementing the Nursing Process*. London: Royal College of Nursing.

Schulz R (1976) Effects of control and predictability on the physical and psychological well-being of the institutionalised aged. *Journal of Personality and Social Psychology*, **33**: 563–573.

Solomon S, Holmes D S and McCaul K D (1980) Behavioural control over aversive events: does control that requires effort reduce anxiety and physiological arousal? *Journal of Personality and Social Psychology*, **39**(4): 729–736.

Stember M L (1977) Familial response to hospitalisation of an adult member. *Communicating Nursing Research*, **9**: 59–75.

Taylor S and Levin S (1977) The psychological impact of breast cancer: theory and practice. In: *Psychological Aspects of Breast Cancer. Technical Bulletin No. 1*, eds. Enelow A J and Panagis D M. San Francisco: West Coast Cancer Foundation.

Tiffany R (1979) Quoted in a news item in *Nursing Times*, **75**(8): 314.

Tryon P A and Leonard R C (1965) Giving the patient an active role. In: *Social Interaction and Patient Care*, eds. Skipper J K and Leonard R C. Philadelphia: Lippincott.

Wilkinson P R and Raftery E B (1978) Patients' attitudes to measuring their own blood pressure. *British Medical Journal*, **1**: 824.

Williamson J A (1981) Mutual interaction: a model of nursing practice. *Nursing Outlook*, **29**: 104–107.

Wilson-Barnett J (1979) *Stress in Hospital: Patients' Psychological Reactions to Illness and Health Care*. Edinburgh: Churchill Livingstone.

Wing J K and Brown G W (1970) *Institutionalism and Schizophrenia: a Comparative Study of Three Mental Hospitals, 1960–1968*. London: Cambridge University Press.

Yura H and Walsh M S (eds.) (1967) *The Nursing Process*. Washington, DC: Catholic University of America Press.

Zola I K (1971) Medicine as an institution of social control. In: *A Sociology of Medical Practice (1975)*, eds. Cox C and Mead A. London: Collier Macmillan.

Chapter 12

Patients' Perceptions
of Acute Pain

Kate Seers

The care of patients in pain is an important part of nursing. Nurses have the unique opportunity to be constantly with the patient and are thus well placed to assess pain and its relief. Prescriptions for analgesics often give the nurse flexibility to decide what type of painkiller is appropriate, whether and when to give it and at what dose. The nurse should thus be a key person in providing pain relief.

BACKGROUND

Pain has been described by Melzack (1984, p. 332) as an '. . . endless variety of qualities that are categorised under a single linguistic label'. This suggests the complexity of pain, influenced by a mixture of physiological, psychological, social and cultural factors. Pain is thus a unique subjective experience, and can be interpreted and expressed in many different ways. Since pain is so complex, McCaffery's (1972, p. 8) definition of pain seems appropriate:

'Pain is whatever the experiencing person says it is and exists whenever he says it does.'

Painful stimuli may occur in any damaged tissue. After surgery, cutaneous pain, involving skin and superficial tissues, may arise from the surgical incision and from the site of any tubing. Deep somatic pain, involving muscles, tendons and ligaments, may arise from muscle stretching during surgery and from muscle spasms after surgery. Visceral pain can occur after organ handling and displacement, and after the stretching and tearing of internal tissues during surgery. After surgery, viscera can be stretched by, for example, the build up of gas, causing pain. Pain arising from different tissues may be of different intensity and unpleasantness, and may even respond differently to analgesic drugs (Dodson, 1985). After surgery patients may thus have different types of pain at different times.

While the actual surgery is an obvious cause of postoperative pain, Melzack and Wall (1982) emphasise that there is not a linear relationship between the stimulus (such as type of surgery) and pain intensity. Rather, any or all of a number of factors can interact, changing the nature or intensity of the pain experience. For example, patients' past experiences of pain, or the meaning of the pain to them, may affect how they experience pain. Pain always occurs against a background of experience, or in the context of other experiences (Chapman, 1978), so each person's response is subjective and unique.

How important is it to relieve postoperative pain? Pain can delay recovery by making the patient reluctant to mobilise, increasing the risk of stasis complications such as deep vein thrombosis and urinary tract infection. Deep breathing and coughing may also be avoided, increasing the risk of respiratory infection (Dodson, 1982). The patient in pain may also become fatigued and demoralised. In a study of 14 men undergoing herniorrhaphy, Fordham (1982, and chapter 14 in this volume) concluded that pain and fear of pain were major deterrents to deep breathing and exercise.

The expectation of unrelieved pain can be stressful for the patient, as Volicier and Bohannon (1975) discovered when they asked 261 short-term medical and surgical patients to rank 49 different items from least to most stressful. Not getting relief from pain medications and not getting pain medication were in the top nine most stressful items.

Pain may thus retard recovery and be stressful for the patient, so adequate control of pain to help the patient recover seems to be important; but what is adequate control?

Patients and health professionals may differ in what they think is a realistic level of relief. Weis et al (1983, p. 72) state: 'In theory the goal of treatment should be complete relief'. They sent a questionnaire to 142 surgical nurses, 70 of whom completed it. They found that only 21 per cent of nurses aimed for complete relief of pain, 54 per cent for enough relief so the patient noticed it but was not distressed, 11 per cent for moderate relief with small distress and 9 per cent for relief at peak periods of pain only. Similarly, Cohen (1980) asked 121 surgical nurses their overall aim of administering analgesics on the first 2 days after surgery. She found that 3.3 per cent aimed for complete relief of pain, 57.5 per cent to relieve pain as much as possible, 38.3 per cent to relieve pain just enough for the patient to function and 0.8 per cent to relieve pain so the patient could just tolerate it. Using the same categories with 64 nurses, Sofaer (1984) found that responses were divided between categories as 9, 79, 9 and 3 per cent respectively.

So, in all these studies, a degree of endurance was expected by some nurses, but most tended to aim for 'as much relief as possible'. Are these aims actually put into practice?

Johnston (1976, p. 41) in a study of 43 postoperative patients and 19 nurses, concluded:

> 'The data would suggest that nurses do so badly on the assessment of pain that analgesics might more reliably be given to patients in greatest pain by distributing them randomly, nurses performing worse than chance.'

Further support for less ideal postoperative pain control comes from a study of 81 patients by Sriwatanakul et al (1983). They found that 90 per cent of patients had pain that disturbed their sleeping, eating, concentrating, talking and moving around. Similarly, Cohen (1980), in her study of 109 surgical patients, found that 75 per cent had moderate or marked pain distress after surgery.

It would seem that pain remains a problem for many postoperative patients. Since less than ideal pain relief after surgery has been well documented, why is it still a problem?

Patients may have low expectations of pain relief. Although 75 per cent of patients in Cohen's (1980) study were in moderate or marked pain distress, nearly 80 per cent felt that analgesia was adequate. Similarly, 75 per cent of Weis et al's (1983) sample said that relief was adequate, despite 41 per cent being in moderate or severe pain at the peak of analgesia.

Patients may be unwilling or unable to communicate their pain to the nursing staff. Smith and Utting (1976) concluded that patients thought nurses would give them a painkiller if they needed one, yet Cohen (1980) found that 32 per cent of nurses would wait for a patient to request medication. This suggests a potential area for a breakdown in communication between nurse and patient. That nurses do not always assess pain was illustrated by Camp and O'Sullivan (1987), who studied 84 nurse–patient pairs and found that nurses documented significantly less than 50 per cent of the patients' description of pain to a researcher. They concluded: 'It appears that nurses have not found pain sufficiently important to merit complete assessment and documentation' (p. 598).

Even if the nurses know the patient is in pain, they may not administer painkillers. Fagerhaugh and Strauss (1977) suggested that the discrepancy between actual and possible pain relief was due to the work demands of the clinical setting, instititutional accountability surrounding pain management, or lack of it, and the complexity of staff-patient and staff-staff relationships.

Inadequate knowledge of analgesics could also hinder adequate pain relief. Cohen (1980) concluded: 'nurses grossly overestimated the addictive potential of narcotic analgesics' (p. 273).

Sofaer (1984) addressed the question of inadequate knowledge of pain and its relief when she implemented a ward-based education programme for nurses. The effectiveness of this programme was assessed in terms of patient outcome. She interviewed 47 patients before and 52 after the programme was implemented. All patients were female and had had surgery for non-malignant conditions. Patient outcome was determined by interviewing the patient on average on the third postoperative day and by using graphic rating scales, asking them to rate retrospectively their average pain intensity and duration on the day of the operation and for the 3 succeeding days. Patients were also interviewed at home about their pain relief experiences. Those patients interviewed after the educational intervention had lower pain intensity and shorter duration of pain on the day of surgery and the first postoperative day than those interviewed before, and said that their pain was noticed by the nurse and felt that nurses cared about pain relief.

This brief review of the literature suggests that postoperative pain relief is not always ideal, and some reasons for this have been outlined.

Methods

This study focused on the nurses' and patients' ratings of pain and pain relief, and included an assessment of anxiety and recovery in order to examine the interrelationship between these variables.

Aims of the study

These were to:

1. assess any differences between the patient's and the nurse's ratings of the patient's postoperative pain and pain relief;
2. identify any pain-relieving strategies used by the nurses and patients;
3. assess whether pain and/or pain relief affect recovery;
4. determine whether anxiety affects pain, pain relief and/or recovery.

A full description of the findings for each of these aims can be found in Seers (1987), but this chapter will focus on the first and second aims only.

Sample

The sample was one of convenience, and consisted of all patients admitted to the study wards for an elective abdominal operation under general anaesthesia during the period of data collection, who were aged 18 years or over and had given written consent to take part in the study.

Instruments used

Ratings of pain

Pain was assessed using the patients' subjective report of their pain. A review of the literature suggested that a verbal rating scale might be more useful for postoperative patients than a visual analogue scale, because it is easy to understand and complete (Kremer et al, 1981). Although arguably insensitive, because pain would be assessed frequently after surgery, it was felt that a simple tool was vital as it is quick to administer and easy for patients to understand (Figure 12.1).

  The nurse looking after the patient was asked to rate the patient's pain up to 5 minutes before or up to 5 minutes after the patient had been interviewed.

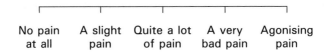

Fig. 12.1   Pain scale used. Patients were asked to put a cross on the line to indicate the point that best represented their pain at that time. The distance to this cross was then measured from the left-hand-side of the scale. This measurement represented their pain score

Ratings of pain relief

This was assessed in a similar way to pain, using a pain relief scale (Figure 12.2).

Pain-relieving strategies

These were assessed by asking the patients, each time their pain was assessed: 'Does anything make the pain better?', and if so, 'What?'. This question was designed to elicit any strategies

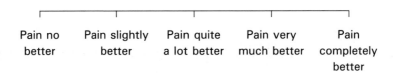

Fig. 12.2   Pain relief scale used. Patients were asked to put a cross on the line to indicate the point that best represented their pain relief at that time. The distance to this cross was then measured from the left-hand-side of the scale. This measurement represented their pain relief score

the patients might have for pain relief. During their last interview they were also asked: 'Did you know what to do if you had pain?', and if so, 'What?'.

The nurses' strategies were assessed as part of a questionnaire for trained nurses on the ward. The nurse was asked: 'What would you do if a patient complained of pain and it was not time for them to have another painkiller for an hour?'

Procedure

All interviews were carried out by one researcher. Patients were interviewed preoperatively, then twice a day postoperatively, for 7 consecutive days.

The patient's name was obtained from the admissions list, and they were approached on the day of admission. The purpose of the study was explained to them, and it was emphasised that if they decided not to take part, it would in no way affect their treatment, and if they decided to take part and later changed their mind, they could withdraw at any time. They were reassured that all information would be treated as strictly confidential. If the patient agreed to take part in the study, their signed consent was obtained. They were also given a letter to keep that restated the verbal explanation. Before each postoperative visit, all analgesic, sedative and anti-emetic drugs that had been administered were recorded on the interview schedule; then the patient interview took place. At the end of the entire study, all enrolled and registered nurses who had been working on the study wards were given a questionnaire to elicit their opinions on some aspects of pain and pain relief.

Ethical clearance

Permission to carry out the study was obtained from the hospital ethical committee.

The setting

This consisted of three general surgical wards in a London district general hospital. Each ward had 28 beds for male and female patients, divided into four single rooms and four six-bedded cubicles. All wards had nurse learners allocated to them.

Pilot work

Two pilot studies were carried out prior to the main study. Main study data collection took 12 months to complete, during which time 80 patients were interviewed.

FINDINGS

Since the data were mainly ordinal or ranked, non-parametric tests of statistical significance were used.

The patient sample consisted of 38 males and 42 females, whose ages ranged from 18 to 85 years, with a mean age of 54 years. Nearly 89 per cent of the sample were Caucasian. The nurse sample consisted of the 18 registered and 10 enrolled nurses from the study wards.

Pain

The findings revealed that over 43 per cent of patients had 'quite a lot of pain' (as rated on the pain scale, see Figure 12.1) or more when questioned on the first postoperative day. Also nearly 22 per cent rated their pain as 'very bad' on this day. One patient said, 'I didn't know if it would ever finish, it just went on for ever'. Another patient said, 'I can't stop the pain - it's all the time'. Over 86 per cent of patients had reported 'quite a lot of pain' or more at least once by their seventh postoperative day.

The spread of reports over time was interesting: although 57 per cent of all reports of 'quite a lot of pain' or more were made during the first 3 postoperative days, 43 per cent were made during days 4–7. It thus appeared that pain persisted well beyond the first 2 or 3 days after surgery.

Interestingly, nearly 9.5 per cent of patients with 'quite a lot of pain' or more did *not* want a painkiller when questioned. They frequently feared addiction. One said, 'I don't want to get attached to them', and another, 'once you get used to them, you've had it'. These patients felt that this fear of addiction was often reinforced by the nurse: 'They're trying to keep me off them' and 'The nurses convey that it's a bit naughty to take a painkiller'. Nearly 86 per cent of nurses overestimated the risk of addiction, a risk that Porter and Jick (1980) described as less than 1 per cent from their review of 11 882 medical patients receiving at least one narcotic. Some patients did not like the effects narcotics had on them, or they wanted to see what they could stand.

Looking at the effect of painkillers for all patients throughout the first 7 days after surgery, over 38 per cent of ratings described painkillers as making the pain slightly better, while over 27 per cent described them as making the pain very much better.

Nurses' and patients' ratings of pain

There were problems in obtaining the nurses' ratings, the numbers of which were as low as 10 per cent of the total possible at times. However, Figure 12.3 includes the averages of 221 separate pairs of nurse and patient ratings.

A Wilcoxon signed rank test revealed that nurses significantly and consistently rated the patients' pain lower than did the patient: $T = 0$, $p < 0.001$. A more detailed study of the scores provided further insight into these ratings. (For 77 per cent of the time, nurses and patients did not agree; 54 per cent of nurses rated the patients' pain as less and 13 per cent as more than did the patient.) The most common type of comment made by the nurse when making the rating was, 'He hasn't complained of any'.

A question to enable direct comparisons between nurses' and patients' ratings of pain relief was dropped after pilot study work, since the nurses often did not know how much pain relief patients had obtained from painkillers. However, all 28 trained staff on the study wards were asked a question adapted from Cohen (1980): 'In general, do you think analgesics on this ward are: more than the patient needs; meet the patient's needs; or are less than the patient needs?'. None thought they were more than the patient needs and 75 per cent felt that they met the patients' needs. When looked at from the patients' perspective, although 61 per cent of patients found pain control as or better than expected, pain disturbed the sleep of 66 per cent of patients on the first postoperative night. Looking back on their stay, almost a third of patients felt that they could not have a painkiller when they wanted one. Although 68 per cent of the nurses felt that patients often or almost always would ask for

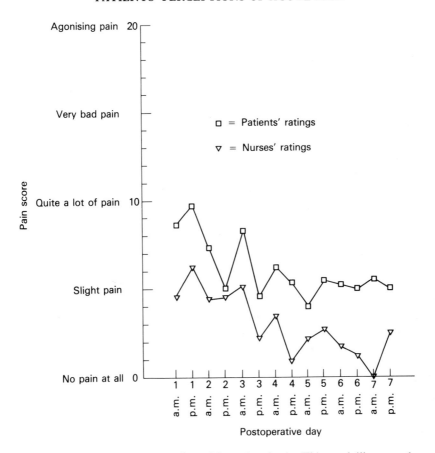

Fig. 12.3 Nurses' and patients' mean ratings of the patients' pain. This graph illustrates the patients' and nurses' mean pain scores, as rated twice a day during the first postoperative days. The nurses' ratings were consistently lower than the patients' ratings and this difference was significant using a Wilcoxon signed rank test (T=0, p<0.001)

a painkiller if they needed one, only 37.5 per cent of patients said that they would ask; 42 per cent expected the nurse to know. One patient said, 'I expect the nurse to know automatically'.

Thus, the nurses' and the patients' views on pain relief were not necessarily the same.

Strategies for pain relief

Patients' strategies at home were varied; in hospital this range was reduced. Over 88 per cent of patients felt that they knew what to do if they had pain in hospital. Of these, nearly 70 per cent said that they would ring for the nurse or take a painkiller. When asked if anything made the pain better, nearly 39 per cent of the responses mentioned drugs, although 28 per cent said that nothing made the pain better.

The 28 nurses were asked, 'What might you do if a patient reported pain, but it wasn't time for them to have another painkiller for an hour?' (all responses were recorded). There were 42 responses that involved the doctor (telling the doctor, recommending a different analgesic, or increased dose or reduced time interval). Six responses involved making the patient comfortable, four involved talking to the patient and reassuring him and four involved telling the patient that he was unable to have another painkiller. These responses were thus mainly directed towards painkillers, and no nurse specifically mentioned any alternative method of pain relief.

IMPLICATIONS FOR NURSING

This study found that 86 per cent of patients had 'quite a lot of pain' or more at least once when interviewed, and thus supported Cohen (1980) and Weis et al's (1983) findings that pain relief after surgery is not ideal. Nurses in this study tended to assess the patients' pain as less than did the patient, which confirmed the findings of Johnston (1976) and Hunt et al (1977). What could account for the difference between the nurses' and patients' assessment of pain?

The care plans suggested that nurses acknowledged pain as a potential problem after surgery, often with the stated goal of a 'pain-free patient', but, for various reasons, this goal was not realised. Graffam (1981) concluded that nurses' assessment of pain was minimal, and no evidence was found in this study to contradict her conclusion. Pain and its relief were infrequently recorded in the Kardex, a finding also noted by Sofaer (1984). Even if a painkiller was given, it was not always effective, as Bourbonnais and Mackay (1981) found, emphasising that not only pain, but pain relief, needs to be assessed.

Why was pain and its relief not systematically assessed? The nurses were often under pressure to complete their work, much of which centred on tasks for which they were accountable. This pressure of work at times pushed pain relief down the list of priorities.

Fear of addiction was another reason for less than ideal pain relief. In the present study, nurses overestimated the risk of addiction. From the patients' perspective, painkillers were avoided for many reasons. Before surgery, over 75 per cent of patients said that they disliked taking painkillers or would take them only if the pain was bad. Fears of addiction, at times reinforced by the nurse, were very apparent. One patient said, 'I'd rather suffer in silence than rely on them', and another, 'It's better not to have anything – I've stuck it out so far, so I might as well for the last bit'. So, attitudes of nurses and of patients towards painkillers are important to consider when assessing pain and its relief.

A breakdown in communication between the nurse and patient may have contributed to poor pain relief. The interactions between the nurse and patient surrounding pain and its relief are complex. The patients must want and be able to communicate their pain to the nurse. The nurse has to ask the right questions and listen to the answers, believe the patient, take appropriate action to relieve the pain and evaluate this relief. At any one of these steps, communication can break down. For example, Ley (1976) found that patients were reluctant to interrupt a 'busy' nurse. The patient may be in pain, but not want to take another painkiller. The patient may not be able to attract the nurse's attention, and the nurse may not ask the patients about their pain, believe the patients, take appropriate action to relieve the pain, or evaluate the extent to which pain has been relieved.

In this study, while nearly 68 per cent of nurses felt that patients would often or almost always ask for a painkiller if they needed one, only 37.5 per cent of patients felt that they would ask; 42 per cent expected the nurse to know. It seems that the problems associated with relying on the patient to ask for a painkiller could be reduced by systematically assessing pain with the patient.

At times, nurses seemed to be controlling pain expression rather than pain. One nurse in this study remarked, 'He's very good and hasn't had many painkillers. He's got the right attitude'. The control that equating 'good' with 'few painkillers' exerted was summed up by another patient who remarked, 'I keep quiet even if the pain is severe. I don't want to get into the nurses' bad books'.

Low expectations of pain relief may also have contributed to less than adequate pain control. Although 86 per cent of patients had 'quite a lot of pain' or more at least once, and nearly a third felt that they had been unable to have a painkiller when they wanted one, almost 61 per cent felt that their pain control had been as good or better than they had expected.

Perhaps the most important reason for lack of systematic pain assessment is the lack of accountability surrounding pain management, highlighted by McCaffery (1979) and Fagerhaugh and Strauss (1977). Nurses are accountable for other aspects of their care. For example, if a temperature, pulse or blood pressure recording is omitted, or a fluid chart is incomplete, the nurse is likely to be held responsible for that omission. These observations are recorded on a chart and it is easy to see if information is missing. Pain could be systematically recorded in the same way. This would also provide a record for other health professionals to consult.

Being accountable encompasses much more than only being held responsible for omissions on a chart: an understanding of the complexities of pain, its assessment and relief, and recognition of one's own opinions and attitudes are essential.

Although current nursing practice emphasises total patient care, for many of the reasons already discussed some patients still remain in pain after surgery.

The aim of adequate pain relief is not an oversedated patient. Controlled drugs are not *the* answer to better pain relief, but in this study it seemed that more could have been used. The effectiveness of non-narcotic analgesics for some pains should not be underestimated. However, in this study it appeared that non-narcotic analgesics were at times given more or less when the patient was able to take tablets, rather than when the type and intensity of the pain warranted this change. Complementary methods of pain relief, such as relaxation and distraction, could be used, especially on later postoperative days when painkillers tended to be less effective. Patients may have already developed their own methods of pain relief, which could be used and built upon.

Since this study found that there were large individual variations in pain between patients, which did not appear to be predictable, it is important to assess pain individually and not by, for example, operation or sex.

The complex, subjective and unique nature of pain needs to be recognised, and, thus, pain and pain relief should be discussed with the patients. Their preferences and usual methods of coping need to be considered, and they should be advised on complementary methods of pain relief. The disadvantages of poor pain relief and any fears of addiction could be discussed as appropriate. Whenever the patient is able, the nurse and patient should reach a decision about pain relief together.

The individual, unpredictable nature of pain and thus the importance of believing the patient needs to be recognised. A pain chart, completed with the patient, will allow for systematic assessment of pain and provide a record of pain and its relief. It will also show the patients that their pain is taken seriously. The effectiveness of pain relief measures can be evaluated and changes made as necessary.

This study demonstrated that pain relief needs to be given a higher priority in nursing care. Each nurse must take responsibility for assessing the pain of patients in her care, and not leave it to someone else.

The main findings of this study have been incorporated into a research-based video entitled 'Anything for Pain?' available from Public Relations Department, North West Thames Regional Health Authority, 40 Eastbourne Terrace, London W2 3QR.

REFERENCES

Bourbonnais F E and Mackay R C (1981) The influence of nursing intervention on chest pain. *Nursing Papers*, **13**(4): 38-48.
Camp L D and O'Sullivan P S (1987) Comparison of medical, surgical and oncology patients' descriptions of pain and nurses' documentation of pain assessments. *Journal of Advanced Nursing*, **12**: 593-398.
Chapman C R (1978) Pain: the perception of noxious events. In: *The Psychology of Pain*, ed. Sternback R A, pp. 169-202. New York: Raven Press.
Cohen F L (1980) Postsurgical pain relief: patient's status and nurses' medication choices. *Pain*, **45**: 867-873.
Dodson M E (1982) A review of methods for relief of postoperative pain. *Annals of the Royal College of Surgeons of England*, **64**: 324-327.
Dodson M E (1985) *The Management of Postoperative Pain*, Current Topics in Anaesthesia Series, vol. 8. London: Edward Arnold.
Fagerhaugh S Y and Strauss A (1977) *Politics of Pain Management: Staff-Patient Interaction*. California: Addison-Wesley.
Fordham M (1982) The recovery of physical fitness. *International Journal of Nursing Studies*, **19**(4): 205-212.
Graffam S (1981) Congruence of nurse-patient expectations regarding nursing intervention in pain. *Nursing Leadership*, **4**(2): 12-15.
Hunt J M, Stollar T D, Littlejohns D W, Twycross R G and Vere D S (1977) Patients with protracted pain: a survey conducted at the London Hospital. *Journal of Medical Ethics*, **3**(2): 61-73.
Johnston M (1976) Communication of patients' feelings in hospital. In: *Communication Between Doctors and Patients*, ed. Bennett A D, pp. 31-43. Oxford: Oxford University Press.
Kremer E, Atkinson J H and Ignelzi R J (1981) Measurement of pain: patient preference does not confound pain measurement. *Pain*, **10**(2): 241-248.
Ley P (1976) Towards better doctor-patient communications. In: *Communication Between Doctors and Patients*, ed. Bennett A E, pp. 77-98. Oxford: Oxford University Press.
McCaffery M (1972) *Nursing Management of the Patient with Pain*. Philadelphia: Lippincott.
McCaffery M (1979) *Nursing the Patient in Pain*. Adapted for the UK by Sofaer B (1983), Lippincott Nursing Series. London: Harper and Row.
Melzack R (1984) Measurement of the dimension of pain experience. In: *Pain Measurement in Man. Neurophysiological Correlates of Pain*, ed. Bromm B chap. 23, pp. 327-348. Amsterdam: Elsevier.
Melzack R and Wall P D (1982) *The Challenge of Pain*. Harmondsworth: Penguin.
Porter J and Jick H (1980) Addiction rare in patients treated with narcotics. *New England Journal of Medicine*, **302**(2): 123.
Seers C J (1987) *Pain, Anxiety and Recovery in Patients Undergoing Surgery*. Unpublished PhD thesis, King's College, University of London.
Smith J M and Utting J E (1976) Postoperative pain. *British Medical Journal*, **2**(6040): 875.
Sofaer B (1984) *The Effect of Focused Education for Nursing Teams on Postoperative Pain of Patients*. Unpublished PhD thesis, University of Edinburgh.
Sriwatanakul K, Weis O F, Alloza J L, Kelvie W, Weintraub M and Lasagna L (1983) Analysis of narcotic analgesic usage in the treatment of postoperative pain. *Journal of the American Medical Association*, **2501**(7): 926-929.
Volicer B J and Bohannon M W (1975) A hospital stress rating scale. *Nursing Research*, **24**(5): 352-359.
Weis O F, Sriwatanakul K, Alloza J L, Weintraub M and Lasagna L (1983) Attitudes of patients, housestaff, and nurses toward postoperative analgesic care. *Anesthesia and Analgesia*, **62**(1): 70-74.

Chapter 13

Risk Factors and Recovery from Coronary Artery Bypass Surgery

Sally West and Jenifer Wilson-Barnett

BACKGROUND TO STUDY AND REVIEW OF PREVIOUS RESEARCH

The study of recovery from surgery has often concentrated on early outcome, and little attention has been paid to experiences following discharge. However, even after minor procedures, few patients feel completely recovered when they leave hospital. Nurses have a responsibility to assist patients towards health and normal function. This should include preparation for leaving hospital and ensuring that there is adequate support after discharge. This is not possible without detailed knowledge of the kinds of problems and feelings patients may encounter.

Certain patients seem more likely than others to experience difficulties. Mathews and Ridgeway (1981) reviewed research on psychological influences on early outcome and concluded that anxiety was the most important factor. Turning to long-term recovery, considerable work has been done on outcome after myocardial infarction (MI) (Philip et al, 1981; Mayou, 1984). A proportion of these patients experience persistent emotional problems and reduced leisure and sexual activity, which are unrelated to cardiac symptoms. Mental state in hospital and premorbid activity levels can influence subsequent recovery. The research by these authors and their colleagues has contributed much to the knowledge of recovery from MI and has also demonstrated the use of global assessments of outcome.

Coronary Artery Bypass Surgery (CABS)

CABS has become an increasingly common treatment for angina. A minority of patients need surgery for prognostic reasons, but generally life expectation is not increased (Killip et al, 1985). The main indication for surgery is angina uncontrolled by medical treatment, and the operation is generally effective in relieving symptoms (Sloman and Sutton, 1981). However, increased satisfaction with life may not always follow.

Problems can occur as a result of the surgery. Wilson-Barnett (1981) interviewed 60 patients one year after CABS and found that 10 still needed dressing for their leg wounds and 19 continued to experience severe sternal wound pain. Other problems such as muscle stiffness and numbness can also occur, and although often dismissed as minor, these can cause considerable distress.

Quality of life after CABS

Employment status is the one widely studied aspect of quality of life (see Mayou, 1986, for a summary). While many patients are able to carry out their jobs more easily, most researchers have found a decrease in the percentage working after surgery. The most important predictors of postoperative work status are preoperative work status, persistent cardiac symptoms and attitudes of employers, doctors and patients themselves.

The most detailed information about other aspects of outcome after CABS comes from two prospective studies. In the United States, 340 patients (86 per cent men) were assessed before surgery and 6 months later (Jenkins et al, 1983; Stanton et al, 1984b) using interviews and an extensive range of questionnaires. In Britain, Mayou and Bryant (1987) used the Present State Examination, semi-structured interviews and questionnaires to study 79 men before surgery, 3 months and 1 year later.

Severe psychological upset is uncommon after CABS. Two studies using standard psychological interviews (Bass, 1984; Mayou and Bryant, 1987) found general improvement after surgery. Fluctuations in moods, however, are frequent, and Jenkins et al (1983) reported that 40 per cent had experienced depression and 38 per cent anxiety.

Increases in physical abilities are considerable. Prior to surgery, 31 per cent of Mayou and Bryant's sample were rated as having slight or no physical limitations, and this rose to 74 per cent after operation. However, there seems to be little change in involvement with leisure and social activities. Eighteen per cent of Mayou and Bryant's study reported obtaining less satisfaction from leisure after surgery.

Both the frequency of and satisfaction with sex, overall, appear to change little, despite the relief of cardiac symptoms (Kornfield et al, 1982; Horgan et al, 1984). In terms of family contacts there appear to be few problems, with over 90 per cent reporting the same or improved relationships (Kornfield et al, 1982; Jenkins et al, 1983). Comments from patients indicate that most are very pleased with the results. For example, 75 per cent of Wilson-Barnett's (1981) sample said they got more enjoyment out of life.

In summary, the symptomatic improvement after CABS is usually accompanied by general satisfaction, increased physical ability and good psychosocial outcome, although Mayou (1986) concludes that many do not wish to make major life-style changes. However, a minority of patients report deterioration in social function which does not appear to be related to poor cardiac outcome. The next question must, therefore, be: can these patients be identified before the operation?

Preoperative risk factors

Little research has considered preoperative risk factors. In a small study by Ramshaw and Stanley (1984), 21 patients were assessed before and after CABS and divided into good and poor outcome groups. Out of a wide range of preoperative measures, only neuroticism and coping style were related to outcome.

Mayou and Bryant (1987) reported that the best predictor of any specific outcome was the presurgical measure of that function and the individual's expectation. They produced a global social outcome by summing changes in four areas (work, leisure, family and sex) and found that the best predictors were variables associated with mental state and a passive, cautious approach to illness.

Advice given to patients

In Wilson-Barnett's study (1981), 29 (49 per cent) did not recall receiving any information and advice prior to discharge and a further 16 (27 per cent) were given only 'a few blanket phrases'. Stanton et al (1984a) asked 249 cardiac patients about preparation for recovery. In terms of sex, symptoms and emotional change, many felt unprepared, although most were happy with advice regarding activities. This is clearly an area of nursing care that needs more attention.

Cardiac rehabilitation

It might be anticipated that rehabilitation would improve outcome. There is some evidence that exercise training can increase functional capacity and cardiac performance after CABS (Froelicher et al, 1985). However, as there appear to be no randomised studies attempting to influence psychosocial outcome after CABS, studies with MI patients will be considered.

Although generally appreciated by participants, there is little evidence that either exercise or advice sessions can produce significant psychosocial changes (Mayou, 1981; Stern and Cleary, 1982). This is partly because outcome after MI (like CABS) is generally very good and leaves little scope for overall improvement. Second, some participants do not complete rehabilitation programmes, and it appears that those most at risk are also those most likely to drop out (Stern and Cleary, 1982; Oldridge et al, 1983).

Such results are likely to be repeated with cardiac surgery patients, and it follows that rehabilitation might be most usefully concentrated on the minority who have poorer outcomes, if these can be identified, and that care should be tailored to suit the individual's needs.

AIMS OF THE STUDY

From the above literature review, a study of recovery from CABS was designed with four main aims:

1. To describe the range of recovery and problems experienced from the patients' viewpoints.
2. To consider medical, emotional and social outcomes and their interrelationships.
3. To establish whether patients at risk of a poor recovery could be identified preoperatively using simple assessments of psychosocial factors previously found to influence recovery.
4. To assess the support, information and advice received in relation to patients' perceived needs both in hospital and after discharge.

METHODS

The sample consisted of 85 patients undergoing CABS for the first time. Patients of both sexes and any age were included. All had to live reasonably near the hospital and be available for the preoperative interview. Assessments were carried out before surgery and 6 months later.

Preoperative assessment

The preoperative assessment took place in hospital on the day before the operation. Data were obtained from the medical notes, a semi-structured interview and three questionnaires.

The interview covered cardiac history, work, leisure activities, psychiatric history, social situation, support anticipated and expectations.

Two psychological scales were administered. These were the trait anxiety scale of the State–Trait Anxiety Inventory (Spielberger et al, 1969) and a mood adjective check-list (MACL; Lishman, 1972), which rates anxiety, depression, hostility, vigour and fatigue. The third questionnaire assessed restrictions in 20 everyday activities (adapted from Mayou and Bryant, 1987).

After the interview, the researcher wrote comments about the patient. The most important observation concerned patients' responses to the research study that seemed to be associated with their attitudes towards the operation and illness. This was termed *interest expressed* and three categories were formed. 'Interested' patients asked most questions and wanted to be involved with their treatment. The 'friendly' group seemed pleased to be in the study and welcomed someone to talk to but asked few questions. The third and smallest group were termed 'wary' and these patients were reluctant to talk about themselves or the operation. They were either passive and withdrawn or suspicious and critical.

Interview at 6 months

Six months after the operation, patients were contacted and visited at home where another semi-structured interview was carried out.

Medical data included treatment since surgery, cardiac symptoms, wound healing and any other problems. The severity of wound pain was rated by the patient as 'slight', 'moderate' or 'severe'.

The interview also covered changes and restrictions in work, leisure, social life, everyday activities, social support, memory, concentration and mood changes. Patients were asked to give a percentage rating (out of 100) to their present health and when (if at all) they had felt completely recovered.

Finally, the interview covered advice and information received in hospital and asked about further support they would have liked.

Analysis

In addition to descriptive information obtained, many of the data were analysed using the Statistical Package for the Social Sciences (Nie et al, 1975). Non-parametric tests were mainly used as most of the data were nominal or ordinal.

FINDINGS

Preoperative characteristics

The sample consisted of 69 men and 16 women aged 34 to 76 years (mean 58.3 years). Nearly all had severe angina and about half also experienced dyspnoea. Most were very restricted in their normal activities. Eight lived alone but just two patients anticipated little social support. The scores on the psychological scales were unremarkable and these were unrelated to the interviewer's rating of 'interest expressed'.

Outcome at 6 months

Seventy-nine patients were interviewed again after 6 months. Two had died, two moved away and two could not be traced.

Only eight still experienced angina and this was always mild. There was also an overall reduction in dyspnoea. Wound pain varied a lot. Most (59 per cent) had occasional discomfort while 18 per cent still experienced pain. Other problems included delayed wound healing, tiredness and numbness.

Overall, patients were less restricted in work, leisure and everyday activities, with 48 per cent reporting no restrictions at all. However, in all areas a few individuals had problems and 16 per cent were rated as severely restricted.

The mood scales showed overall improvement, but for at least one factor on each scale, between 10 and 44 per cent of patients had poorer scores than before surgery. Depression and irritability were common and for some this had been severe.

Views of the operation and percentage rating given to health were also good. However, 9 per cent expressed some disappointment with outcome and 4 per cent regretted having the operation.

Social support was widely praised, with only two reporting this to be inadequate.

Relationships between outcomes at 6 months

There were no significant associations between mood scores at 6 months and cardiac symptoms. However, those with more negative mood scores had more severe wound pain and visited their GP more often. Restrictions in activities and variables that assessed patients' views of health were strongly related to cardiac symptoms, wound pain and mood scores.

Preoperative data and outcome at 6 months

Cardiac outcome

Women had poorer cardiac outcomes, but otherwise there were only modest associations between preoperative factors and cardiac outcome.

Emotional outcome

The severity of wound pain was related to preoperative psychological data, especially depression and fatigue ($\chi^2 = 12.03$ and 12.88 respectively, both $p < 0.005$).

Age, sex and preoperative medical variables had little influence on mood scores at 6 months. However, emotional outcome was closely associated with preoperative psychological data, especially trait anxiety and depression.

Restrictions in activities

Patients who reported no restrictions in activities were compared with those who were restricted. Both cardiac and psychological preoperative variables were significantly associated with restrictions, the most important being 'interest expressed', fatigue, dyspnoea and heart failure (Table 13.1).

Table 13.1 Associations between restrictions in activities at 6 months and preoperative factors (n = 79)

χ^2		Mann-Whitney (z)	
d.f. = 1			
Sex	3.21	Age	1.76
Severity of dyspnoea	7.86**	Trait anxiety	2.15*
Heart failure	9.68†	MACL anxiety	2.32*
Previous MI	0.55	MACL depression	2.23*
		MACL hostility	1.49
d.f. = 2		MACL vigour	0.98
Severity of angina	0.01	MACL fatigue	2.84‡
Interest expressed	14.75‡		

($*=p<0.05$, $**=p<0.01$, $†=p<0.005$, $‡=p<0.001$)

Expectations and outcome

There was a weak correlation between expected time for complete recovery and actual time (Spearman, $r=0.22$, $p<0.5$). However, the predictions for specific activities were not very useful as the majority of patients expected to resume all activities.

Social support

Social support had only modest associations with outcome. Low support was significantly related to depression (Mann-Whitney, $z=2.28$, $p<0.05$) and low vigour (Mann-Whitney, $z=2.60$, $p<0.01$).

Percentage rating to health

The percentage rating patients gave to their own health at 6 months had little association with preoperative demographic or cardiac data. However, it was strongly associated with preoperative psychological measures (Table 13.2). Eight patients felt unable to make this assessment.

Table 13.2 Associations between percentage rating of health at 6 months and preoperative factors

Mann-Whitney (z)		Spearman (r)	
Sex	1.36	Age	−0.03
Severity of dyspnoea	1.48	Trait anxiety	−0.37‡
Heart failure	1.87	MACL anxiety	−0.42‡
Previous MI (associated with lower % rating of health)	2.13*	MACL depression	−0.32†
		MACL hostility	−0.04
Kruskal Wallis, χ^2 approximation		MACL vigour	0.05
Severity of angina	3.33	MACL fatigue (higher scores	−0.28**
Interest expressed (those expressing more interest were more likely to give higher % ratings to their health)	13.41†	on negative moods preoperatively were correlated with lower % ratings of health)	

($*=p<0.05$, $**=p<0.01$, $†=p<0.005$, $‡=p<0.001$)

Advice and information

Most patients were happy with the preparation for discharge, although 20 per cent would have liked 'a little more' and 6 per cent 'a lot more'. Some had been unsure about commencing activities and were unprepared for the problems and feelings encountered. Most were satisfied with support after discharge, although 15 per cent would have liked additional help such as a nurse visiting. Some said that their families needed more support.

DISCUSSION

The overall picture of recovery from CABS was very positive. The excellent cardiac outcome was generally accompanied by improvement in other areas of life-style, and many patients were enjoying a new lease of life. However, it would be misleading to consider only overall changes, as the range of experiences was extremely wide. Some patients felt that their lives had changed little, and a minority had encountered major problems. When staff are preparing patients for discharge, they must understand that there is no 'normal' recovery. They should encourage return to active life-styles but outline possible problems and not give unrealistic expectations.

Cardiac factors were independent of psychological measures and had only limited relationships with variables such as activity levels. This emphasises the need for holistic assessment of recovery. The severity of wound pain was closely related to all aspects of psychosocial outcome. While it is generally realised that pain can persist for many months, its influence on other aspects of recovery has not been examined previously. If pain could be reduced using medication or treatments such as relaxation, corresponding improvements in other areas might occur.

Assessing pain in a global way poses methodological problems because concepts such as 'satisfaction' are difficult to quantify. Mayou and Bryant (1987) employed detailed interviews from which researchers rated changes in different areas. However, this is time consuming and requires experienced workers. The activity questionnaire used in the present study proved useful as it produced a wide range of responses and the items were relevant to most patients. There remains a need for development of other appropriate research tools.

Identification of risk factors

The present study found that certain preoperative factors predisposed to a poorer outcome. The most important factors were trait anxiety, depression, fatigue and 'interest expressed'. Anxiety and depression have previously been found to be influential, although often using more detailed assessments. Those employed here were quick and simple to complete and could feasibly be routinely administered prior to surgery. Alternatively, trained staff could assess patients during an interview. Research would be needed to ascertain the accuracy of such judgments and to discover what form of assessment would be most acceptable to patients.

An unexpected finding was the importance of the variable 'interest expressed', rated according to the interviewer's observations. The 'wary' group may correspond to those described by Mayou and Bryant (1987) as cautious and passive. This variable also identified 'interested' patients who had particularly good outcomes. It is not clear exactly what this variable is measuring or how it influences recovery, but these results suggest that it would be fruitful to explore this concept further.

The other two factors previously suggested as being important – expectations and social support – had limited influence. The assessments may not have been detailed enough to bring out individual differences. However, levels of social support were very high for almost all patients and only two patients reported little support. Both of these had experienced a very poor recovery with many problems. Despite the limited influence in this study, social support must remain an important factor to assess before surgery.

Next, the implications of these findings will be considered. Although highly significant relationships were found, these were not strong enough to predict individual outcome with any confidence. Preoperative factors only accounted for about a quarter to a third of the variance in outcome measures. It would, therefore, not be possible to recommend that certain patients are psychologically unsuitable for surgery, especially when symptoms are severe. However, psychological factors could be useful when the decision to operate is difficult. In addition, there would be reservations if moves were made to make the operation more readily available to patients with mild or moderate angina and no prognostic indications.

The other and perhaps more important reason for preoperative assessment is to identify patients in need of extra support. A system whereby this could be done will be described next.

Proposed care of cardiac patients

Although pre-discharge preparation has increased since Wilson-Barnett's (1981) study in the same cardiac unit, there is still a need for further improvement. In hospital, the nursing process aims to provide individualised care, and it is proposed that such a system could be extended to the preoperative and post-discharge periods. An initial psychosocial interview could be carried out at the cardiac clinic. This could be done by nurses rotated from the wards and, ideally, each patient would be allocated to a small team who would provide continuity of care. Detailed notes would be made and relatives would be involved. The first meeting would include assessments of the factors previously found to increase psychosocial risk. Problems would be discussed and further care and support planned accordingly, for instance additional counselling. The nurse could telephone the patient occasionally during the waiting period and he or she would be encouraged to contact the team if there were any problems or queries. When the patient was admitted for surgery, his/her team would be involved with the nursing care as much as possible. After discharge, contact would be continued at out-patient clinics and by phone for as long as necessary. Home visits could also be arranged where practical. By building up a relationship with the patient, minor problems might be prevented or soon solved, and if severe difficulties developed, referral to appropriate professionals, such as psychiatrists and social workers, could be made. While most patients would probably require minimal support, a system such as this could promote good recovery for those who need extra help.

Summary

The recovery of a sizeable minority of CABS patients can be impeded by psychosocial factors, and many others may have temporary concerns that could be avoided. There is now some indication of psychological factors that can predispose patients to a poor recovery. A system is suggested whereby a small group of nurses would keep in regular contact with the patients throughout the recovery period. Individual assessment, planning and support might help to prevent psychosocial factors and promote recovery.

ACKNOWLEDGEMENTS

This research was carried out with support from the DHSS Nursing Studentship scheme and the Band Trust.

REFERENCES

Bass C (1984) Psychosocial outcome after coronary artery by-pass surgery. *British Journal of Psychiatry*, **145**: 526-532.

Froelicher V, Jensen D and Sullivan M (1985) A randomised trial of the effects of exercise training after coronary artery bypass surgery. *Archives of Internal Medicine*, **145**: 689-692.

Horgan D, Davies B, Hunt D, Westlake G W and Mullerworth M (1984) Psychiatric aspects of coronary surgery. *Medical Journal of Australia*, **5**: 587-590.

Jenkins C D, Stanton B, Savageau J, Denlinger P and Klein M D (1983) Coronary artery bypass surgery: psychological, social and economic outcomes six months later. *Journal of the American Medical Association*, **250**: 782-788.

Killip T, Passaman E, Davis K and the CASS principal investigators and their associates (1985) Coronary Artery Surgery Study (CASS) - a randomised trial. *Circulation*, **72**(suppl. V): V102-V107.

Kornfield D S, Heller S S, Frank K A, Wilson S N and Malm J R (1982) Psychological and behavioural responses after coronary artery bypass surgery. *Circulation*, **66**(suppl. III): 24-28.

Lishman W A (1972) Selective factors in memory. Part 2: affective disorder. *Psychological Medicine*, **2**: 248-253.

Mathews A and Ridgeway V (1981) Personality and surgical recovery: a review. *British Journal of Clinical Psychology*, **20**: 243-260.

Mayou R (1981) Effectiveness of cardiac rehabilitation. *Journal of Psychosomatic Research*, **25**: 423-427.

Mayou R (1984) Prediction of emotional and social outcome after a heart attack. *Journal of Psychosomatic Research*, **28**: 17-25.

Mayou R (1986) The psychiatric and social consequences of coronary artery surgery. *Journal of Psychosomatic Research*, **30**: 225-271.

Mayou R and Bryant (1987) Quality of life after coronary artery surgery. *Quarterly Journal of Medicine*, **63**: 639-248.

Nie N H, Hull C H, Jenkins J G, Steinbrenner K and Bent D H (1975) *Statistical Package for the Social Sciences*. New York: McGraw-Hill.

Oldridge N B, Donner A P, Bock C, Jones N L, Andrew G M, Parker J O, Cunningham D A, Kavanagh T, Rechnitzer P A and Sutton J R (1983) Predictors of dropout from cardiac exercise rehabilitation. *American Journal of Cardiology*, **51**: 70-74.

Philip A E, Cay E, Stuckey N A and Vetter N J (1981) Multiple predictors and multiple outcomes after myocardial infarction. *Journal of Psychosomatic Research*, **25**: 137-144.

Ramshaw J E and Stanley G (1984) Psychological adjustment to coronary artery surgery. *British Journal of Clinical Psychology*, **23**: 101-108.

Sloman J G and Sutton L D (1981) Coronary artery graft surgery. *Medical Journal of Australia*, **2**: 489-491.

Spielberger C D, Gorusch R L and Lushene R (1969) *The State-Trait Anxiety Inventory Manual*. Palo Alto: Consulting Psychologists Press.

Stanton B-A, Jenkins C D, Savageau J A, Harker D E and Aucoin R (1984a) Perceived adequacy of patient education and fears and adjustments after cardiac surgery. *Heart and Lung*, **13**: 525-531.

Stanton B-A, Jenkins C D, Savageau J A and Thurer R L (1984b) Functional benefits following coronary artery bypass surgery. *Annals of Thoracic Surgery*, **37**: 286-290.

Stern M J and Cleary P (1982) National exercise and heart disease project. *Archives of Internal Medicine*, **141**: 1463-1477.

Wilson-Barnett J (1981) Assessment of recovery: with special reference to a study with post-operative cardiac patients. *Journal of Advanced Nursing*, **6**: 435-445.

Chapter 14

Recovery from Surgery

Morva Fordham

INTRODUCTION

Occupational health and ergonomics aim to optimise the relationship between man's physical and mental capacities and the demands of his work and leisure activities. Illness and surgery may alter this match between capacity and habitual life-style. This study aimed to investigate the relationship between physical fitness, work and leisure activities and the existence and treatment of an inguinal hernia. The basic tenet that underlies the research is that the goal of recovery from the point of view of the patient undergoing elective surgery is the ability to resume his or her habitual life-style of work and leisure activities, and that to achieve this it is necessary for him/her to retain or regain both muscular strength and stamina.

Physical fitness or 'the ability to do muscular work satisfactorily' as defined by the World Health Organisation (Shepherd et al, 1968) makes demands upon almost all systems of the body. The physiological and psychological determinants of fitness are well summarised by Shepherd (1969). If illness or operation interferes with the ability to meet any of the physiological demands of muscular work or reduces the motivation to be active or the skill in co-ordination of movement, then a downward spiral of decreasing activity and physical fitness may be set in train, as illustrated in Figure 14.1.

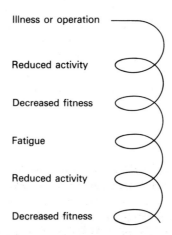

Illness or operation

Reduced activity

Decreased fitness

Fatigue

Reduced activity

Decreased fitness

Fig. 14.1 Deconditioning spiral

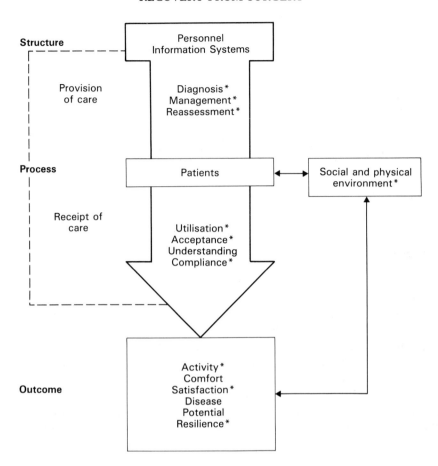

Fig. 14.2 Dynamics of health outcome (adapted from Starfield, 1973)

It was hypothesised that the fitness or condition of patients would not only be determined by their physical status at the onset of illness or surgery but also by their level of activity during and following illness, and, furthermore, that the care and advice they received from nurses and doctors during illness would influence this activity at least in part.

Conceptually this study fits into a framework of structure, process and outcome as described by Starfield (1973). The aspects of his 'Dynamics of Health Outcome', which were investigated in this study, are shown in Figure 14.2, specifically those marked with an asterisk.

RESEARCH METHODS

The research design was a longitudinal study with intermittent repeated measurements of objective and subjective physical fitness parameters. These were used, first, to investigate the extent of conditioning, deconditioning and reconditioning that occurred during the time awaiting surgery and during convalescence, and, second, to elucidate the relationship between objective and subjective criteria of fitness. As activity is a major intervening variable between changes in conditioning, estimations of the activity of the subjects prior and subsequent to surgery were made. A two-pronged attack was used to elicit these data. First, information about habitual work and leisure activities before and after operation was sought by questionnaire, including the number of days or weeks after surgery when key activities were resumed, the experience or not of fatigue following return to work, and advice received from nurses, doctors, family and others. Second, the level of activity at work preoperatively, in hospital postoperatively and at home during convalescence was monitored using 24-hour heart rate recordings on Medilog recorders (Smith and O'Brien, 1976) plus self-kept diaries of activities. The overall sequence of data collection is depicted in Table 14.1.

Aspects of this study, including the choice of fitness tests and the normative findings, have been published elsewhere (Fordham, 1982; Wilson-Barnett and Fordham, 1982), as has the entire thesis (Fordham, 1985). This chapter focuses on two points: first, the ethical and practical considerations in undertaking a longitudinal study in which physical demands were made on the subjects, and, second, the use of individual case studies or vignettes to examine and elucidate normative findings.

Table 14.1 Data collection timing

	Questionnaire/ interview	Physical fitness tests and self-rating	24-h ECG and activity diary
OPD	Personal medical history, work and leisure activities	X	
W/L			X
O/A	Preoperative advice	X	
OPERATION DAY			
PO day			X
Day before discharge		X	
Convalescence	Postoperative advice, convalescent activities		X
OPD F/U		X	
Return to work	Hours and nature of work. Felt fatigue		

Key: OPD Out-patient department
      W/L   Waiting list
      O/A   On admission
      PO   Postoperative
      F/U   Follow-up

Physical fitness tests: 1. Submaximal bicycle exercise test
                         2. Tilt-table posture test
                         3. Grip strength
                         4. Lung capacity

ETHICAL AND PRACTICAL CONSIDERATIONS

Patients were first seen at the out-patient visit when the consultant decision to operate was made, and were followed up until they returned to work. This time span ranged from 2 to 12 months.

Piloting

As data collection from any one patient might have covered months or years, it was expedient for the pilot study to be undertaken in piecemeal fashion. Most of the physiological tests, including the bicycle exercise test, had been learned and rehearsed in a previous study (Fordham et al, 1978). Other tests, including the tilt-table test, were rehearsed with students and colleagues, and the whole battery of tests was performed by one surgical in-patient. Questionnaires were tested on surgical in-patients and modified as a result. This piloting could give little indication of the likely loss of subjects or data in the main study.

Ethical considerations

Biomedical research ethics seem to be primarily based on utilitarian theories of morality, the aim being to promote such values as health by maximising benefits and minimising harms. Members of ethics committees and researchers are expected to describe the risks and benefits for potential subjects prior to the subjects' consent to participate in the research (Beauchamps and Childress, 1983). When the benefits to the subjects are non-existent or negligible, as in this study, the costs or risks should also be negligible. The requirement to obtain voluntary informed consent from human subjects is based on respect for autonomy.

The declaration of Helsinki (1964, 1975), which deals with non-therapeutical biomedical research involving human subjects (non-clinical biomedical research), states:

'1. In the purely scientific application of medical research carried out on a human being it is the duty of the doctor to remain the protector of the life and health of that person on whom biomedical research is being carried out.

2. The subjects should be volunteers – either healthy persons or patients – for whom the experimental design is not related to the patients' illness.

3. The investigator or the investigating team should discontinue the research if in his/her or their judgement it may, if continued, be harmful to the individual.

4. In research on man, the interest of science and society should never take precedence over considerations related to the well-being of the subject.'

These principles were applied in the present study as follows:

1. The consultant surgeon responsible for the patient was the first person to screen the suitability of potential subjects, following a medical history and examination. He was fully aware of the nature of the research as he was also a member of the ethics committee that gave permission for the research, and the physical fitness tests were undertaken in a laboratory of his surgical unit.

2. There is always a possibility of undue pressure or coercion on potential subjects, particularly when they are in the role of patient confronted by medical or paramedical staff. The voluntary

nature of the research was fully explained to each potential subject both orally and in writing by the investigator before commencement of the study and prior to each physiological testing session.

3. Both the investigator unilaterally and the patient unilaterally recognised the option to discontinue the research at any stage. Monitoring of heart rate, blood pressure, general appearance and comments of subjects were used as criteria to judge the likelihood of harm during the exercise and tilt-table tests. The patient and researcher discussed the potential problems that might arise before each repeated session of testing, and did not proceed when any risk to the patient was apparent. Concern for the safety and autonomy of the subjects is not the only motive for taking ethical factors into consideration. The particular research, as well as future research, would founder if any harm ensued.

4. Discussion of the willingness and well-being of the patient before each test session was used to determine whether the patient should or would continue with the research. Consequent loss of data was recognised as a necessary sequel.

Informed voluntary consent was obtained following an explanation of the following:

That the research was unrelated to the herniorrhaphy surgery and that this surgical procedure would be carried out whether or not the person agreed to participate in the research; that they were being asked to participate because they represented healthy people who underwent elective surgery and not because of any other particular personal characteristics; that the aim of the study was to further understanding of how people recovered from operations and how physically fit they were, and that although the study would not be of direct benefit to them, the findings might be useful to help future patients to recover more quickly. Each aspect of the research – the questionnaires, diaries of activities, medilog recorders and physical fitness tests – were described and the potential subjects were shown the apparatus and protocol of fitness tests. If the subject agreed to participate he was then asked to sign a written consent form and was given a written summary of the research to keep and read again at leisure.

Risks of harm and benefits

There was no benefit to the research to be gained by deception as to the nature or reason for the study, so this dilemma was not posed by the research.

There were no a priori benefits to the patient who participated. The exercise testing sessions, which could potentially improve the fitness status of the patient, were undertaken at such long-time intervals that this benefit was not likely to accrue. If the subjects enjoyed the extra interest taken in them by the researcher, this would be a fortuitous benefit. The potential physical risks to the subjects arose from the physical fitness tests. On rare but documented occasions, subjects have collapsed during maximal physical exercise tests. The statistical risk of collapse or heart attack during submaximal work was not known exactly, but from the total lack of reporting of such mishaps in all the texts and articles read during the literature review and the knowledge that similar tests carried out on patients following more serious surgical procedures (Carswell, 1975) had not resulted in any documented casualties, it was assumed that the risk was minimal and could be further minimised by continuous ECG monitoring during these tests and by assuring the patients that they, as well as the researcher, could decide when they wanted to stop the test. Disruption of the herniorrhaphy during cycling was not thought likely by the surgeon or researcher. The leg movement involved would increase the approximation of the wound edges when the leg was raised and would not stretch the suture line further than in standing and walking when the leg was in its lowest position. Discomfort or pain could potentially be exacerbated by cycling as well as by the tilt-table saddle and by deep breathing for the lung capacity tests. However, this would be a subjective judgment of the patient, which he could use as a criterion to avoid or discontinue the tests.

Regarding the use of medilog recorders for 24-hour recording of heart rates, the subjects had the option of refusing to wear the apparatus. They were in control and were taught how to disconnect temporarily or remove the apparatus completely. If they did not wish certain periods of heart rate to be recorded or found that the wearing of the recorder and leads impeded their activities, they were at liberty to remove them. However, there is little risk involved in the use of these recorders apart from the possibility of developing a skin rash under the electrodes, or knocking into something by misjudging the minimally extended body image. Many people are monitored at home and work with this apparatus for diagnostic reasons.

It is not usual to obtain written consent for interview or questionnaire data. Refusal to answer or failure to return questionnaires are taken as unwillingness to participate. The biographical, occupational and activity data sought in this study were either straightforward, unambiguous, factual information or the subjective judgment of the patient. No psychological tests were used. The possibility of doing any psychological or material harm to the participants was thought to be negligible provided that the requirements of confidentiality were adhered to.

Data collection

A summary of the data collection is shown in Table 14.2. Twenty persons were approached at the initial out-patient visit. Two of these evinced signs of high anxiety and declined to take part. This was heartening as it suggested that the patients did understand the voluntary

Table 14.2 Summary of data collected

Questionnaire	Personal history		Preop. advice	Postop. advice
	14		14	13
24-hour ECG	Preop. at work		Postop. in hospital	Postop. convalescence
	9		14	4 (2 failed)
Fitness Tests	Preop. OPD	Preop. OA	Postop. IH	Postop. FU
Exercise test	12	12	3	8
Tilt-table	8	11	1	4
Vitalograph	13	12	7	9
Grip strength	8	11	5	8
Self-rating	12	12	12	12

Abbreviations:
Preop. OPD = Preoperative out-patient visit
Preop. OA = Preoperatively on admission, the day before operation
Postop. IH = Postoperatively in hospital, the day before discharge (usually second or third postop. day)
Postop. FU = Postoperative follow-up: out-patient visit 1 month after discharge

nature of the research. Four were omitted as the experimenter was unaware of their admission. Thus 14 subjects took part in the study. No subject withdrew from the study once he had consented. One subject who was willing in principle, and did participate on admission to hospital, declined to do so at the initial out-patient visit because he did not have time to stay. He was in fact afraid he would lose his job if his employer discovered his absence and diagnosis. This was a potential advantage to the research as high heart rates due to anxiety could result in spuriously low fitness estimates from the submaximal exercise test (Thompson, 1977).

Other data lost at the preoperative out-patient visit were due to problems with the apparatus. Overall the major data loss in the immediate postoperative period was due to patients' fear of pain or other symptoms. No patient was pressed to perform a test if he or she was reluctant to do so.

The major reason for failure to obtain postoperative follow-up data was that eight of the 14 patients both lived and worked outside the health authority region, and five of these were followed up by their local doctors.

Data analysis

There were two methods of presenting and dealing with the result:

1. Collated data from all subjects were examined using a repeated measures analysis of variance, correlated t-test and correlational statistics to confirm or refute hypotheses and reveal trends.
2. Vignettes of each individual were examined to compare the extent to which the progress of individuals fitted with group findings.

One accusation commonly made against studies such as this is that the sample size is too small to ensure that a type 1 error [rejecting the null hypothesis (H_o) when it is true] is not made. The level of statistical significance (α) decided a priori affects this situation in that the smaller the figure of probability taken as acceptable, the less likelihood there is of making a type 1 error. However, in addition to the above and other statistical arguments there are other considerations that are important to the interpretation of physiological data. In any estimation or measurement of physiological parameters there is variability that is not necessarily attributable to genuine change in that parameter. This can arise because of a standard error in the calculation of the data or because of day-to-day fluctuation in the variable under scrutiny. Random variation is large in data from untrained subjects at a low level of performance according to Karvonen (1974). If the magnitude of conditioning or deconditioning is not greater than the standard error and the day-to-day fluctuation, it is arguably not valid to make too strong a claim about the data, whether a statistically significant difference is found or not. The judgment of clinical significance depends partly on the above arguments about variability but also upon the practical consequences to the subject of increasing or decreasing their fitness status. Here we are obliged to consider not only the magnitude of change in absolute or percentage terms but also the relationship of the difference to the initial state of this variable. One way of tackling this is by looking at each individual separately to examine their actual status on each test occasion, plus their subjective view of their fitness and the effect this had on their life-style and activities. The following account of the consequences of a hernia and surgical repair on the life of one patient illustrates these points.

THE USE OF A VIGNETTE TO EXAMINE NORMATIVE FINDINGS

Subject X

This subject was 46 years old, 1.8 m tall and weighed 76 kg. His wife was his sole financial dependent. From the age of 12–32 years he had suffered from pulmonary tuberculosis, spending a month in hospital and 8 months in a sanatorium when first diagnosed, and being readmitted to the sanatorium when 21 and 28 years of age. He had been clear of TB for 14 years when seen for his hernia. He currently attended an osteopath for 3-monthly checks on cervical spondylosis, and was admitted to hospital for 1 week for removal of a lipoma on his arm when aged 44 years.

This gentleman was an accountant who lived in the countryside and travelled 2½ hours per day by car and train to work. His work was mainly sedentary with some walking involved and occupied him about 36–37 hours per week. He was first seen in June and stated that he undertook strenuous gardening daily amounting to more than 24 hours per week, including tree felling. Otherwise his main leisure activity was reading. He smoked half an ounce of pipe tobacco per day.

This subject did not recall any preoperative advice but advised himself, so to speak, to 'lift the proper way'. His work and leisure activities continued and he had no sick leave in the 7½ months (32 weeks) awaiting surgical admission.

Strenuous and regular gardening would lead to an expectation of high muscle strength, though not necessarily to high oxygen capacity. His mean 24-hour heart rate on a working day was 76 b.p.m., being 79 during the day and 86 during the evening. The latter included 2½ hours of gardening. These are not suggestive of aerobic training levels. TB might or might not have left a legacy of low lung capacity. Little change in fitness would be anticipated except that the latter months of waiting for admission were mid-winter, when presumably gardening would have been less frequent and possibly less strenuous. On testing, this man's aerobic power was reasonably high at 38 ml/kg body weight in June, but had fallen to 33 ml/kg by late January when admitted to hospital. His grip strength was, as anticipated, high when first tested and had fallen 10 kg in the right hand and 14 kg in the left by admission. He correctly judged his muscle strength as well above average for age and sex, but regarded his endurance capacity to be below average. These judgments remained identical on admission in contradistinction to the fall in objective measurements. His lung capacities (FEV_1 and FVC) improved between the two preoperative occasions. When first seen, his FEV/FVC percentage was 65 per cent, suggestive of some obstruction, but it was 79 per cent on admission. He had not given up his pipe and had no history of summer asthma, so there was no obvious clinical explanation of this change. Response to tilting was marginal. His systolic blood pressure was low, though normal, on both occasions (118 mmHg resting). It failed to rise when tested initially and fell 8 mmHg on the day of admission. He did not faint so the heart rate rises presumably compensated adequately.

On admission this patient had his left inguinal hernia repaired under general anaesthesia, made a good recovery and was discharged 44 hours postoperatively. He did not feel well enough to repeat the cycle or tilt-table test so soon, fearing that he might faint. In view of his poor postural responses before surgery this was possible, though he was mobile around the ward. His grip strength had fallen a further 7 kg and both his FEV_1 and FVC were 1 l less than prior to surgery, though the percentage was only slightly lower. Both residual anaesthesia effects and fear of pain could account for the lowered lung capacities. This patient estimated a seven-point fall in muscular strength (on a 13-point scale) over the 3 days in hospital. This was the largest subjective fall estimated by this group of patients.

He also felt that his endurance capacity was lowered. His postoperative heart rates were not higher in hospital than on a work day, except for a small rise from 71 to 74 b.p.m. in night-time rates. Nonetheless, his activity levels were lower in hospital, sedentary (bed and chair) time rising from 66 per cent on a work day to 84 per cent in hospital. On discharge this patient sought advice. Friends had told him to be cautious when coughing and wary of lifting after operation: 'if he had to lift, to keep his feet and legs together'. He asked for corroboration of this from the doctors, but did not record any advice on other topics such as driving or general activity level. His convalescence was short as he returned to work 3 weeks post surgery, having sought specific permission to return from the surgeon prior to his official follow-up visit. He received help from his wife in caring for himself throughout his convalescence. He climbed stairs on the day of discharge, but did not walk out of doors for 1½ weeks. He resumed driving after 2½ weeks, much sooner than other patients, but at 1 month had resumed neither gardening nor lifting heavy objects. It was interesting to note that his idea of a heavy object changed according to his condition. Prior to developing a hernia he thought that ½ cwt (56 lb) was heavy; when he knew that he had a hernia he revised this down to 14 lb and took care to use two hands and a straight back for lifting, but after the operation he defined a heavy weight as less than 14 lb.

At his 1-month postoperative check-up he repeated all tests other than the tilt-table. He declined to attempt the latter because of left abdominal pain, but was willing to cycle. His aerobic power had declined, falling by 50 per cent of the preoperative level to 17 ml/kg, and his heart rate at a standard workload of 75 W was 45 b.p.m. higher than on admission to hospital. His muscular strength was as low as it had been on the second postoperative day and he rightly estimated his strength and endurance capacity to be below preoperative levels, though slightly higher than immediately after surgery. The only physical measure to have recovered fully was his lung capacities.

Although he had returned to work a week before this session of testing, his work was sedentary and he only worked part-time, going home when he felt tired. This usually meant working 1½ hours less per day. He certainly felt more tired after work than he had done prior to surgery. This accords with his reduced fitness status.

This articulate man, who had had numerous previous hospital experiences, made copious remarks about the advice received, or rather not received. He would have liked written advice on what to do and when to do it. He felt he was 'not at his articulate best just after operation' and failed to gain information about the care of his wound, when to bath and how to protect the operation area from his dog, who was accustomed to climbing over him. He did not know whether to go to his own doctor or await surgical out-patient follow-up for advice, and had a long discussion with his wife on return home as to what had or had not been advised.

He had a strong incentive to return to work as he was changing to a new job 5 weeks after surgery and wished to leave his current work in good order before leaving. He also had sedentary work and hours that he could arrange to suit himself, both important factors for these herniorrhaphy patients. However, he apparently was not advised to, nor did he, spontaneously do anything that would have hastened his recovery of physical fitness, and consequently suffered the penalty of fatigue.

CONCLUSIONS AND RESEARCH SUGGESTIONS

The use of vignettes thus enabled examination of the clinical and personal significance of herniorrhaphy to individuals, so revealing findings that may be masked by group means and statistical significance levels. In particular, this method is useful to examine extreme cases and exemplars who do not conform to the main findings. In this study two subjects did not lose subjective or objective fitness status for more than a few days. This provided some evidence that the group mean response of prolonged loss of fitness ($p < 0.05$ at 1 month) was not obligatory, and examination of the behaviour of the exceptions suggested possible ways of maintaining fitness by pre- and postoperative activity.

Overall, the physical fitness of these herniorrhaphy patients did not change while awaiting surgery, nor on the whole did their work and leisure activities. Light duties at work and, in one instance, sick leave had been instituted by general practitioners and employers before the first out-patient visit, so it is possible that some patients were already deconditioned. It does not follow that other groups of patients maintain fitness over the prolonged time awaiting elective surgery. Conditioning or deconditioning will depend in part upon the effect of pathology on the ability to remain active. In this study, pre- and postoperative fitness were positively correlated ($r = 0.72$, $p < 0.05$); the most fit persons regained their fitness most quickly, and the least fit most slowly, following surgery. It would seem from observation and self-reports that the most fit preoperatively were also the most active postoperatively in a situation where neutral or negative activity advice during convalescence was received. It could be argued that advice to achieve a high level of fitness prior to surgery is desirable, not only as Carswell et al (1978) suggest, because this is the best preparation for withstanding physical insult, but also because the person who feels fit and is accustomed to exercise is more willing and/or able in unsupervised convalescence to resume habitual activities. Longitudinal studies of those who have more incapacitating conditions seem desirable. If, as is likely, such persons incur a loss of fitness while awaiting surgery, this might provide evidence for the need for systematic preoperative advice, and in some instances for more urgent admission.

In the days immediately following surgery, the majority felt that their strength and endurance capacity had fallen dramatically. This attitude was reflected in the patients' level of activities, and was one reason why they were loath to repeat the exercise test prior to discharge. However, this research does not provide evidence of cardiorespiratory or muscle deconditioning resulting from the few days of restricted activity in hospital. Along with other similar studies such as Bassey et al (1973), many factors, including dehydration, drugs, anxiety, pain and sleep disturbance, are thought likely to contribute to the acute feeling of deconditioning. Many of the subjects would have had high scores on Yoshitaki's fatigue check-list (1971). Moreover, the subjective maintenance and minimal loss of objective conditioning of two subjects suggests that prolonged loss of fitness is not an obligatory response to herniorrhaphy. Nonetheless, the main findings suggest that inguinal herniorrhaphy – relatively minor, trivial, elective surgery to the most commonly weakened part of the anatomy of males (and occasionally females) – has drastic and long-term effects on work capacity. Indeed, the mean percentage fall in predicted maximum oxygen uptake at 1 month of 29 per cent was similar to the fall in this measure following 20 days of bedrest (Saltin et al, 1968).

This study confirms the findings of Morris et al (1968) that return to work, and hence length of convalescence, is logically related to the physical content of the job, not to the recovery of fitness of the patient. Fears are not of overtaxing the cardiorespiratory or locomotor systems but of excessive strain on the wound, causing a recurrent hernia. However, the potential outcome of this delay in resumption of work plus generally cautious or negative activity advice is that the ex-patient eventually returns to work in a deconditioned state and suffers the penalty of fatigue. Advice may necessarily have to remain vague regarding weight-lifting and aerobic exercise, but there is no doubt that it could be vaguely positive (Bourke et al, 1981) rather than vaguely negative and could be tailored to the individual's life-style.

The use of case and situation studies to enhance understanding of the process of patient recovery or to supplement normative findings would seem to be a potentially fruitful research ploy (Mitchell, 1983) when attempting to evaluate the outcome of multiple influences on health and fitness status. Current early discharge policies may be increasing the contribution of the patient and his social and physical environmental to recovery. As Given et al (1979) state: 'A comprehensive and systematic evaluation of patient care includes both patient and health care professional contributions to the process and overall outcome and care'.

REFERENCES

Bassey E J, Bennett T, Birmingham A T, Fentem P F, Fitton D, and Goldsmith R (1973) Effects of surgical operation and bed-rest on cardiovascular responses to exercise in hospital patients. *Cardiovascular Research*, **7**(5): 588–592.

Beauchamps T L and Childress J F (1983) *Principles of Biomedical Ethics*, 2nd edn. Oxford: Oxford University Press.

Bourke J B, Lear P A and Taylor M (1981) Effects of early return to work after elective repair of inguinal hernia: clinical and financial consequences at one year and three years. *Lancet*, **ii**: 623–625.

Carswell S (1975) Changes in aerobic power in patients undergoing elective surgery. *Journal of Physiology*, **251**: 42–43.

Carswell S H, Holman B D, Thompson J and Walker W F (1978) Acceptable level of aerobic power for patients undergoing elective surgery. *Journal of Physiology*, **285**: 16P.

Declaration of Helsinki (1964, 1975) *The World Medical Association Declaration of Helsinki*. 18th World Medical Assembly, Helsinki 1964. Tokyo 1979: 29th World Medical Association.

Fordham M (1982) The recovery of physical fitness. *International Journal of Nursing Studies*, **19**(4): 205–212.

Fordham M (1985) *Deconditioning and Reconditioning following Elective Surgery. An Investigation of Physical Fitness and Activity Patterns in Herniorrhaphy Patients*. PhD thesis, King's College University, London.

Fordham M, Appenteng K, Goldsmith R and O'Brien C (1978) The cost of work in medical nursing. *Ergonomics*, **21**(5): 331–342.

Given B, Given C W and Simoni L E (1979) Relationships of process of care to patient outcomes. *Nursing Research*, **28**(2): 85–93.

Karvonen M J (1974) Work and activity classifications. In: *Fitness, Health and Work Capacity*, ed. Larson L A, pp 38–54. New York: Macmillan.

Mitchell J C (1983) Case and situation analysis. *The Sociological Review*, **31**: 187–211.

Morris D, Ward A W M and Handyside A J (1968) Early discharge after hernia repair. *Lancet*, **i**: 681–685.

Saltin B, Blomquist G, Mitchell J H, Johnson R L, Wildenthal K and Chapman C C (1968) Response to exercise after bed-rest and after training. *Circulation* XXXVIII, supp. VII, 1–55.

Shephard R J (1969) *Endurance Fitness*. Toronto: University of Toronto Press.

Shephard R J, Benade S M, Davies C T M, di Prampero P E, Hedman R, Merriman J E, Myhre K and Simmons R (1968) The maximum oxygen uptake: an international reference standard of cardiorespiratory fitness. *Bulletin of the World Health Organisation*, **38**: 757–764.

Smith W S and O'Brien C (1976) A system for rapid analysis of longterm recordings of heartrate and other physiological parameters. *Biomedical Engineering*, **11**(4): 128–131.

Starfield B (1973) Health services research. A working model. *New England Journal of Medicine*, **289**: 132–136.

Thompson J (1977) The repeatability of the measurements of aerobic power in man and factors affecting it. *Quarterly Journal of Experimental Physiology*, **62**: 83–97.

Wilson-Barnett J and Fordham M (1982) *Recovery from Illness*. Developments in Nursing Research, vol. 1. Chichester: Wiley & Sons.

Yoshitaki H (1971) Relations between the symptoms and the feelings of fatigue. *Ergonomics*, **14**(1): 175–186.

Chapter 15

Relatives' Participation in the Care of the Stroke Patient in General Medical Wards

Lynn Batehup

BACKGROUND TO THE STUDY, AND PREVIOUS RESEARCH

There is as yet a lack of research that is concerned with the relative's perspective of the caring situation. This is especially so for the relatives of stroke patients. The majority of patients admitted to acute hospital wards with a stroke, who have been living with a relative and who survive, will return home to live with and be cared for by that relative. Brocklehurst et al (1981) found that by 1 year 49 out of 69 stroke survivors were living with their relative again. The majority (75/92) of the relatives were women, mainly wives and daughters.

Impact of the stroke on the relative/carer

The residual effects of the stroke on patients are well known and can include loss of independence in carrying out usual daily activities (walking, dressing, eating, attending to personal hygiene); social life, hobbies and work are usually curtailed to some degree (Holbrook, 1982), and the patient's personal relationships with family and friends may also suffer (Coughlan and Humphrey, 1982). The impact of the stroke on relatives is less well recognised, but the short- and long-term effects on family life, work and general life-style can be very disrupting. A study by Holbrook (1982) shows that stroke disrupts almost all aspects of the life of the nearest family members, with over 70 per cent of the spouses and main carers reporting problems related to their social mobility and social life. Additional problems reported by relatives included depression (Wade et al, 1986), frustration, stress and tension. As time passes, problems experienced by relatives are seen to persist. A study by Coughlan and Humphrey (1982) of relatives' experiences 8 years after the stroke found that depression and tension affected one-third of them. Unhappiness over the loss of their companion in social activities and feelings of being tied to the home were all frequently voiced by spouses.

The relative's influence on the stroke patient's recovery and level of functional activity

Most patients discharged from acute medical wards after a stroke go home to live with a relative (Brocklehurst et al, 1981), and most of these patients and relatives are in a two-person household, usually patient and spouse (Schmidt et al, 1986; Wade et al, 1986). Since the work of Richardson (1945), cited by Litman (1966), the notion that the family may play an integral part in determining a patient's response to treatment has been given some recognition. One of the earliest studies to explore this relationship in stroke patients and their families was undertaken by Litman (1966). This and other early studies (Overs and Belknap, 1967; New et al, 1968) assumed that the family could have a beneficial influence in helping the patient in attaining and maintaining high levels of functional activity during hospitalisation and following discharge. Their results are inconclusive and relatives are seen to have some beneficial effects, but negative effects such as overprotection are also evident.

More recent studies have tried to clarify the situation. Garraway et al (1980), in a randomised controlled trial, compared the rehabilitation of stroke patients in a stroke unit with medical wards. The outcome measured was level of independence in activities of daily living before discharge, and 1 year later at home. Stroke unit patients' relatives were encouraged to be involved in care in an effort to help the patient to maintain or gain even higher levels of function once at home. Findings showed that although more stroke unit patients than medical ward patients were independent at discharge, 1 year later more medical ward patients were independent. It appeared that the relatives of stroke unit patients were being overprotective and were not allowing their relative to carry out activities of which they were capable. Other studies comparing levels of independent activity of stroke patients who live with a relative and those who live alone do not come to firm conclusions that would explain why stroke patients who live alone appear to function at a higher level than those who live with a relative (Townsend, 1965; Brocklehurst et al, 1978; Schmidt et al, 1986). Possible explanations include:

1. Overprotection by relatives not allowing the stroke patient to carry out activities of which he/she is able, and not encouraging movement to higher levels of independence because of fear of further stroke or ignorance.
2. Over-reliance by stroke patients on their relatives because of fear of further stroke or poor motivation.
3. Patients discharged home to care by relatives are more disabled than those discharged to live alone.
4. Stroke patients who live alone are forced to become more independent because there is nobody there all the time to help them.

More recently, studies have been carried out that have looked at involvement and education of stroke patients' relatives during the rehabilitation process, with the assumption that this active relative participation, education, and support will help the patients to achieve their highest level of independent function (Wells, 1974; Field et al, 1983; Dignan et al, 1986). There is little support from these studies for the contention that relative participation and education has a measurable effect on the patient's level of functional activity, or that relatives perceive the support and education given in the hospital as a benefit in the long term. The reasons for these findings are numerous and may include lack of systematic relative participation and education during the study, restricted and limited outcome measures and inappropriate follow-up periods.

To date, assumptions that the education of relatives and their participation in care can benefit both the patient and relative have been made by the various researchers whose work has been discussed here. The greatest proportion of this work, with a few exceptions (Garraway et al, 1980; Field et al, 1983), has been carried out in North America, where relatives' and nurses' attitudes to participation in hospital may not reflect those of relatives and nurses in the United Kingdom. Brooking's (1986) study of relative and patient participation in care has highlighted the fact that, although some patients and relatives want more opportunity to take part in care, others clearly indicated negative attitudes to participation, which may make it stressful and difficult for them. It may, therefore, not be appropriate to transfer these ideas directly, but rather to explore the situation as it exists in British hospitals. Consequently, it was the intention of this study to discover the relative's attitudes to participating in the patient's hospital care, and to identify what type of participation is taking place at the present time in general medical wards. By doing so it was hoped that this would provide some basic data that may be useful for future programmes aimed at stroke patient care.

METHODS AND DESIGN OF STUDY

The research design chosen to answer the study questions was a descriptive correlational study (Polit and Hungler, 1982). This allows the study of several variables and their interrelationships in a natural setting. The research was carried out in one London health district, and included five general medical wards in two general hospitals, the out-patient physiotherapy department and the homes of patients and relatives. Data were collected via self-completion questionnaires and semi-structured interviews.

Description of study instruments

1. Patient characteristics

This form was used to record demographic information and information related to the stroke, and its effects on the patient, and levels of therapy received by the patient.

2. Relative/carer characteristics

This form was used to record demographic information and other information regarded as important in relation to the relative's attitudes to participation in care.

3. Participation in care as reported by the relative/carer

This instrument was designed for this study and used to record the relative's reported participation in eight activities of daily living that are important for a stroke patient's independence. Content validity of these three instruments was assured by including only factors that had a sound basis in the relevant literature.

*4. Occurrence of problems following the discharge of the stroke
patient, as reported by the relative/carer*

This is a 29-item check-list devised from a published and tested check-list (Gilleard, 1984), and was used to record predetermined problems as reported by the relative 4 weeks after discharge.

5. Barthel index of activities of daily living (Mahoney and Barthel, 1965)

This is a 10-item scale for recording a patient's level of independence in activities of daily living (ADL) and mobility. This was recorded soon after admission, before discharge, and 4 weeks after discharge.

6. Relative's attitudes towards participation in care scale

This is a 20-item Likert-type attitude scale devised for the study and including eight statements that were taken from an attitude scale devised by Brooking (1986). This scale was intended to measure at an ordinal level the relative's attitudes to carer participation in stroke care.

The three parts of the study

The study was divided into three parts. The first was carried out to develop and test the 'attitude to participation scale'. The sample included 18 relatives of stroke patients who had been caring for their relative since the stroke occurred. Reliability testing focused on the internal consistency of the scale. Spearman rank order correlation coefficients were used to calculate inter-item correlations and corrected item index correlations. Each item also underwent analysis by visual inspection and reporting of subject's comments.

The second part of the study describes the total population of stroke patients admitted to the study wards during the data collection period. During the pilot study it became obvious that the number of subjects (patients and relatives) who would be suitable for inclusion in the third part, or main study, would be very small. The criteria for inclusion called for stroke patients with relatives who would eventually be discharged home. When such factors as early deaths, early spontaneous recovery and severe disability resulting in long-term institutional care are accounted for, the numbers of patients discharged home are small. For these reasons the researcher decided to record all patients admitted to the study wards with a confirmed diagnosis of stroke in an effort to describe the population demographically and to identify each patient's outcome.

The third part and 'main study' was carried out to answer the main study questions. Patients and relatives were seen in hospital and interviewed. The instruments as described previously were applied. Four weeks after discharge, patient and relative were seen again and interviewed at home.

MAIN FINDINGS

**Development and testing of the 'relative's attitude to
participation in care' scale**

According to Oppenheim (1966), analysis of a Likert-type attitude scale requires at least 100–300 subjects. As this study had only a sample of 18 subjects, a conventional item analysis may not be appropriate. However, it was decided to undertake item analysis using non-parametric tests. The scale was subjected to visual inspection of the data for questions that failed to discriminate well among subjects, and to inter-item correlation and corrected item index correlations. Each of 20 items could be scored 1–5, with higher scores representing a more positive attitude. The actual range of mean scores for each item was 2.3–4.5 (n = 18). Cumulative scores were calculated for each subject, giving a possible range of 0–100 (no answer scored 0). The mean score was 69.4 and the standard deviation was 9.17 (n = 18). The actual range of scores was 56–89, covering 33 per cent of the possible distribution. Following visual inspection of each item and the subject's comments, 9 items were retained, 10 items required revision and re-testing, and one item was discarded.

Description of total population of stroke patients admitted to the study wards

A total of 53 stroke patients was admitted to the five medical wards (three female, one male and one mixed ward) during the 6 months of data collection. Out of this number, seven were found to be eligible for the 'main study'. The average age of all patients was 74.4 years (n = 53). Fifty-two per cent had a relative to care for them. The majority of relatives were spouses, of whom 63 per cent were wives. Twenty patients (38 per cent) were discharged home. Patients with relatives went home earlier than those patients who lived alone. Fifteen patients (28 per cent) died in hospital, eight of these in the first 2 weeks. Eighteen patients were either transferred to other institutions, or were still in hospital at the end of the study. Twelve patients were eventually regarded as only being capable of long-term institutional care. Those patients transferred spent, on average, 15.2 weeks in hospital. Three patients were still waiting to move 9 months after admission.

Main study: relatives' participation in the care of the hospitalised stroke patient

Only seven pairs of subjects fulfilled the necessary criteria. Six patients were women, of whom three were married. The other three women were widows; one lived with her son and the other two women lived next door to their carers. The male patient was married. The average age of the patients was 69.4 years, with four patients over 69 years of age. The average age of the relatives was 61 years; the youngest, who was a daughter, was 31, and the oldest a husband of 81. Relatives' reported frequency of participation in care was low. All relatives reported helping with eating and drinking, but only one relative was active in helping the patient with activities such as getting dressed, personal hygiene, getting in and out of bed, doing exercises and walking. Most relatives were not involved in helping with these activities, and most demonstrated a positive attitude to participation. The possible range of scores was 0–100, and the actual range was 39–71, with a mean of 60.9 and a standard deviation of 10.4 (n = 7). After discharge, relatives were asked about problems they had experienced with caring. Almost all relatives had experienced disagreements with the patient about various matters. Almost all relatives reported feeling worried or anxious at some time since the patient's discharge. Another problem was that relatives reported that they were unable to leave the patient alone for any length of time, and so were tied to the home. This caused a sense of isolation, and reflected an overwhelming commitment by the relatives.

IMPLICATIONS FOR NURSING

This study was on a very small scale, and it is with this in mind that the following discussion takes place.

Little participation in care was reported by relatives of stroke patients. On the whole a passive role was adopted. Reasons for this are speculative and may include a feeling that this is not their role. A recent study by Brooking (1986), which examined patient and relative participation in nursing care, found that none of the wards studied had formal or informal policies about patient and family participation; and although many nurses claimed to organise care to help patients and family to take part, there was little actual evidence of this. As in this study, Brooking (1986) found that relatives reported little participation in care and expressed a desire for increased participation. Not all relatives may want to participate in direct care, but the opportunity should be given to them. The effects on the relative of a loved one having a stroke can be devastating and can make them passive and distant. It is, therefore, important that their feelings and wishes about participating be reviewed regularly. Not all relatives want or are able to take an active role, so they should be given the choice as to the extent to which they wish to be involved.

Patients may be discharged to the sole care of just one elderly relative. Teaching relatives how best to help with activities such as dressing, washing or getting in and out of bed, or up from low chairs, should be seen as an important part of the nurse's role. Teaching plans for relatives should become a routine part of early discharge planning for stroke patients. A series of home visits, supervised by nurses for a day and progressing to overnight stays, should lead up to discharge. A female patient in this study found that although she could get out of the hospital bed unaided, when she got home she could not get out of her own bed until her friend from next door came in to help her. The reason for this was that her own bed was soft and sagged in the middle. Between them they put a board under the mattress, and she could then get up unaided – another small step to independence. This situation could have been avoided had preparatory supervised overnight stays been part of the planned discharge. Assessment of the relatives' skills in managing the stroke patient should be carried out at regular intervals.

Support and counselling for relatives and patients should begin when the patient is still in hospital. It may be appropriate, considering the numbers of stroke patients in general medical wards, to employ a nurse specialist in this field to take on this role. Continuing support and contact after discharge may go far to reduce the feeling of isolation felt by relatives and patients. An educative role for the stroke nurse specialist in teaching and informing nursing staff would be envisaged.

The use of the Barthel index of ADL in this and other stroke rehabilitation studies has confirmed its ability as a useful tool to monitor return to independence in self-care and mobility of stroke patients. Routine use of this scale by nurses could provide a more objective assessment of return of function over time than is generally carried out now in medical wards. The tool is simple and quick to use, and has some demonstrated reliability and validity. Relatives could be taught to use the tool, thereby involving and motivating the patient and relative.

REFERENCES

Brocklehurst J C, Morris P E, Richards B and Laycock P (1978) *Medical Social and Psychological Aspects of Stroke. Final Report.* University of Manchester, Department of Geriatric Medicine.

Brocklehurst J C, Morris P, Andrews K, Richards B and Laycock P (1981) Social effects of stroke. *Social Science and Medicine*, **15**: 35-39.

Brooking J (1986) *Patient and Family Participation in Nursing Care: The Development of a Nursing Process Measuring Scale*. Thesis submitted for the degree of PhD, Department of Nursing Studies, University of London (KQC).

Coughlan A K and Humphrey M (1982) Presenile stroke: longterm outcome for patients and their families. *Rheumatology and Rehabilitation*, **21**: 115-122.

Dignan M B, Howard G, Toole J F, Becker C and McLeroy K R (1986) Evaluation of the North Carolina Stroke Care Programme. *Stroke*, **17**(3): 382-386.

Field D, Cordle C J and Bowman G S (1983) Coping with stroke at home. *International Rehabilitation Medicine*, **5**: 96-100.

Garraway W M, Akhtar A J, Hockey L and Prescott R J (1980) Management of acute stroke in the elderly: follow up of a controlled trial. *British Medical Journal*, **281**: 828-829.

Gilleard C J (1984) Problems posed for supporting relatives of geriatric and psychogeriatric day patients. *Acta Psychiatrica Scandinavica*, **70**: 198-208.

Holbrook M (1982) Stroke: social and emotional outcome. *Journal of the Royal College of Physicians*, **16**: 100-104.

Litman T J (1966) The family and physical rehabilitation. *Journal of Chronic Diseases*, **19**: 211-217.

Mahoney F I and Barthel D W (1965) Functional evaluation: the Barthel Index. *Maryland State Medical Journal*, **14**: 61-65.

New P, Ruscio A T, Petritsi R P and George L A (1968) The support structure of heart and stroke patients. *Social Science and Medicine*, **2**: 185-200.

Oppenheim A N (1966) *Questionnaire Design and Attitude Measurement*. London: Heinemann.

Overs R P and Belknap E L (1967) Educating stroke patients' families. *Journal of Chronic Diseases*, **20**: 45-51.

Polit D F and Hungler B P (1982) *Nursing Research. Principles and Methods*, 2nd edn. Philadelphia: J B Lippincott.

Richardson B H (1945) *Patients have Families*. New York: The Commonwealth Fund.

Schmidt S M, Herman L M, Koenig P, Leuze M, Monahan M K and Stubbens R W (1986) Status of stroke patients: a community assessment. *Archives of Physical Medicine and Rehabilitation*, **67**: 99-102.

Townsend P (1965) The effects of family structure on the likelihood of admission to an institution in old age. In: *Social Structure and the Family: Generational Relations*, eds. Shanas E and Streib G F. New Jersey: Prentice Hall.

Wade D T, Legh-Smith J and Langton Hewer R (1986) Effects of living with and looking after survivors of a stroke. *British Medical Journal*, **293**(6544): 418-420.

Wells R (1974) Family stroke education. *Stroke*, **5**(3): 393-396.

Section 3

Preparation for Practice: Aspects of Basic and Post-basic Education

Chapter 16

The Quality of Care and Students' Educational Experience in Hospital Wards

Pamela Smith and Sally J Redfern

BACKGROUND TO THE STUDY

This study arose from a longstanding interest in the dual and potentially conflicting role of student nurses as learners and as principal care-givers. Previous research had shown that, in British hospitals with nursing schools, as much as 75 per cent of direct patient care may be provided by nurses in training (Moores and Moult, 1979). This statistic confirms what is well known: that students constitute the main workforce in British hospitals. Their status as learners is based on the twin assumptions that trained nurses teach in the ward and students learn as they work (Fretwell, 1982). Since students work in the wards and learn as they nurse, it could be inferred that there is an association between the learning environment and quality of nursing on a ward. Revans (1964), for example, suggested that hospitals with high morale had effective communication systems, 'good ward atmospheres', a stable nursing workforce and rapid patient recovery. Orton (1981) specified the characteristics of 'good ward atmospheres' or 'learning climates' and proposed that students and patients benefited from ward sisters who were interested in teamwork and consultation, and who were aware of subordinates' needs. Orton (p. 61) concluded that on wards with 'good' learning climates, '. . . not only did students see their own physical and emotional needs amply met, but also those of the patients'.

Other researchers confirmed the importance of positive working relationships between permanent ward staff and students in creating a good learning environment (Fretwell, 1982; Lewin and Leach, 1982; Ogier, 1982). Ward specialty has also been identified as an important variable.

The use of medical specialties to organise nurse training was shown by Roper (1975) to be an unreliable way of predicting learning experiences available to students. Not only were patients' diagnostic labels often different from the designated specialty of the ward, but patients, irrespective of diagnosis, provided nurses with unexpected opportunities for teaching and learning (see chapter 17 for further exploration of this topic).

Attempts to define quality of nursing have proved more controversial. On the one hand, quantitative researchers believe that quality of nursing can be operationalised into objective

147

measures of patient care (Jelinek et al, 1974; Wandelt and Ager, 1974; Goldstone et al, 1983); on the other, qualitative researchers such as Evers (1982) suggest that the 'essence' of quality is a relative concept which defies quantification. Hawthorn (1974), in a study of nurses' activities in paediatric wards, also identified the lack of a universally accepted definition of quality of nursing. In the light of the literature on the hospital care of children, Hawthorn selected consideration of the emotional needs of young patients as a necessary component of quality of nursing.

An early British study recognised that nurses' work included 'affective' as well as 'technical' and 'basic' components (Goddard, 1953). Affective nursing was defined as meeting the patient's psychosocial and, by implication, emotional needs. Basic nursing was described as the care of patients' physical needs, and technical nursing referred to nurses' work associated with the medical treatment of disease.

McFarlane (1976) believed that the categorisation of nurses' work in this way led to an undervaluing of their role in caring for patients' affective and basic needs by attributing higher status to technical nursing. McFarlane asserted that nursing was about 'helping, assisting, serving, caring' rather than working as doctors' assistants. In a later paper McFarlane (1977) promoted the nursing process as a way of formalising the caring role of the nurse, particularly in relation to its affective and basic components, by providing a methodology for organising nursing knowledge and practice and improving patient care.

Armstrong (1983) noted a reinterpretation of the nurse's role in general nursing textbooks, following the introduction of the nursing process. Patients were no longer described in strictly biological terms. Psychology and communication skills were emphasised, and 'subjectivity' and emotions entered the nurse–patient relationship.

Macleod Clark (1981), in a study of verbal communication between nurses and patients, found that, despite the rhetoric of the nursing process, patients' emotional needs were inadequately met. Recent studies of nurse training found that students valued technical nursing and saw basic nursing as low status work (Fretwell, 1982; Melia, 1982; Alexander, 1983). Affective or 'social' nursing was described by Melia's students as 'not really nursing'. Thus, the literature illustrates a gap between the professional rhetoric of caring and nurses' own work priorities and preferences.

Not only have nurse leaders and educationalists failed to grapple with the gender divisions of labour within the health service (Friedson, 1970; Oakley, 1984) but also they have failed to acknowledge the emotional complexity of care (Menzies, 1970; Strauss et al, 1982) and its relationship to women's work (Ungerson, 1983a). The importance of the emotional component of caring and its relationship to the power relations within an institution are raised in Hochschild's analysis of emotional labour in the USA airline industry (Hochschild, 1983). She concluded that the quality of a service is judged by the emotional style in which it is given.

On the basis of the findings outlined above, the present study aimed to reassess the concept of quality of nursing and explore the way in which it related to the learning environment in a variety of wards and from a number of nursing and patient perspectives. The study also investigated the extent to which the nursing process and communication skills had become part of the practice and learning of nursing. The subjective experiences of students as learners and principal carers, at different stages of training, were also described.

Hochschild's definition and analysis of emotional labour in the workplace was used as a conceptual means to understanding the emotional complexities of the nursing labour process and the training and supervision of students in school and ward.

RESEARCH STRATEGY AND METHODS

The setting for the study was a London teaching hospital. The fieldwork was conducted from January 1984 to June 1985. January to June 1984 was used as an exploratory period for preliminary observation and interviews in the wards and nursing school, following which it was decided to narrow the study to medical nursing in the first and third year of training. Three months were spent on the first study ward (March–June 1984). In the in-depth study (July 1984–June 1985) 14 contact weeks were spent in the nursing school and 8 weeks on each of three study wards. A first- and third-year group of students (two sets, 20 and 30 students respectively) were observed during classes in the school of nursing. A number of them were also interviewed. In addition, other students and trained nurses were observed and/or interviewed on the four wards. A total of 392 first- and third-year students completed questionnaires following allocation to 12 medical wards.

Research strategies included 'triangulation' or a multimethod approach advocated by Denzin (1970) using both qualitative and quantitative methods, and the application of grounded theory (Glaser and Strauss, 1967), by which the data were gathered, handled and analysed concurrently. In this way, working hypotheses related to the research problem were developed and explored as the study progressed (Smith, 1987). A summary of methods as defined by Denzin (1970) is outlined below.

Observer participation

The core research method was that of participant observation used during fieldwork on four medical wards and in the school of nursing, supplemented with interviews. Collins's (1984) notion of 'participant comprehension' was applied, in which the researcher enters the research setting seeking to maximise rather than minimise her interaction so as to grow both in competence and comprehension of the 'native culture'.

Survey interviewing

Interviews were constructed around topics and questions, which were discussed with everyone according to the group (i.e. student, tutor, sister, patient). Additional topics and questions also evolved during individual interviews, and were integrated into further data collection. Interviews with students and teachers included issues such as the theory and practice of nursing, the use of the nursing process and the identification of key people and incidents in the learning process.

The ward sister interview was based on Pembrey's (1980) semi-structured schedule and check-list of work priorities and problems with additional questions about student nurse learning. Coser's (1962) patient interview guide was used to explore patients' perceptions of quality of nursing.

Fretwell's rating questionnaire of the ward learning environment was completed by students (Fretwell, 1983, 1985). Questions were grouped under headings related to the ward learning environment, such as ward atmosphere, ward teaching and learning, patient care, staffing levels, workload and stress. Responses were on a five-point Likert scale from 'strongly agree' (5) to 'strongly disagree' (1). There were also five open-ended questions, which asked students for general comments on ward learning.

Direction observation

The Patient Dependency Check-list (Barr, 1967) and the Quality Patient Care Scale (QualPacs) (Wandelt and Ager, 1974) were used. QualPacs sets out to measure the multidimensional concept of quality of care by non-participant observation of patients for 2 hours, followed by 2 hours spent collecting data from case notes, nursing records and patient charts or listening to nurse handover reports. Nursing dimensions being observed relate to physical and psychosocial care of patients, staff communication and professional implications covering 68 items. The standard of care expected is that of a first level (newly qualified) staff nurse, described as 'safe, adequate, therapeutic and supportive' to the patient (p. 45). The content and tone of each interaction is considered and rated on a five-point scale of 'Best' (5), 'Between' (4), 'Average' (3), 'Between' (2) and 'Poorest' (1) care given.

Non-participant observation was made of selected classes in the school of nursing.

Document analysis

Existing documents were consulted for student biographical information, patient turnover, death and discharge, and the planning of nurse training, timetabling, prospectus and school progress reports.

MAIN FINDINGS

The findings describe patients' and nurses' perceptions of the quality of nursing in relation to its physical, technical and affective components. Even though students preferred technical nursing and valued it as learning material, they were able to identify the importance of their physical and emotional labour to patients. Findings suggested that patients judged the quality of nursing by the emotional style in which it was given, irrespective of their diagnosis and technical care required. Our experience with the quality patient care scale (QualPacs) and participant observation confirmed that quality of nursing was extremely difficult to measure objectively. Strauss et al's (1982) classification of sentimental work offered a conceptual framework for describing the type of emotional labour that nurses undertook.

The characteristics of a 'good' ward learning environment, according to nurses, were found to be based on the assumption that formal teaching was necessary for learning to take place. Despite the predominance of this formal teaching/learning paradigm, students described the ward rather than the classroom as the place where most of their learning took place, and the ways in which they learnt as informal.

The relationship of quality of nursing and the ward learning environment was explored and explained by three hypotheses or clusters of conceptual categories. These hypotheses suggested that the quality of nursing and student learning in a ward were influenced by the nature of the work and the learning material, the sister's management style and the students' personal and learning trajectory. It was concluded that the relationship between quality of nursing and ward learning is articulated through the sister's emotional style of management.

The nature of the work and the learning material

Findings suggest that students associated 'good' learning environments with wards that had a high patient turnover, and patients with a variety of diagnoses requiring acute, technical nursing and specialist medical intervention. Wards that had a higher percentage of elderly patients with chronic medical conditions and high dependency were viewed less favourably by students as providing good learning environments. Despite identifying technical nursing and specialist medical intervention as valuable to their learning, students associated quality nursing with those wards where the affective components of nursing were both visible and valued by the sister and trained staff.

Since meeting patients' affective needs was recognised as neither work nor learning material (unless legitimised by a medical specialty), students did not believe that they needed to be taught how to do emotional labour. Rather, they believed that they were able to meet patients' affective needs because of their interest in people, which had brought them into nursing.

The promotion of the nursing process as a problem-solving, individualised approach to patient care was not evident in the students' school-based teaching programmes and ward-based learning objectives. The students described the nursing process as a work method rather than in conceptual terms and as a means of carrying out patient-centred tasks. Consequently, they did not accept it as a viable means of gaining knowledge and acquiring skills, preferring instead to use a medical rather than a nursing approach to patient care.

Ward management styles

Sisters and trained staff who were regarded by students as demonstrating favourable management styles were described as: happy; approachable; interested in students as people; accessible both in physical and personal terms; giving positive feedback, which made students feel appreciated; clear about what they expected from students as well as encouraging initiative; and allowing students to be involved in decision-making and discussion about patient care.

Students valued ward sisters who showed that they cared about patients by talking to them and their relatives and staying on duty longer than they should to do this. Management styles that created positive ward atmospheres and staff relations motivated students to care more for patients. Some ward sisters created stress or anxiety for students and staff nurses through their management styles, by being unappreciative and/or critical. An explicit commitment to the nursing process appeared to be associated with sisters who valued interpersonal communication with patients and nurses, interpreted as the recognition of patients' affective needs and doing emotional labour.

The characteristics of the 'good' nurse valued by patients bore similarities to some of the characteristics of sisters and trained staff regarded by students as demonstrating favourable management styles both towards themselves and patients, i.e. being happy, cheerful and showing interest in others.

Students as workers and learners

Students were the primary workforce and saw their ward activities as work that they might also identify as learning material depending on ward specialty and stage of training. Stage of training was also important in determining what a student was expected to do, irrespective of the content of previous ward experiences. Student learning was also influenced by their personal and emotional needs throughout training. The findings show, however, that first-year students were seen to be given more emotional support than were students in their third year.

Student learning was shaped by the hierarchical structure within nursing, which determined not only whom the students worked with, but also whom they learnt from. They preferred to work with other students rather than with trained staff. Students believed that they were best able to learn from others who did not threaten them hierarchically and who also did emotional labour on their behalf.

IMPLICATIONS AND RECOMMENDATIONS

Hochschild (1983) found that, in the US airline industry, certain conditions, such as reduction in staffing levels and quicker turnaround of aircraft flights, militated against the production of emotional labour. Similarly, in the NHS, the cutback of resources on an already limited resource allocation circumscribes the amount of emotional labour that nurses are able to do. Furthermore, nurses are among lower income workers, and their salaries do not reflect payment for the emotional component of their labour. By comparison, flight attendants' higher wages represent the airlines' recognition that the production of emotional labour has financial implications, since passengers are more likely to use an airline where emotional labour is explicit. It is interesting to speculate as to whether the Thatcher government (1979 to the present), with its commitment to privatisation of the public sector, will lead to a commercialisation of nurses' emotional labour in the private health industry. Already the images used for advertising private health insurance bear similarities to those used by the airline industry for attracting custom.

Demographic changes have resulted in a reduction of the number of 18-year-old girls and a nursing recruitment crisis (Committee of Public Accounts, 1987). There is also evidence to suggest that nurses are leaving the NHS because they are becoming increasingly dissatisfied with what they are able to do physically and emotionally for patients under the present conditions. Correspondence in *The Guardian* newspaper in 1985 bears witness to this (Black, 1985; Pearmain, 1985) and is confirmed by a study of nursing drop-out factors (West and Rushton, 1986). An article in *The Independent* newspaper (Timmins, 1987) reported the findings of a study that discovered that trained staff, especially those with specialist skills, are also leaving the NHS, and are abandoning it for the more attractive conditions of the private sector. The study concluded that the drift of staff to the private sector could be prevented if the NHS conditions were made more attractive for nurses.

Feminist research explains why technical nursing holds higher status as work and learning material than as physical and affective nursing. Both physical and affective aspects of nursing, like any care work, are taken for granted as something that women automatically do and derive fulfilment from. Oakley (1974) and Ungerson (1983b) have both described women's work related to mothering and housewifery as a 'set of skills'. Many of the skills associated with women's work, such as the creation of a positive ward atmosphere, approachability, accessibility and ability to communicate, were described by students in the present study as important components of quality of nursing and ward learning environments. Students recognised that they learnt such skills informally from observing other people who were adept at them.

The need to recognise and support the emotional and physical components of caring advocated by McFarlane (1976) becomes even more urgent in the battered NHS of the 1980s. However, there is already a possibility that because of their technical skills, nurses such as those working in theatre and intensive care will be given financial incentives to stay in the NHS.

The physical and emotional labour demanded by elderly and chronically ill patients continues to go unrecognised by politicians and by nurses themselves.

The present study suggests that in order to go beyond the rhetoric of nursing leaders it is necessary to redefine nursing work, learning material and the way in which students learn. Until the importance and complexity of emotional labour to the quality of nursing and ward learning is recognised, supported and adequately rewarded, any recommendations for change will be limited.

ACKNOWLEDGEMENTS

We are indebted to Bloomsbury Health Authority for sponsoring and supporting the study, and to the patients and nurses who participated in it.

REFERENCES

Alexander M F (1983) *Learning to Nurse*. Edinburgh: Churchill Livingstone.

Armstrong D (1983) The fabrication of nurse–patient relationships. *Social Science and Medicine*, **14B**: 3–13.

Barr A (1967) *Measurement of Nursing Care*. Operational Research Unit Report No. 9. Oxford: Oxford Regional Hospital Board.

Black G (1985) When nurses feel ill-at-ease. Letter to the editor. *The Guardian*, 7 May.

Collins H M (1984) Researching spoonbending: concepts and practice of participatory fieldwork. In: *Social Researching – Politics, Problems, Practice*, eds. C Bell and H Roberts. London: Routledge & Kegan Paul.

Committee of Public Accounts (1987) 11th report from the Committee of Public Accounts, session 1986-87: *Control of National Health Service Manpower*. Chairman: Robert Sheldon. London: HMSO.

Coser R L (1962) *Life on the Ward*. East Lansing: Michigan State University Press.

Denzin N (1970) Strategies of multiple triangulation. In: *The Research Act in Sociology*. London: Butterworth.

Evers H (1982) Key issues in nursing practice: ward management 1 and 2. *Nursing Times*, Occasional Papers, **78**(6): 21–24; (7): 25–26.

Fretwell J E (1982) *Ward Teaching and Learning: Sister and the Learning Environment*. London: Royal College of Nursing.

Fretwell J E (1983) Creating a ward learning environment: the sister's role – 1. *Nursing Times*, Occasional Papers, **79**(21): 37–39.

Fretwell J E (1985) *Freedom to Change*. London: Royal College of Nursing.

Friedson E (1970) *The Profession of Medicine: a Study of the Sociology of Applied Knowledge*. New York: Dodd, Mead and Co.

Glaser B and Strauss A (1967) *The Discovery of Grounded Theory*. London: Weidenfeld and Nicolson.

Goddard H A (1953) *The Work of Nurses in Hospital Wards: Report of a Job Analysis*. Oxford: Nuffield Provincial Hospitals Trust.

Goldstone L A, Ball J A and Collier M (1983) *Monitor, an Index of the Quality of Nursing Care for Acute Medical and Surgical Wards*. Newcastle: Newcastle upon Tyne Polytechnic.

Hawthorn P (1974) *Nurse I want my Mummy*. London: Royal College of Nursing.

Hochschild A R (1983) *The Managed Heart: Commercialisation of Human Feeling*. Berkeley: University of California Press.

Jelinek R, Haussman R K D, Hegyvary S T and Newman J E (1974) *A Methodology for Monitoring Quality of Nursing Care*. Bethesda, Maryland: US Dept of Health, Education and Welfare.

Lewin D C and Leach J (1982) Factors influencing the quality of wards as learning environments. *International Journal of Nursing Studies*, **9**: 125–137.

McFarlane J K (1976) A charter for caring. *Journal of Advanced Nursing*, **1**: 187–196.

McFarlane J K (1977) Developing a theory of nursing: the relation of theory to practice, education and research. *Journal of Advanced Nursing*, **2**: 261-270.

Macleod Clark J (1981) Communication in nursing. *Nursing Times*, **77**(1): 12-16.

Melia K M (1982) 'Tell it as it is' - qualitative methodology and nursing research: understanding the student nurses' world. *Journal of Advanced Nursing*, **7**: 327-335.

Menzies I E P (1970) *The Functioning of Social Systems as a Defence against Anxiety*. London: Centre for Applied Social Research, The Tavistock Institute of Human Relations.

Moores B and Moult A (1979) Patterns of nurse activity. *Journal of Advanced Nursing*, **4**: 137-149.

Oakley A (1974) *The Sociology of Housework*. London: Martin Robinson.

Oakley A (1984) The importance of being a nurse. *Nursing Times*, **80**(50): 24-27.

Ogier M (1982) *An Ideal Sister*. London: Royal College of Nursing.

Orton H D (1981) *Ward Learning Climate: a Study of the Role of the Ward Sister in Relation to Student Nurse Learning on the Ward*. London: Royal College of Nursing.

Pearmain B (1985) Nursing a few doubts about hospital work. Letter to the editor. *The Guardian*, 18 April.

Pembrey S E M (1980) *The Ward Sister - Key to Nursing*. London: Royal College of Nursing.

Revans R W (1964) *Standards for Morale: Cause and Effect in Hospitals*. Oxford: Oxford University Press for Nuffield Provincial Hospitals Trust.

Roper N (1975) *Clinical Experience in Nurse Education: a Survey of the Available Nursing Experience for General Student Nurses in a School of Nursing in Scotland*. MPhil thesis, University of Edinburgh.

Smith P (1987) The relationship between quality of nursing care and the ward as a learning environment: developing a methodology. *Journal of Advanced Nursing*, **12**: 413-420.

Strauss A, Fagerhaugh S, Suczek B and Wiener C (1982) Sentimental work in the technologized hospital. *Sociology of Health and Illness*, **4**(3): 254-278.

Timmins N (1987) NHS losing 1,000 nurses a year to private sector. *The Independent*, 16 March.

Ungerson C (1983a) Why do women care? In: *A Labour of Love: Women, Work and Caring*, eds. Finch J and Groves D. London: Routledge & Kegan Paul.

Ungerson C (1983b) Women and caring: skills, tasks and taboos. In: *The Public and the Private*, eds. Gamarnikov E, Morgan D, Purvis J and Taylorson D. London: Heinemann.

Wandelt M and Ager J (1974) *Quality Patient Care Scale*. New York: Appleton Century Crofts.

West M and Rushton R (1986) The drop-out factor. *Nursing Times*, **82**(52): 29-31.

Chapter 17

The Clinical Learning of Student Nurses

Keith Jacka and David Lewin

This chapter describes a two-phase project that investigated factors facilitating the clinical learning of student nurses and factors inhibiting this process. One of the main aims of the project was to provide criteria for the evaluation of hospital wards as learning environments that could be used to monitor and assess, and if needs be modify, the experience of learners.

BACKGROUND

The majority of state registered nurses in the United Kingdom qualify after a 3-year apprenticeship. Most of this period is spent on hospital wards and the rest mainly in the classrooms of the associated school of nursing. Over the whole course of training the ratio of totals of time spent (hospital : school) is approximately 5 : 1. This kind of training, in which a student is on the job as a junior nurse, much of the time participating in the giving of care, means that her learning career, her sustained attempt to develop into a competent and knowledgeable practitioner, will depend greatly on two elements:

1. The quality of the training wards as educational environments, the variety and frequency of opportunities to learn and the extent to which such learning is facilitated, and
2. The harmonising of ward experience with classroom teaching, i.e. the degree to which these elements complement and reinforce each other.

These general conditions for effective training have long been recognised. In 1966, for example, the General Nursing Council stipulated that:

'the hospital, or group of hospitals, must satisfy the Council that adequate clinical experience is available . . .'

and that:

'satisfactory arrangement must be made for the supervision and teaching of the student nurses by registered nurses in all wards and departments both day and night.'

This policy statement was later replaced by a more substantial declaration of educational policy (GNC, 1977). Unlike the 1966 policy statement, the 1977 document attempted to specify the characteristics of 'a good climate for learning'. These, it advised, included the identification of learning objectives, with written worksheets available for learners, and the ideals that the ward sisters should be, or should want to be, GNC examiners and assessors, and that opportunities were given for continuing professional education. The council further recommended that schools of nursing define overall aims for their course (suggesting, in this connection, that the nursing process offered a helpful framework for nursing practice) and that nurse teachers should involve themselves more closely with the clinical setting. Training schools were required to draw up written statements of learning objectives for each area of clinical experience.

Very few studies, however, have focused directly on the problem of developing criteria for assessing wards as learning areas. Martin (1976) offered some very general guidelines about converting the learner's daily work into 'clinical learning experiences'. Strohmann (1977), discussing student clinical experiences in the United States, similarly provided a series of broad pointers for 'establishing a better and stronger clinical programme'. Skeath et al (1979) attempted, in a local study, to establish criteria for selecting areas for basic nurse training, focusing in particular on the assessment of attitudes of those involved in the teaching process. Schrock (1973), in a more substantial piece of research, aimed to describe more precisely the clinical areas in a large hospital caring for mentally handicapped and mentally ill patients, and to develop a method of ongoing evaluation of a clinical area's suitability as a training area. The data suggested that learners' needs were often better met in long-term than in admission wards. Since too many learners tended to be present in admission wards at one time, trained staff were often unable to meet their teaching needs.

One of Schrock's main conclusions – that wards with a common designation do not necessarily have similar characteristics – was given supporting evidence by the work of Roper (1976). She found that 39 per cent of patients in the general hospital, 18 per cent in the maternity hospital, 23 per cent in the psychiatric hospital and 38 per cent in the community had more than one medical diagnostic label. Ward 'labels' such as paediatric and geriatric were found to be misleading, since there were children and elderly patients in most wards in the general hospital. Roper made the point that her data suggested a wider variety of possible learning experiences, in particular 'kinds' of ward, than might have been expected, and she recommended, on the basis of this, fewer clinical allocations of longer duration.

Roper's work on wards as learning areas was, in many respects, complemented by that of Pearson's on ward teaching (Pearson, 1979). Her data suggested that learners most appreciated wards where the sister played an active teaching role. They appreciated teachers who put pressure on them to work and generally controlled their learning to some extent. Pearson pointed out, however, that her data suggested that not all ward sisters were prepared to undertake such a teaching role and that those who were had received little training for such a role.

The hospital context as a learning environment for nurses in training was explored in more detail by Dodd (1973). Her work, in two hospitals, convinced her that neither constituted a learning environment. Learners experienced difficulties in the application of knowledge, and the ideal description of skills in the school did not always correspond with the reality of ward practices. The most detailed study of wards as learning environments was undertaken by Fretwell (1978), who concluded that the key person in the learning environment was the ward sister. The 'ideal' sister was democratic, patient-orientated and fulfilled an active teaching role.

Ogier (1980), in a small but methodologically imaginative study, also investigated the role of the ward sister with regard to trainee learning. The results of her work indicated that sisters who appear to have a 'style' that is 'open and inclusive to the nurse learner' are more highly rated by the latter, and that a course in interpersonal skills might be beneficial to ward sisters as part of their preparation for taking charge of a ward.

Marson (1981), undertaking an exploration of the teaching and learning of nursing in the work environment, investigated the behavioural characteristics of effective ward teachers. She concluded that 'on the job' teaching of nurse learners is a complex global act in which the role model presented to the learner is a powerful influence. Nurses perceived as effective teachers generally expressed an attitude of care and concern for the welfare of others and a commitment to the training of nurses in particular.

It is apparent that there has been concern for many years about the adequacy of the clinical education received by student nurses. As we have seen, however, there has been relatively little research into student nurse clinical learning and, in the absence of data derived from systematic enquiries, few guidelines have been available to assist those concerned with improving the educational quality of clinical allocations. The need for such research was one of the topics discussed at a workshop organised by the DHSS in December 1977, and provided the impetus for the research described here.

For many years the Royal College of Nursing (RCN) has pressed the case for radical reorganisation of nurse training, advocating a shift from apprenticeship to full student status, to a situation where the trainee would be supernumerary, not a member of the nursing workforce, and where her living and training expenses would come from educational funds entirely separate from those used for patient services. Supporters of apprenticeship on the other hand have argued that nurses can learn their craft only by caring for patients in real rather than controlled situations. The RCN Commission on Nursing (1985) states that trainees 'march to the drumbeat of service', i.e. that manpower demands of the hospital – for workers able to give patient care – characteristically dominate the activities of trainees. Is this a fact, and if it is, does it hinder the educational development of trainees? On the other hand Michael Polanyi, a noted writer on apprenticeship, views it benignly as a system in which the trainee learns by example by being close to an expert in action (Polanyi, 1958). To what extent does this kind of osmotic learning actually happen throughout the 3 years of training? The project provided findings bearing upon each of these questions.

PART 1: EXPLORATORY WORK

The first part of the project comprised three stages. Within the confines of this chapter the methods and findings can only be briefly summarised, and for further details the reader is referred to Leach and Lewin (1981) and Lewin and Leach (1982, 1983).

Methods

The first two stages of the first part of the project were concerned with investigating, in 10 schools of nursing, the activities of various grades of nurse in respect of student nurse clinical learning. Data were obtained by questionnaire and semi-structured interview schedules.

The third stage, a 'case study', considered in more detail the factors influencing student nurse clinical learning in the wards of one hospital. Three intakes (sets) of student nurses were investigated; a two-thirds random sample was drawn from each set, giving an average sample size of 20:

1. a group of first-year student nurses experiencing their first ward placement;
2. a group of second-year student nurses experiencing their third ward placement;
3. a group of third-year student nurses experiencing their second ward placement.

The first- and second-year student nurses were working in 10 medical wards, and the third-year students in 11 surgical wards.

Information about these wards was obtained in several ways. Each student nurse was interviewed, at the end of the ward placements specified, in order to record certain of her experiences in the ward (for example, the extent to which her clinical work had been supervised by trained staff) and her evaluation of the ward as a learning area. The sisters in charge of the wards were also interviewed, particular attention being paid to their teaching activities. The data were supplemented by information obtained from a 'ward profile', a schedule designed to record details about the ward as an 'environment' – its level of staffing, patient turnover, 'geography' and so on.

Findings

Clinical teaching and supervision

According to the students, theoretical instruction was fairly common, practical demonstration less so. They worked infrequently with trained staff and consequently they were seldom supervised in any nursing performance, particularly second-year students. On the other hand, ward sisters saw themselves as closely involved in teaching and supervising students. There was a clear discrepancy between students' and sisters' perceptions; independent observation inclined the researchers towards the student view. School tutorial staff had little contact with training wards.

Quality of allocations

Students were asked to rate their current ward placement as a clinical learning environment. The behaviour and attitude of trained staff appeared to be the discriminating elements. On highly rated wards the trained staff gave more practical demonstrations, worked more with the students, supervised them more, quizzed them more (on theoretical knowledge) and were more approachable; also, on these wards the sisters were typically older, more experienced, better qualified and more overtly committed to teaching.

Implications

Findings were not unexpected, but they were nonetheless useful. The most important finding was that problems in clinical learning were similar, regardless of type of hospital, training scheme or geographical location; i.e. there was a core of problems common to all programmes, and quality of training available to students was much affected by how well these problems were handled.

There was also the methodological finding that most students appeared to be effective estimators of at least the quantitative aspects of their own ward experiences. Together these two findings decided the design of the main study. The first finding led to the central decision: to opt for an intensive design, an investigation of the clinical learning careers of three cohorts of student nurses from beginning to end of training, as opposed to the cross-sectional design used in the exploratory work. The second finding supported the decision to use the students themselves as the main recorders of experience.

PART 2: THE MAIN STUDY

The primary aim of the main study was to devise ways of improving arrangements whereby students are enabled to acquire knowledge and skill necessary for competence in nursing practice within a hospital setting. The three schools from which the cohorts were drawn were selected to provide examples of different ways of organising nurse training: modular, modified modular and block programmes.

Research design

Figure 17.1 displays both the research design and training system.

Structure (AA) refers to the training scheme as designed and constituted by the architects of the course: the broad outline of the academic programme, the training wards selected, the tutors and the ward sisters. This is a structure of promise only, a static potential. For the student it exists not as experience but as a dimly perceived system of opportunity.

Structure (AA)	Structure/ experience (AB)	Experience/ learning (BC)	Learning (CC)
AA1. Academic programme (formal specification of aims/ objectives/syllabus)	AB1. Academic instruction of student set (content, sequence, methods of instruction from tutorial staff and others; detailed timetables for 3 years)	BC1. Clinical instruction and oversight of individual student (mainly by ward staff: quantity and sequence)	CC. Clinical learning by student (as a result of AA, AB and BC)
AA2. Academic milieu (teachers; school organisation)			
AA3. Clinical programme (formal specification of course of clinical training)		BC2. Clinical experience of individual students	
AA4. Blocks, modules, placements (interweaving of elements of AA1 and AA3)	AB2. Placement sequences of *individual* students (groups of clinical conditions sequentially available)	(range, quantity and sequence of nursing procedures practised)	
AA5. Clinical potential (clinical conditions on wards/departments selected as training areas)			
AA6. Clinical milieu (training wards: sisters, staff, organisation)	AB3. Sequence of theory and practice (individuals: interrelation of AB1 and AB2)		

Fig. 17.1 Analytic schema

Structure/experience (AB) refers to the actualisation of possibilities implicit in structure (AA), e.g. the detail of timetables for the set of students, and the sequence of placements for an individual student. In this element there are aspects of both structure and experience. For example, a sequence of placements can be seen as structure in that it is an external framework and it is about opportunity; also, information about it can be obtained from the allocation officer without asking the student. On the other hand, it is experiential in that it is peculiar to that student, and could have been otherwise.

Experience/learning (BC) refers mainly to the experience of students in school and ward. The focus is on variety and quantity of teaching received by the student, including being in learning situations, and the student's response to this teaching.

Learning enters since there is experience with a view to learning, but here we do not attempt to record learning directly. We are registering the external (teaching) aspect (mainly from the students' point of view) of the dynamic teaching–learning situation.

Learning (CC) refers to the crystallised deposit of experience-structure (AA) finally made fully manifest and incarnate in the person of the student who, having been subject to the constraints and having used the facilitations of the training system as she has experienced it, has undergone a self-transformation into a qualified nurse.

Data collection

Data consisted of:

1. case studies of three training schemes, concentrating on structural elements: course content (school of nursing), clinical conditions on training wards, significant persons in the training programmes;
2. biographical studies of the clinical learning careers of 71 student nurses.

Methods employed included interviews, questionnaires, informal discussion and ward observation. The overall aims of the fieldwork were to acquire a deep and detailed understanding of the working of each training scheme and to generate a body of empirical data sufficiently large and various that quantitative analysis could be used to establish benchmarks and to reveal any underlying patterns.

The main aggregates of data are described below.

Ward sister questionnaire

All sisters on all training wards used by cohort students were interviewed once and a questionnaire completed. Interviews averaged about 1¼ hours. Information gathered related both to the sister and to the ward itself, as described by the sister, and covered items relating to age, qualifications, time in post, time spent on teaching and administration, views on factors inhibiting or facilitating teaching of students, adequacy of staffing levels, patient throughput and distribution of clinical conditions on the ward.

Ward observation

Apart from specialist wards and departments, most wards were visited by the researchers, usually more than once. Visits were made during the morning, and typically lasted from 7.30 a.m. to 1.00 p.m. The researchers observed and recorded the detail of activities on the ward during that morning, examined the Kardex and recorded the clinical conditions of patients, and noted the numbers and types of nursing staff on duty.

Tutorial staff questionnaire

Postal questionnaires were sent to tutorial staff of the three training schools and included items relating to age, qualifications, time in post, time spent on teaching, time on administration and opinions on facilitating and inhibiting factors.

Student nurse questionnaire

The activities of data collection outlined so far relate to structural elements of the training schemes, but the heaviest burden of data gathering was associated with the student nurse questionnaire; these data were concerned with experience rather than structure. Since each student was interviewed at the end of each of 15 placements, the total of questionnaires was approximately $15 \times 71 = 1065$.

The questionnaire was in two parts. The first part consisted of 42 questions relating to the student's instructional and environmental experience of that particular placement. For example:

1. For how much of your time on duty was the ward understaffed?
2. How much of your time did you spend working with a trained member of staff?
3. How often were you questioned about the physical or psychological state of one of your patients?

The second part related to a large number of individual items of nursing procedure. For each item the student was asked several questions, for example whether she had actually performed the procedure on that placement.

Data analysis

In a cohort of this kind a vast amount of data is generated over the the 3-year period, and a major problem is that of condensation and aggregation in order to try to see the wood instead of the trees.

Numerical values computed included:

1. Simple descriptive statistics. These were usually mean values or proportions; for example, in Hospital 3, throughout the 3 years of training, the proportion of lecture time allotted to 'respiratory nursing' was 3.9 per cent.
2. Values calculated by further aggregation. Many items of data, however much initially qualitative, were ultimately quantified in some fashion. A general technique, often used to condense information, was to construct a single index aggregated from repeated answers to several questions.

Precise details of quantification and condensation – scoring systems for each question and the computation of a particular index by aggregation of weighted scores on an appropriate set of items – can be found in the Jacka and Lewin (1987) reference.

Findings

The findings from this part of the project fall into two main sections: first, the academic and clinical opportunity provided by each scheme and the degree of integration between the two, and second, the actual learning experiences of students on the wards.

Academic and clinical opportunity

Using information supplied mainly by tutorial staff of the three schools, an analysis was made of classroom instruction (academic opportunity) received by the students. An example of such analysis is shown in Table 17.1, which refers to the entire 3 years of training. Content of instruction was classified into 27 categories, the first five of which are shown. As can be seen, there is substantial variation between schools in the amount of time spent on a given item (e.g. 'alimentary nursing').

Table 17.1 Syllabus : aggregate analysis (examples of categories)

Topic	Hospital 1		Hospital 2		Hospital 3		Total	
	Hours	%	Hours	%	Hours	%	Hours	%
Aims, objectives, tests, assessments, evaluations	82	13.7	78	13.4	62	11.5	222	12.9
Study, project work, progress reports, counselling	49	8.2	31	5.3	41	7.6	121	7.0
Alimentary nursing	31	5.2	23	3.9	53	9.8	107	6.2
Obstetric nursing	28	4.7	42	7.2	32	5.9	102	5.9
Cardiovascular, circulatory, thoracic nursing	30	5.0	22	3.8	45	8.3	97	5.6
Total	597	100.3	584	99.8	539	99.4	1720	99.6

'Clinical opportunity' refers to the potential for clinical observation and nursing practice on wards to which an individual trainee is assigned. Unlike academic opportunity, which is invariant within each cohort, there are possibilities of substantial individual variation in content and sequence of clinical opportunity, especially when a large number of wards is used.

Diagnostic information was collected and categorised by researchers, and checked with ward sisters. Table 17.2 is an example of collation and analysis.

About half of the cohort are represented, together with five out of a total of 13 diagnostic categories. The figures in the body of the table are sums of percentages. For example, for the category 'Alimentary', Nurse 201 has a score of 184 made up as follows: on her first placement she was assigned to a ward assessed as typically having 5 per cent of patients with alimentary conditions; on her second placement the figure was 3 per cent, the third was 9 per cent, the fourth 64 per cent and so on. The total for all placements was 184.

The natural criteria for examining these figures are:

1. approximate equality of opportunity for individuals within a cohort;
2. minimum levels of opportunity for individuals for each diagnostic category.

'Eye, ear, nose and throat' is the most extreme case: a glance along the row of figures shows clearly that the two criteria are not being satisfied.

Table 17.2 Hospital no. 2 – analysis of data collected

Category	Nurse 201	203	205	207	209	211	213	215	217	219	221	223	225	227	229	231	233	x̄	s.d.	C.V.
Psychiatry	41	38	35	39	64	36	49	14	44	37	34	45	49	33	43	34	34	39.4	10.22	0.26
Social admissions	0	18	21	6	14	11	9	25	9	21	16	9	24	10	13	26	15	14.5	7.25	0.50
Dermatology, plastics, burns	61	68	94	28	51	69	47	77	58	42	35	69	44	68	69	32	31	55.5	18.67	0.34
Eyes, ear, nose & throat	18	63	115	12	96	150	136	51	87	25	90	11	76	29	11	96	3	62.9	47.19	0.75
Alimentary	184	200	150	154	163	164	154	159	167	129	169	144	210	132	206	144	167	164.5	23.83	0.14

x̄ = mean
s.d. = standard deviation

The underlying pedagogic assumption of the 'modular system' of nurse training is that both understanding and practical skill with regard to an item of nursing care are facilitated when theoretical presentation of this item in the classroom and relevant clinical experience on the ward are close together in time. In such a system, the course consists of a series of modules, each made up of certain elements of theory, and closely related practical experience.

A simple scoring procedure was devised: one point was awarded to a trainee each time an element of class instruction was immediately preceded or followed by an essentially similar element of clinical opportunity. Each trainee accumulated a total integration score for the whole course. The average score for each hospital was:

Hospital 1 : 29.2 points
Hospital 2 : 69.9 points
Hospital 3 : 33.1 points

Clearly, the score for Hospital 2 is by far the greatest, in accord with expectations, since the training scheme for Hospital 2 was a modular one, whereas the other two were not. Scores for individual students demonstrated considerable intra-cohort variation with regard to the integration of academic and clinical opportunity. The scoring system devised to measure this integration provides tutors with a means of monitoring individual students' progress and making adjustments to subsequent placements if necessary.

Learning experiences of students

Indices of apprenticeship. Towards the end of every placement each trainee was interviewed, and a questionnaire was completed about experiences in that placement that directly or indirectly related to educational aspects of her apprenticeship.

We took it that, within an effective apprenticeship milieu, one can distinguish a variety of modes of learning:

1. Observing an expert in action.
2. Working alongside an expert.
3. Working as a principal, but under some degree of supervision.
4. Being explicitly instructed by an expert.
5. Working with more experienced fellow learners.
6. Working alone, consolidating skill and gaining confidence.

These modes of learning are not mutually exclusive; several may occur together. We tried to record the occurrence of most of these events from which learning might ensue.

As noted, a small set of indices was calculated for each student. Data on two of these indices are presented here: the *core index* (AICORE), focusing on learning by association with clinical experts, and the *clinical experience index* (AICE), focusing on clinical procedures practised by the trainee.

The core index. The core index was constructed from the answers to six questions in the student nurse questionnaire:

1. With which grade of ward staff have you worked most during this placement?
2. How often do trained nursing staff demonstrate practical procedures to you?
3. How often do trained nursing staff pose questions to test your theoretical knowledge?

4. How often do trained nursing staff ask your opinion about patients' physical and psychological states?
5. For how much of your time in the ward did trained nursing staff perform practical procedures with you?
6. For how much of your time in the ward were you personally supervised by trained staff?

Responses were translated into numerical scores. An example is shown below:

With which grade of staff have you worked most during this placement?			
Grade	Score	Grade	Score
Ward sister	100	Third-year student nurse	40
Staff nurse	75	Second-year student nurse	20
Enrolled nurse	60	First-year student nurse	10

A summary of all answers to this question for all students throughout the course of training is given in Table 17.3.

Answers to the other five questions were quantified in a comparable way, and finally all were combined to give a single composite index (AICORE). The index is weighted towards practical instruction, by example and supervision; questions 2, 5 and 6 are each given twice the weight of the others. Final values were as in Table 17.4.

The mean score for H3 (51.3) is markedly higher than the score for H1 and H2. This substantial difference accords with the independent observations of the researchers. All values in this table derive from a very large database, the last percentage (44.9), for example, being calculated from about 6000 items of information (71 students, six questions each repeated about 15 times).

Table 17.3 Summary of answers to sample question of student nurse questionnaire

	Grade worked with			
	Hospital 1	Hospital 2	Hospital 3	All hospitals
Mean	42.8	37.3	61.4	44.8
Standard deviation	12.9	5.9	11.7	14.2
Maximum score	75	51	75	75
Minimum score	23	22	25	22
Coefficient of variation	0.30	0.16	0.19	0.31

Table 17.4 AICORE values

	Hospital 1	Hospital 2	Hospital 3	All hospitals
Mean	44.0	42.2	51.3	44.9
Standard deviation	9.11	7.9	11.6	10.0
Maximum score	60	60	73	73
Minimum score	26	29	35	26
Coefficient of variation	0.21	0.19	0.22	0.22

Table 17.5 Clinical experience: cardiac resuscitation

Assisting with cardiac resuscitation	H1	H2	H3
Mean no. of experiences	2.32	0.53	2.16
Standard deviation	0.95	0.63	1.57
Coefficient of variation	0.40	1.19	0.73
Maximum no. of experiences	4	2	5
Minimum no. of experiences	1	0	0
No. of students with no experience	0	16	2
Percentage of students with no experience	0	53.3	10.5

We consider that 55 per cent or above would be a good score. The overall score of 44.9 per cent would count as fair. Within each cohort there is moderate variation, of similar magnitude in all three cases.

The clinical experience index. Seventy-seven items of nursing procedure were selected for analysis. Towards the end of each ward placement a student would record (for each item) whether or not she had been involved, at least once, in the specified procedure or situation. Therefore, for a nurse whose training scheme included 15 placements, the maximum possible score for each item of clinical experience was 15. Table 17.5 gives an example of analysis for one item. With this item there is a clear difference between H1 and H3 on the one hand, and H2 on the other. For most students, in H1 and H3 cardiac arrest is relatively uncommon, but it does happen, whereas in H2 more than half the cohort are never involved at all in this situation during training. (We are *not* suggesting that in this respect the H2 training scheme is inferior to the others; there is room here for difference of opinion. We *are* saying, however, that there is value in accurate knowledge of what is happening.)

All 77 items were analysed similarly. Scores were combined to generate a single clinical experience index (AICE), and other conflation analyses were made. For example, rank orderings were constructed: it emerged that 'checking/administering drugs' was the most common procedure, and 'Care of peritoneal dialysis' the least common.

Wards as units of analysis. In the previous section the primary unit of analysis was the individual student (her total experience), leading to cohort indices, and each cohort was taken to be indicative of the corresponding training scheme.

Table 17.6 AICORE values by type of ward

Type of ward	H1	H2	H3	All
Medical	37.1	30.1	47.7	37.6
Surgical	33.6	40.4	51.7	39.1
Gynaecology	43.9	33.3	77.7	42.6
Orthopaedics	44.7	37.3	44.1	41.8
Geriatrics	43.3	41.6	39.6	41.2
Obstetrics	74.3	64.7	57.7	65.6
Paediatrics	43.9	39.6	46.7	42.4
Operating theatres	72.7	75.9	73.9	74.3
Accident & emergency	63.0	41.0	62.5	55.1

Table 17.7 Apprenticeship indices – selected wards

Hospital	Ward	Type	AICORE
1	111	Medical	56
1	110	Medical	33
3	308	Paediatric	64
3	321	Paediatric	30
3	332	Geriatric	52
3	329	Geriatric	28

However, we can proceed differently, attending only to happenings and experiences of those students assigned to a particular training ward, and by aggregation and analysis we can construct indices for each ward. An example of this type of analysis is given in Table 17.6. Looking at the column headed 'All' we can see that the two specialty areas, 'Obstetrics' and 'Operating theatres', have notably high scores, as one would expect because of the continuously critical nature of the work in these areas and the consequent necessity for oversight of student performance.

In Table 17.7 we show figures for three pairs of training wards, indicating the large differences that can occur. (The high and low numbers accorded closely with researchers' and tutors' expectations.)

CONCLUSIONS

We have given a few examples of findings of Part 2 of this project, and of methods devised for generating and analysing data. We see the findings as useful in that they provide bench marks in a relatively unexplored area, but we consider methods to be the project's main contribution. Those involved in the education of nurses need detailed information about individual student careers and wards as learning environments, and a means to monitor progress and identify those areas where improvement is needed. The authors are currently working with staff in several schools of nursing, helping them to implement the techniques devised in the monitoring of their own student nurse programme.

ACKNOWLEDGEMENTS

We wish to acknowledge the contribution made by colleagues who worked with us on the Clinical Learning Project: John Leach – research fellow responsible for Part 1 of the project; Susan Hewins, Karen Bowman and Julia Hedley – research assistants on Part 2.

REFERENCES

Dodd A P (1973) *Towards an Understanding of Nursing.* Unpublished PhD thesis, University of Warwick.
Fretwell J E (1978) *Socialisation of Nurses: Teaching and Learning in Hospital Wards.* Unpublished PhD thesis, University of Warwick.

General Nursing Council for England and Wales (1966) *Conditions of Approval of Training Schools.* London: GNC.

General Nursing Council for England and Wales (1977) *Educational Policy 1977:* 77/19/A, 77/19/B, 77/19/C, 77/19/D. London: GNC.

Jacka K and Lewin D (1987) *The Clinical Learning of Student Nurses.* NERU Report No. 6. King's College, University of London.

Leach J and Lewin D (1981) *A Study of the Factors Influencing the Clinical Learning of Student Nurses.* A pilot study of the Clinical Learning Project, Report submitted to the Department of Health and Social Security. King's College, University of London: Nursing Education Research Unit.

Lewin D and Leach J (1982) Factors influencing the quality of wards as learning environments for student nurses. *International Journal of Nursing Studies,* **19**(3): 125-137.

Lewin D and Leach J (1983) A clinical learning project. *Nursing Times,* **79**(47): 61-65.

Marson S N (1981) *Ward Teaching Skills - an Investigation into the Behavioural Characteristics of Effective Ward Teachers.* MPhil thesis, Sheffield City Polytechnic.

Martin J L (1976) Learning through experience. Nursing Times, **72**: 546-548.

Ogier M E (1980) *The Effects of Ward Sisters' Management Style upon Learner Nurses.* Unpublished PhD thesis, University of London.

Pearson J (1979) *Educational Encounters in the Ward.* Unpublished MPhil thesis CNAA (available from RCN library).

Polanyi M (1958) *Personal Knowledge: Towards a Post-critical Philosophy.* London: Routledge and Kegan Paul.

Roper N (1976) *Clinical Experience in Nurse Education.* Edinburgh: Churchill Livingstone.

Royal College of Nursing (1985) *The Education of Nurses: a New Dispensation* (Judge Report). London: Royal College of Nursing.

Schrock R A (1973) No rhyme or reason; a clinical area identification project. *International Journal of Nursing Studies,* **10**: 69-80.

Skeath W A et al (1979) Criteria to be used in selection of clinical areas for basic nurse training. *Journal of Advanced Nursing,* **4**: 169-180.

Strohmann R (1977) Improving student clinical experiences. *Nursing Outlook,* **25**: 460-462.

Chapter 18

An Experimental Training Scheme for Ward Sisters

Judith Lathlean

BACKGROUND

'The ward sister is the head of the ward . . . and upon her rests the management of the ward and the direction of ward staff.' (From a memorandum, dated 1879, quoted in Cope, 1955)

'The ward sister . . . is the only person in the nursing structure who actually and symbolically represents continuity of care to the patient. She is also the only nurse who has direct managerial responsibilities for both patients and nurses.' (Pembrey, 1980)

Despite 100 years separating these two quotations, they are surprisingly similar in their description of the nature of the ward sister's role and her importance in nursing. Yet although the last 40 years has seen many attempts to highlight the sister's unique position in nursing, and to make recommendations for her training and preparation, many feel inadequately prepared for their first sister's post and lack confidence in the skills required to undertake the job (Farnish, 1983, and chapter 19).

The Horder report (RCN, 1943) recognised the sister as the 'lynchpin' in the system of nurse education and thus in need of training to impart her knowledge in the best way, and the Wood report (Ministry of Health, 1947) recommended a post-graduate preparation for ward sisters 'including principles and methods of teaching, administration and social psychology'. The King Edward's Hospital Fund for London established a residential training centre for ward sisters in 1949, but it was not until the implementation of the recommendations of the Salmon Committee (Ministry of Health, 1966) that management training became available for large numbers of sisters rather than the 'privileged few' who were catered for by the King's Fund courses.

However, provision of places on first-line management courses did not meet the needs, and although there was evidence that staff who attended courses generally enjoyed the experience, sisters in one research study (Farnish, 1983) described their experiences using terms such as a 'conveyor belt' and a 'sheep-dip' approach. Indeed, 'there was little apparent relationship between theory and practice (in the ward situation) and sisters were alienated by the emphasis on the academic and industry-orientated approach to management' (Lathlean and Farnish, 1984).

In a major evaluation of such courses in one particular region (Manchester), Davies (1972) found that the factors that inhibited the achievement of course objectives included:

1. the physical distance of the course members from their 'organisational realities' (the hospitals);
2. the gap between the lecturers and the course members;
3. the difference in the value systems of the two groups.

She concluded that a new strategy was needed for management training, which fitted the courses to the requirements of the organisation.

Disenchantment set in with many of the externally led courses and some hospitals started their own management training in an attempt to remedy the deficiencies.

RESEARCH ON THE ROLE OF THE WARD SISTER

Research highlighting the difficulties and complexities inherent in the sister role is not new. For example, both Menzies (1960) and Revans (1964) identified the high level of anxiety associated with nursing work, with sisters deprived of potential satisfaction because they want 'more opportunity to use their nursing skills directly but much of their time is spent initiating and training student nurses . . .' (Menzies, 1960). The Briggs Report (DHSS, 1972) stressed the managerial role of the sister, and stated that the key figure in the ward team was, and would continue to be, the ward sister. There were also studies in the Royal College of Nursing's series of research reports that were relevant to the sister, such as the work of Lelean (1973), who identified the ward sister as 'the key person on the ward controlling all communication coming into and out of the ward, as well as that within the ward itself' (Lelean, 1973).

The importance of the sister as teacher and role model for her staff was emerging strongly with studies of this aspect of the sister's job reaching a peak in the late 1970s and early 1980s, exemplified by the work of Orton (1979) and Ogier (1980). Furthermore, the fragmented nature of the sister's role, and the problems encountered in undertaking the full role, were highlighted (Runciman, 1983), these being factors that can lead to role conflict and diminished job satisfaction (Redfern, 1981).

These studies, and others, were beginning to focus considerable attention on the complex and difficult task of being a sister. But the research that was perhaps most influential in encouraging the King's Fund to turn its energies yet again to the provision of training for sisters was that of Pembrey (1980). Pembrey's study centred on the nature of the ward sister role and how this might be developed. It was based on the assumption that patient allocation and individualised patient care are likely to result in better quality care for patients.

Pembrey identified a 'daily management cycle of activities' comprising:

1. assessment of patient's needs (the daily ward round);
2. work prescription;
3. work allocation;
4. receiving accountability reports;

and observed whether sisters completed these sequential activities in relation to each patient and each nurse. She found that only nine sisters (18 per cent of her sample of 50) did manage the nursing on an individualised patient basis, that is they undertook at least three out of the four activities. She argued that this reflected the failure 'over the years to analyse the nature of this role . . . and to provide necessary preparation for nurses holding posts as ward sister' (Pembrey, 1980).

Pembrey concluded that 'consideration [should] be given to designated training wards for ward sisters, in which the opportunity to work with role models and to learn to manage the nursing in its operational environment could be combined with theoretical work' Pembrey, 1980).

AN EXPERIMENTAL TRAINING SCHEME FOR WARD SISTERS

Stimulated by its own experiences and the work of others, particularly Pembrey (1980), the King's Fund decided in the late 1970s to set up an experimental scheme for the preparation of ward sisters. This was established in two hospitals – a central London teaching hospital and a non-teaching hospital on the outskirts of London. In the former a mixed (male and female) surgical ward was used, in the latter a female medical ward.

Underlying principles

There were four major premises:

1. That there is a need for *specific training* for ward sisters.
2. That this training should be *ward-based*.
3. That a *joint* service/education approach is required.
4. That nurses learn how to become ward sisters by *observing the behaviour* of other, more experienced sisters (the notion of role modelling).

It was suggested that 'the best and quickest method for [ward sister] preparation is in the real-life situation: where the nurse will encounter the day-to-day problems and challenges of running a ward, but will have the advantage of the support of a tutor to guide her studies and an experienced ward sister to act as a role model' (Davies, 1981). These principles informed the setting up of the scheme.

Design of the scheme

Figure 18.1 illustrates the main features of the scheme at the beginning of the experimental period. Each course lasted 6 months; the first 3 months' module was based in the designated training ward, and the second 3 months' in the course member's own ward. A ward sister and tutor (known as preceptors) were specially appointed for the scheme, the ward sister acting as a role model and facilitator, the tutor assuming the main responsibility for organising and running the programme. Course members (trainees) were selected for the course, usually as newly appointed ward sisters in their first sister post (though some were night and departmental sisters and others were senior staff nurses).

The course was based on a curriculum (King Edward's Hospital Fund for London, 1982) and covered five areas: management of patient care, ward management, personnel management, teaching and research. Teaching methods included seminars, discussions, visits, written assignments, observation of sisters at work, and practice with advice and assessment.

As the scheme progressed changes were made; some of the major changes are illustrated in Figure 18.2. A total of 62 trainees undertook the course during the experimental period – 24 in one hospital, 35 in the other and three on a combined hospitals course.

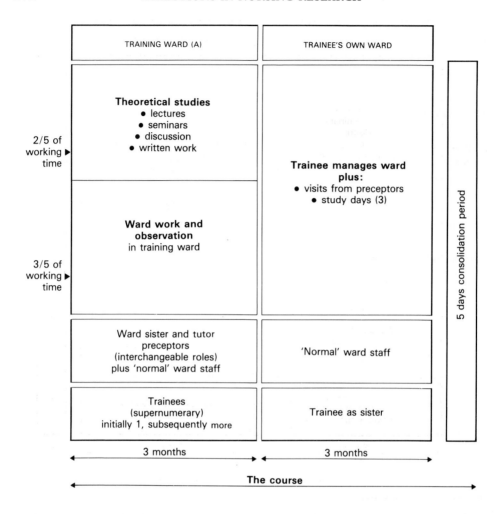

Fig. 18.1 Planned structure and design of the ward sister course

APPROACH TO EVALUATION

The evaluation project, which was funded jointly by the King's Fund and the DHSS, commenced in February 1979 and was completed in December 1983. Since the aim of the research was to assess the effectiveness of the scheme in achieving its aims, and to assist in the modification and development of the scheme, an action research approach was used which facilitated both of these aspects.

Action research has been described as a strategy which 'aims to contribute both to the practical concerns of people in an immediate problematic situation and to the goals of science by joint collaboration within a mutually acceptable framework' (Rapoport, 1970). There are different concepts of action research but mostly it aims either to solve problems or to assist development, as well as to advance knowledge.

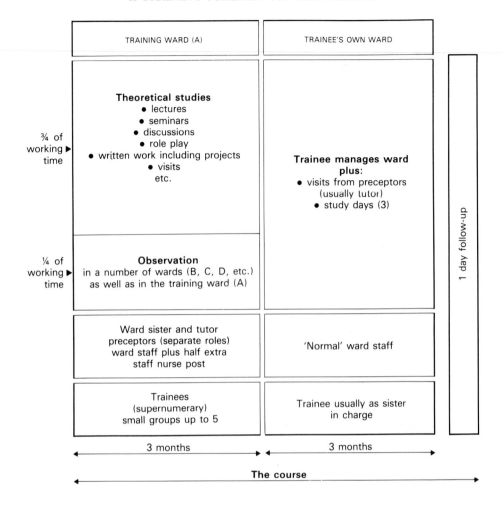

Fig. 18.2 Structure and design of the ward sister course at the end of the experimental period

Greenwood (1984) has argued that it is the approach that is most appropriate for nursing research since it is 'situational, collaborative, participatory and self-evaluative'. Yet it has been little used in nursing research, perhaps in part because it is – to the 'classical', experimental researcher – subjective and lacking in generalisability. Nevertheless, it is a strategy 'which does not pretend to be objective and which involves the objects of the research in the process itself' (Pedler, 1974). It is an approach where subjectivity is valued rather than criticised, and a mode of inquiry which can 'base its legitimacy . . . in philosophical traditions that are different from those . . . [of] positivist science' (Susman and Evered, 1978).

The features of this project included:

1. an early exploratory phase where issues were identified;
2. a subsequent series of cyclical stages where issues were identified, recommendations made, and changes implemented and reviewed, often resulting in further recommendation for change (see Figure 18.3);
3. evaluation at each stage of the programme, the process and the product (outcomes);

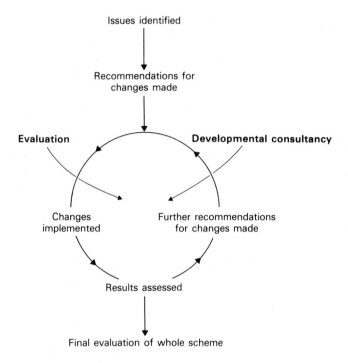

Fig. 18.3 The cyclical nature of the action research approach

4. a collaborative relationship between the researcher team and the clients (those involved in the organisation and running of the programme);
5. continual feedback to the clients, the organisers and the policy makers;
6. researcher involvement in the discussion of policy so that the research formed an integral part of the process for making decisions about the scheme.

RESEARCH DESIGN AND METHODS

The phases and the different parts of the project – including the main study and complementary studies – are summarised in Figure 18.4. In addition to the main research on the developing programme, four other studies were undertaken. These were a survey of three health districts to investigate the preparation available to sisters and charge nurses for their role (Farnish, 1983, and chapter 19), a follow-up survey by postal questionnaire of former trainees, an observation study of former ward sister trainees (looking at how the ward sisters performed on their wards), and a survey of training provided for ward sisters and experienced staff nurses throughout UK health districts. These helped to expand the information collected in the main study but were all self-contained projects.

Although action research is an approach that favours certain types of data collection, it does not prescribe methods. In the main study, a whole range was used including interviews (both open-ended and semi-structured), observation in various settings (e.g. hospital, ward and training events), documentary analysis, attendance at meetings (informal, committees and purposely established groups) and questionnaires (including pre-course, trainees' course

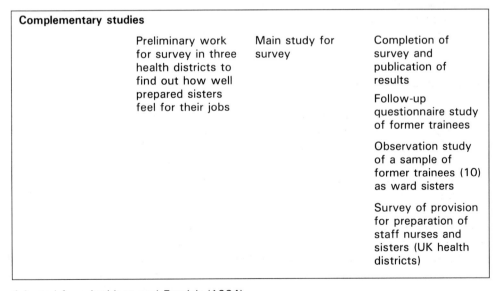

Orientation phase	Early monitoring phase	Further monitoring phase	Final evaluation phase
(1979–1980)	(1980–1981)	(1981–1982)	(1982–1983)
Main study			
Continuous historical account	→ → → → → → → → → → → → → → → →		Completion of historical account
Literature search and review	→ → → → → → → → → → → → → → → →		Completion of literature review
Development of research proposal	Review of research plans	→ → → → → → →	Review of changes required in early plans
Establishment of research role	Further negotiation of research role	→ → → → → → →	Termination of research role
Preliminary identification of factors important in implementing and sustaining schemes	Identification of key issues	Detailed investigation of key issues ↓ Recommendations for change ↓ Implementation of change ↓ Evaluation of results	Review of state of key issues
			Evaluation of relatively stable programme

Complementary studies			
	Preliminary work for survey in three health districts to find out how well prepared sisters feel for their jobs	Main study for survey	Completion of survey and publication of results
			Follow-up questionnaire study of former trainees
			Observation study of a sample of former trainees (10) as ward sisters
			Survey of provision for preparation of staff nurses and sisters (UK health districts)

Adapted from Lathlean and Farnish (1984)

Fig. 18.4 The phases of the project and the research activities: main and complementary studies

evaluations, assessment of trainees by tutors/managers). A number of measurement tests and existing tools were also used. These were not found to be *extensively* useful but more specific to certain parts of the research [for example, Pembrey's (1980) check-list was the basis for the observation study of former trainees].

The training programme changed and developed throughout the evaluation period as a result of the experience gained, informed by the feedback of findings from the research. In the last year of the period, when the programme was relatively stable, it was possible to undertake a complete review of it in its entirety – the implementation, the processes it went through and the results.

RESEARCH FINDINGS AND IMPLICATIONS

The findings of the project were presented by discussing a large number of issues related to elements of the scheme (such as plans, location, staff and participants), to the course (e.g. the framework, contents and teaching methods) and to the outcomes (including the effects on the trainees and other staff on wards and hospitals involved). These are detailed in the project report (Lathlean and Farnish, 1984); some of their main implications are discussed in this chapter.

It is possible to conclude from the research that certain conditions and features are vital whereas others remain debatable. Essentially, the sister must be recognised as important in ensuring effective clinical management in hospitals, otherwise there is little rationale for a programme of this kind, which deliberately sets out to reinforce such a role. Nevertheless, there remains the need to examine critically various sister roles since, despite common principles and responsibilities, there are differences related to specialty, environment and organisation structures. Specific investment must be made in the preparation for, and development within, the sister role if sisters are to achieve the extended role of an autonomous clinical manager, as envisaged by the Royal College of Nursing (RCN, 1983) and others.

Learning by observing and working with other more experienced nurses was found to be beneficial, and ways should be explored of maximising and facilitating such learning. And as well as needing certain knowledge and skill, sisters require support in developing their own practice, particularly when newly appointed. Above all, the prerequisite for the successful implementation and sustenance of a programme for sisters, as well as the provision of support, is management commitment. 'If managers believe that the ward sister role is crucial in ensuring effective clinical management, and if they have a clear and realistic conception of this role, then they will be prepared to allocate resources for specific training' (Lathlean and Farnish, 1984).

The issues that are open to debate include the participants, the location, the programme structure and the theoretical input. For example, should the programme be for newly appointed sisters, for those with some experience so that they are more aware of the role, or even for staff nurses prior to taking on the role? Should the programme be ward based, school based or a combination of the two? There appeared to be merit in a programme with two parts – one concentrating on the more formal elements of learning and the other on the application of this learning in a supportive environment. But how should this best be organised? And what should be the theoretical input, bearing in mind the different and changing roles?

The research provided considerable data to allow others to examine the advantages and disadvantages of the decisions made and the action taken, and to match the situations under study against their own particular settings. But, additionally, the action research approach enabled the twin components of developmental consultancy and evaluation to take place, at times a challenging and difficult combination to achieve without conflict.

THE WAY FORWARD

There has been no lessening of interest in the sister role since completion of this study, with all the major statutory and professional nursing bodies reinforcing the importance of the role and supporting the greater provision for the training and development of sisters and charge nurses. Indeed, in a memorandum sent to all regional general managers, the Chief Executive of the NHS Management Board recommended strongly that, 'in view of the crucial importance of the leader of the ward nursing team in maximising the quality and cost-effectiveness of patient care, authorities should make every effort to provide the necessary training and analytical support to facilitate the work of ward sisters and charge nurses' (DHSS, 1986).

There appears to have been an increase in training and education opportunities for sisters in a number of health authorities, but no co-ordinated source of information exists. However, the NHS Training Authority (NHSTA) has the development of team leader management training as one of its priorities (NHSTA, 1987) and is likely to be identifying the extent and nature of current provision by health authorities as part of this. It is hoped that this kind of information will be widely available – possibly as part of a research-based activity – to inform other health authorities of current initiatives in sister development.

The role of the sister has been subject to change in recent years and this is likely to continue. The major influences could include the further implementation of primary nursing in clinical areas, proposed changes to basic nurse education and the implementation of UKCC Project 2000's recommendations, the development of the support worker role and the conclusions reached about skill mix in clinical settings. Further research is, therefore, needed to examine this changing role, to review the training needs of team leaders (sisters and charge nurses) and to consider the most appropriate and cost-effective ways of meeting these needs.

One of the areas that has been studied indirectly, but about which more needs to be known, is the precise relationship between the performance of the sister and quality of patient care. This would entail a drawing together of much of the existing research and an exploration of the factors necessary for the promotion of good care.

Finally, there are signs that the whole nature of the management of clinical practice is being questioned. For example, Oxfordshire Health Authority have looked at nursing structures, a process that has challenged the viability and appropriateness of the traditional sister role and the lines of accountability between the ward-based nurses and the most senior nurse managers. This is a subject ripe for action. Research should not merely respond to current problems, nor only confirm or promote the status quo. It should also be used to explore alternatives, to develop new perspectives.

The research on the ward sister role from the post-war period until the early 1980s tended to suggest that the role was unfulfilled in some way, often as a result of a lack of time, understanding, preparation and training, or support. The remedy offered tended to be relatively straightforward. If more of what was lacking could be provided, all would be well and sisters could function 'properly' again. However, if knowledge is to be extended, and research strategies used to enhance nursing practice and challenge boundaries, it needs to concern itself with such questions as, 'Is the presently conceived sister role the best way of achieving the management, education and clinical functions necessary for good patient care?'

REFERENCES

Cohen L and Manion L (1980) *Research Methods in Education.* London: Croom Helm.

Cope Z (1955) *A Hundred Years of Nursing at St Mary's Hospital, Paddington.* London: Heinemann.

Davies J (1972) *A Study of Hospital Management Training in its Organisational Context: an Evaluation of First-Line Management Courses for Ward Sisters in the Manchester Region.* University of Manchester Centre of Business Research, Manchester Business School.

Davies C (1981) Training for ward sisters: an innovative research and development project. *Nurse Education Today,* 1(2): 16–18.

Department of Health and Social Security, Scottish Home and Health Department and Welsh Office (1972) *Report of the Committee on Nursing* (Chairman: Briggs). London: DHSS.

Department of Health and Social Security (1986) *Letter to Chairmen and Regional General Managers,* June 13.

Farnish S (1983) *Ward Sister Preparation: a Survey in Three Districts.* NERU Report No. 2. Chelsea College, University of London: Nursing Education Research Unit.

Greenwood J (1984) Nursing research: a position paper. *Journal of Advanced Nursing,* 9: 77–82.

King Edward's Hospital Fund for London (1982) *Ward Sister Preparation: a Contribution to Curriculum Building.* Project Paper 36. London: King's Fund.

Lathlean J and Farnish S (1984) *The Ward Sister Training Project: an Evaluation of a Training Scheme for Ward Sisters.* NERU Report No. 3. Chelsea College, University of London: Nursing Education Research Unit.

Lelean S (1973) *Ready for Report Nurse?* London: Royal College of Nursing.

Menzies I E P (1960) A case study in the functioning of social systems as a defence against anxiety. *Human Relations,* 13: 95–121.

Ministry of Health, Department of Health for Scotland, Ministry of Labour and National Service (1947) *Report of the Working Party on the Recruitment and Training of Nurses* (Chairman: Wood). London: HMSO.

Ministry of Health and Scottish Home and Health Department (1966) *Report of the Committee on Senior Nursing Staff Structure* (Chairman: Salmon). London: HMSO.

National Health Service Training Authority (1987) *Training Products and Services 1987–1988.* Bristol: NHSTA.

Ogier M (1980) *A Study of the Leadership Style and Verbal Interaction of Ward Sister with Nurse Learners.* PhD thesis, University of London.

Orton H D (1979) *Ward Learning Climate and Student Nurse Response.* MPhil. thesis, Sheffield City Polytechnic.

Pedler M (1974) An action research approach to training interventions. *Management Education and Development,* vol. 5.

Pembrey S E M (1980) *The Ward Sister: Key to Nursing.* London: Royal College of Nursing.

Rapoport R (1970) Three dilemmas of action research. *Human Relations,* 23: 499–513.

Redfern S J (1981) *Hospital Sisters: their Job Attitudes and Occupational Stability.* London: Royal College of Nursing.

Revans R W (1964) *Standards for Morale. Cause and Effect in Hospitals.* Oxford: Oxford University Press and Nuffield Provincial Hospitals Trust.

Rogers J and Lawrence J (1987) *Continuing Professional Education for Qualified Nurses, Midwives and Health Visitors.* Peterborough and London: Ashdale Press and Austen Cornish.

Royal College of Nursing (1943) *Report of the Nursing Reconstruction Committee* (Chairman: Horder). London: Royal College of Nursing.

Royal College of Nursing (1983) *Towards a New Professional Structure for Nursing.* London: Royal College of Nursing.

Runciman P (1983) *Ward Sister at Work.* Edinburgh: Churchill Livingstone.

Susman G I and Evered R D (1978) An assessment of the scientific merits of action research. *Administrative Science Quarterly,* 23: 582–603.

United Kingdom Central Council for Nursing, Midwifery and Health Visitors (1986) *Project 2000.* London: UKCC.

United Kingdom Central Council for Nursing, Midwifery and Health Visitors (1987) *Mandatory Periodic Refreshment for Nurses and Health Visitors.* Discussion Paper, London: UKCC.

Chapter 19

Ward Sister Preparation: A Survey in Three Districts

Judith Lathlean and Sally Farnish

INTRODUCTION

At the inception of the National Health Service in the late 1940s, the King Edward's Hospital Fund for London identified one possible reason for the wastage of trained staff as the 'almost universal lack of preparation for ward sister's posts and the example of those who have been appointed to them unprepared, with resultant strain and waste of effort' (King's Fund, 1948). Since then, the problem of lack of preparation has been reiterated many times and some attempts made to remedy the deficits. Nevertheless, 30 years later, concern was being expressed about the appointment of very young and relatively inexperienced sisters, again with little or no preparation for their new roles. As a result the King's Fund set up an experimental scheme for ward sisters, and the innovation was evaluated by the Nursing Education Research Unit (Lathlean and Farnish, 1984). (This project is the subject of chapter 18.)

The experimental scheme was established on the assumption that sisters and charge nurses *do* need preparation for their jobs – an assumption that has some basis in research and much support from anecdotal evidence, but which had not hitherto been the subject of a particular study. Thus a survey in three health districts was undertaken, as an adjunct to the main study, in an attempt to produce answers to the question, 'What do we know about the preparation nurses receive for the role of ward sister?' (Farnish, 1985).

AIMS OF THE STUDY

The study aimed to:

1. discover how nurses are prepared for the role of ward sister;
2. determine how nurses view effectiveness of preparation;
3. discover in which areas of responsibility sisters feel least prepared for their roles (Farnish, 1983).

As such, it was intended both to generate information from the three districts about the preparation of sisters and to examine whether this need for preparation varied across the different parts of their role. Furthermore, it was hoped that it would provide support for training schemes like the ones established by the King's Fund and additional insight into the areas of the role requiring the most development, plus the opportunity for some comparison between the views of those taking part in the scheme and nurses elsewhere.

A subsidiary, but nevertheless important, consideration was that of geography. The ward sister training scheme was operating in two London hospitals. A natural question could be asked: 'How different are the training and preparation needs of nurses in these settings compared with those in the provinces?'. The survey provided an ideal opportunity to explore the different perceptions of nurses in districts outside London. For ease of access, however, the preliminary and pilot work took place in London hospitals, but in ones that were unconnected with the training scheme.

RESEARCH DESIGN AND METHODS

Although the focus of the study was the sister, the views of staff nurses (as prospective sisters) and nursing officers (as former sisters) were considered to be important. Thus all three grades were included in the survey. The information to be gathered from the three groups – sisters, staff nurses and managers – was related primarily to preparation for the role of ward sister. The study started with a period of preparatory work followed by a pilot study, prior to the main survey, which involved postal questionnaires.

Preliminary planning and piloting

In order to expand and clarify the research questions, a series of interviews was carried out with 16 sisters, one senior nursing officer, two nursing officers and two staff nurses in a hospital in the Greater London area. The material from these interviews, together with the curriculum of the King's Fund scheme, formed the basis of questionnaires, which were then piloted in two stages in two other London hospitals.

The main survey

The survey took place in three health districts that had expressed interest in the training scheme: one in the north of England and two in the Midlands. Two were teaching districts with mixed urban and rural populations; the third was non-teaching and mainly rural. They comprised a variety of hospitals and units – large and small, acute and chronic. In order to facilitate comparison between the King's Fund scheme participants and those in the survey, certain specialty areas were excluded. These comprised accident and emergency, out-patients, theatres, maternity, psychiatry and mental subnormality, since staff from such areas were not involved in the scheme at the time of the study.

A total of 204 sisters was eligible, and all were included in the survey. A one-in-four random sample of eligible staff nurses (89) and all the related nursing officers (31) were also included. Access to staff in the three districts was negotiated by telephone, letter and visits. Each grade of staff had a different questionnaire to complete and return by post. The response rates across the three grades and three districts were high – 81 per cent of sisters (166), 91 per cent of staff nurses (81) and 94 per cent (all but two) of the nursing officers – indicating an interest and concern in the topic. Some demographic characteristics of the three groups are shown in Table 19.1.

Table 19.1 Some demographic characteristics of the three groups participating in the study

	Sisters/Charge nurses (N = 166)	Nursing officers (N = 29)	Staff nurses (N = 81)
Sex			
Female	92%	86%	99%
Male	8%	14%	1%
Age			
Mean	37 yr 2 mth	43 yr 6 mth	27 yr 1 mth
Marital status			
Single	32%	48%	37%
Married	60%	48%	58%
Divorced/separated	5%	4%	5%
Widowed	3%	—	—
One or more children	34%	38%	26%
British	96%	83%	97%
Working full time	89%	100%	78%

Eight per cent of the sister/charge nurse group were charge nurses. For convenience, the group as a whole is referred to in the text as sisters.

FINDINGS

In this chapter most of the material presented is that obtained from the sisters, although the views of staff nurses and nursing officers on certain aspects of preparation for the sister's role are also included. The findings presented focus on the following:

1. A profile of the sisters and the wards on which they worked.
2. Sisters' views of their own staff nurse experience as a preparation for the role of sister.
3. Sisters' recollections of how they acquired the knowledge and skills necessary for their role.
4. Professional development: attitudes and opportunities.
5. Experience of management courses.
6. Views of sisters, staff nurses and nursing officers on which aspects of a staff nurse's experience constituted an appropriate foundation for the sisters' role.

Details of all the findings are reported in Farnish (1983).

A profile of the sisters and their wards

The average age of the sisters in the survey was 37 years, with over three-quarters having worked as sisters for more than 2 years. (Five had been sisters for 30 years or more.) Prior to becoming sisters, the average length of time worked as a staff nurse was 3 years, but eight had less than 1 year's experience and a sizeable proportion (36 per cent) between 1 and 2 years. The sisters were asked how many hospitals, other than their training hospital, they had worked in as a sister or staff nurse. One in five had only worked in the hospital where they did their basic or post-basic training, but the average was between one and two. Very few had worked in more than three other hospitals.

The nursing training and professional qualifications of the sisters were considered. It is interesting to note that less than 5 per cent had the Diploma in Nursing Part A (only three had Part B), and one in five had undertaken a JBCNS course. However, four-fifths had attended courses or study days relevant to their jobs since becoming sisters.

The wards of the sisters included all specialties within surgery and medicine, including paediatrics, geriatrics and rehabilitation. Three-quarters of the wards were training wards for student or pupil nurses, but only 43 per cent of the sisters were GNC examiners or assessors. A minority of the sisters (35 per cent) were the sole sister of the ward; 28 per cent were the senior sister of two and one in five the junior sister of two. This is an interesting pattern and one that is not always matched in other districts where, for example, there is only one sister, except in a few specialty areas. The opportunity to work alongside another sister may well have implications for the nurse's feeling of adequacy of preparation.

Staff nurse experience as preparation for the sister role

Sisters were asked the general question, 'How adequate was your experience as a staff nurse in preparing you for the role of sister?', and three-quarters considered that it was adequate or more than adequate. When the responses were analysed according to the length of time that the sister had been a staff nurse, no significant relationship emerged. Many of their remarks indicated that they had been 'lucky' to work with a sister who was interested in teaching and who set a good example; others pointed out that it was adequate then because the role was far less complex than today, or was adequate for their role as a junior sister.

This topic was explored in more depth by considering how adequately the sisters felt prepared when first taking up post for the main areas of the role: management of patient care, methods of teaching and assessment of staff, ward management and personnel management. The areas of responsibility and the responses of the sisters are shown in Table 19.2. The results show the areas of greatest concern to be mobilising community resources, teaching and assessing, industrial relations and counselling members of the ward team. For all these aspects, around half or more of the group felt less than adequately prepared, and in terms of industrial relations this proportion rose to 81 per cent. When analysed by length of time in post there was no significant difference between the relatively newly appointed sisters and those who had been in post for many years, despite the increased emphasis on preparation in the 1970s and 1980s.

Almost exactly the same pattern was found when the King's Fund trainees were asked the same questions about inadequacy of preparation prior to their course, except that most felt confident about mobilising community resources (Lathlean and Farnish, 1984). Lack of preparation for teaching and assessment has been a common finding of other studies too, as highlighted in Lathlean (1987).

Acquiring knowledge and skills

A number of ways in which knowledge and skills can be acquired were identified in the course of the preliminary interviews, and these included:

1. trained by a sister (role model);
2. learned through experience (trial and error);

3. preparation from management courses;
4. in-service training.

Alternatively, 'no specific training' was used as a category to describe situations for which there was no formal training and was linked with 'learned through experience' to indicate a lack of preparation.

Sisters were asked to select one or more of these categories as their source(s) of learning for the items they had been asked to consider in terms of adequacy of preparation (Table 19.2).

Table 19.2 Sisters' views on how adequately they felt their training and subsequent experience had prepared them to cope with the responsibilities of the sister's role (N = 166)

Areas of responsibility	Less than adequate (%)	Adequate (%)	More than adequate (%)
Management of patient care			
1. Organisation and management of clinical care within a ward	10	66	24
2a. Prevention of accidents and incidents	17	74	9
2b. How to deal with those that occur	19	67	12
3a. Identifying the particular needs of the dying	19	55	25
3b. Supporting friends and relatives of the terminally ill	28	46	24
3c. Unexpected death	30	54	17
4. Mobilising community resources	48	42	9
Teaching and assessment			
5. Methods of teaching for various groups	60	33	4
6. Setting appropriate objectives for individual needs of ward staff; learners, trained staff	65	30	4
7a. Continuous assessment of staff	61	36	1
7b. Writing reports	51	45	3
Ward management			
8. Establishing and maintaining good relationships with other members of the health care team	12	65	22
9. The responsibilities of leadership	18	64	18
10. Planning off duty rotas and allocation of nurses	28	50	20
11. Implementing hospital policies and procedures	27	62	10
Personnel management			
12. Issues concerned with industrial relations	81	13	2
13. Dealing with complaints from patients, relatives or visitors	30	60	8
14. Counselling members of the ward team	51	44	4
15. Understanding the role of the nursing officer	31	52	8

NB: Percentages add up to slightly less than 100% as a small proportion of respondents did not answer the question.

Those selected by far the most frequently were informal means, that is no specific training and/or learned through experience. Learning from another sister (role modelling) was important for about one-third or more of the sisters in relation to the management of patient care (particularly the organisation and management of clinical care within a ward) and ward management. But the apparent influence of role models was less overall than might have been expected from the findings of other earlier studies, for example Pembrey (1980) on the role of the ward sister.

Management courses and in-service training were relatively unimportant sources of learning, a finding which is perhaps unsurprising and supported by the work of Heath (1980) and Rogers and Lawrence (1987). This is worrying, however, as learning by trial and error has a tendency to be stressful and to promote previous bad practice (Runciman, 1983).

Attitudes to and opportunities for professional development

All but one of the sisters (and all but one of the staff nurses) felt that continuing education should be available for all registered nurses; the majority considered that it should be a shared responsibility of the individual nurse and management.

The majority of sisters (80 per cent) felt the need personally for further professional development, particularly in relation to keeping up to date with developments in nursing, medicine and drug therapies and with relevant clinical topics. The great majority also considered that developing their skills as a manager was important, though this did not achieve quite the same rating as clinical knowledge. (This has been corroborated by Rogers and Lawrence (1987), who found that clinical topics were more highly favoured than management topics by the group of trained staff, including sisters.) The area that sisters were least likely to rate as important was that of research: 41 per cent said that it was only of minor importance.

Sisters were asked about the opportunities that existed for professional development. The type of provision that sisters were most likely to say was available to them was that concerned with widening their knowledge in a particular area of clinical interest. They were asked to specify factors that prevented the uptake of training opportunities; those cited most frequently by the respondents were shortage of staff in the ward preventing attendance (65 per cent), lack of finance (for local provision or secondment elsewhere; 45 per cent), inadequate advance publicity (59 per cent) and lack of encouragement from management to attend (30 per cent). It is predictable that staff shortage was given as a reason for inability to take advantage of training opportunities; this is, however, related to management encouragement, in that managers are in a position to ensure (or not) adequate staffing levels to allow sisters to participate.

Management courses

Management courses have long been available to sisters. Varying widely in organisation and content, the main criticism levelled at them has been that too often the tutors are industry orientated and do not fully appreciate or understand the situations encountered in a hospital. The sisters taking part in this study were asked a number of questions relating to their experiences of management courses.

Sixty-four per cent of sisters in the survey had attended a management course, but the proportions differed across the three districts; in one district it was over three-quarters, in another under a half, and in the third, 67 per cent. Of those who had attended, 40 per cent had been in their post for more than 2 years when seconded to a first-line management course, yet nearly 70 per cent considered the most appropriate time to attend would have been as a staff nurse.

The majority of sisters (83 per cent) attended courses that were held outside the district, in polytechnics or colleges of further education, and the average length was 3 weeks. Many problems surrounding these courses were identified, both by the sisters themselves and by their nursing officers. They included an inadequate number of places, poor or insufficient information prior to attendance, and sketchy or non-existent feedback and discussion after the course. Almost a quarter of sisters felt dissatisfied with the course. Just under half felt satisfied, but with only some aspects. Forty-six per cent considered that it helped them a little with their performance, but 34 per cent said that it did not help them at all. The favourable comments included 'helpful', 'useful', 'stimulating' and 'enjoyable', whereas the unfavourable often referred to the lack of relevance to the role, the gap between course contents and need, the inappropriate business or industrial orientation and the poor timing. Thus, the picture overall is not encouraging. The majority of sisters in this survey appear not to have been satisfied with their course (Farnish, 1983).

Staff nurse experience

In an effort to ascertain what aspects of a staff nurse's experience might prepare the way for a sister's post, various questions were asked of all three grades. The average length of time needed in a staff nurse's post before taking up a sister's post was considered to be between 2 and 3 years. This average concealed quite a variation in views, however, and while 13 per cent of sisters considered that less than 18 months' experience could be sufficient, all the nursing officers considered that sisters should have 18 months' experience or more as staff nurses. The views of staff nurses more nearly matched those of the sisters, though a slightly higher proportion of staff nurses than sisters felt that between 3 and 4 years' experience was necessary.

When probed about particular experience as a staff nurse, a high proportion of sisters (87 per cent) considered that experience in more than one specialty was fairly or very important, whereas the possession of more than one nursing qualification was thought not to be important by 59 per cent of the respondents. Interestingly, one-third considered that experience in a hospital other than his/her training school was not important, despite the policy of some hospitals, particularly prior to the current concerns about retention, to encourage their trained nurses to gain experience outside the training hospital.

Staff nurses were asked for what reasons they felt a staff nurse might not apply for a sister's post. About half suggested that this would be for reasons of outside commitment or an inability to work full time. Just over 40 per cent said that the responsibility was too great, and about the same proportion said that there was a lack of confidence. Surprisingly few (7 per cent) said that contentment with the staff nurse role would be an inhibitor, despite the often quoted anecdote that many nurses shun management roles and wish to remain 'at the bedside'.

About 70 per cent of all three grades felt that the responsibility for preparing staff nurses should not rest with the sisters alone. One telling comment indicated the sisters' lack of suitability for the sole task since 'they themselves have not had any specific or systematic training in the past'. Reference was made to the need to involve other disciplines and grades, such as nursing officers and in-service education staff. One of the staff nurses saw the benefit of having 'a total view of the role of sister rather than just one person's ideas' and another warned against 'a carbon copy of the previous sister'.

A majority of all grades felt that not enough was done to prepare the staff nurse for the sister's post, though a higher proportion of sisters than the other two groups felt this way. There was considerable support for 'more formal and specific preparation' while in a staff nurse post – a plea that has become increasingly recognised since the survey, in part stimulated by such initiatives as the DHSS encouragement of professional development schemes for staff nurses (DHSS, 1982).

THE IMPLICATIONS AND POTENTIAL OF THE STUDY

Though some caution needs to be exercised with a retrospective survey of this kind in terms of the recall ability of respondents, the transition between staff nurse and sister is such a critical one that views about it are likely to remain vivid for some time. And indeed, many of the findings support previous studies and are reinforced by subsequent work, such as that of Rogers and Lawrence (1987). The validity of case study and small-scale survey research is often tested out by the subsequent judgment that the results seem to fit reality (Walker, 1980). This study has obviously caught the imagination of a wide audience since it has been referred to in a number of publications, and many have deemed it 'to fit reality'. Further-more, from informal contact with health districts, it is known that it has been used to inform the development of programmes for sister preparation, since it highlights those aspects where particular attention appears to be necessary. In addition, it provides 'ammunition' to persuade doubtful managers of the need for specific preparation.

The study also raises issues that have been actively debated in recent years. For example, is the sister role the most appropriate focus for professional and management development, especially when resources are limited, or would a programme commencing with the newly registered nurse make specific training for sisters largely redundant? (The DHSS-funded study of professional development schemes for newly qualified nurses concluded that professional development is necessary for *all* nurses post-registration, and that expecting sisters to participate in the development of their staff nurses without sufficient personal training, development and support is an inefficient use of resources; see Lathlean et al, 1986, and chapter 20.)

Secondly, what are the most helpful ways of preparing for and developing the role, given that relying on experience alone is ineffectual, role modelling can be overestimated and management courses of the past were of limited use to many participants? Since the survey, new or reworked approaches have been increasingly promoted such as open and distance learning, role-based development and training based on an analysis of competencies.

Finally, the role of sister is changing with such influences as the impact of general management, the devolution of budgets to ward level, the problems of recruitment and retention, the need to attend to efficiency and effectiveness, the increased attention to quality of care issues and the changing patterns of the way nursing care is organised, particularly if primary nursing is implemented. Perhaps the key to the developing role is to prepare sisters to manage change, to cope in an unstable environment and one with considerable pressures such as limited resources and competing demands.

It would be of considerable interest to repeat this survey now in order to determine how well sisters feel prepared for their roles today. Even with the increased provision for sisters (as indicated by a recent, unpublished study commissioned by the NHS Training Authority), with many more districts now having specific programmes for sisters, it is unlikely that *all* sisters will feel confident – and prepared – to handle the complexities of the role in the current climate of rapid change. Maybe, though, the profession is expecting too much of this role, and the time is ripe for a reconsideration of how nursing is delivered and managed. There are signs that this is beginning to happen in some health districts, providing a challenge to the traditional role and to the training required.

REFERENCES

Department of Health and Social Security (1982) *Framework for Professional Developmental Programmes for Nurses*. London: DHSS.

Farnish S (1983) *Ward Sister Preparation: a Survey in Three Districts*. NERU Report No. 2. Chelsea College, University of London: Nursing Education Research Unit.

Farnish S (1985) How are sisters prepared? *Nursing Times*, Occasional Paper, 81(4): 47-50.

Heath J (1980) In-Service Training and all that. *Nursing Times*, 76(25): 1081.

King's Fund (1948) *Annual Report of the Fund*. London: King Edward's Hospital Fund for London.

Lathlean J (1987) Training the teacher. *Nursing Times*, 83(40): 36-37.

Lathlean J and Farnish S (1984) *The Ward Sister Training Project: an Evaluation of a Training Scheme*. NERU Report No. 3. Chelsea College, University of London: Nursing Education Research Unit.

Lathlean J, Smith G and Bradley S (1986) *Post-Registration Development Schemes Evaluation*. NERU Report No. 4. Chelsea College, University of London: Nursing Education Research Unit.

Pembrey S (1980) *The Ward Sister – Key to Nursing*. London: Royal College of Nursing.

Rogers J and Lawrence J (1987) *Continuing Professional Education for Qualified Nurses, Midwives and Health Visitors*. Peterborough: Ashdale Press.

Runciman P (1983) *Ward Sister at Work*. Edinburgh: Churchill Livingstone.

Walker R (1980) The conduct of educational case studies: ethics, theory and procedures. In: *Rethinking Educational Research*, eds. Dockrell W B and Hamilton D. Sevenoaks: Hodder and Stoughton.

Chapter 20

Development Schemes for Newly Registered Nurses

Judith Lathlean and Gillian Smith

BACKGROUND

There has been an increasing recognition in the last decade that nurses are often inadequately prepared for new roles, in particular their initial job following registration and their first post as a sister. This has accompanied a growing belief that continuing professional education for nurses is not an expensive luxury but an important necessity, given that the initial training cannot hope to provide all that is required for the complex nursing situations of the present day.

The 1970s and early 1980s also saw a focus in nursing on a number of related issues such as standards of care, the development and clarification of roles of trained nurses and the use of resources in clinical settings. For example, the Royal College of Nursing produced several discussion documents and reports highlighting some of the principles of what constitutes good patient care (RCN, 1979) and how high standards can be gained (RCN, 1981a). It also looked at the professional structure and delineation of roles required in nursing to accomplish the dual goals of good patient care and satisfying career opportunities for all qualified nurses (RCN, 1981b, 1983).

This work on professional structure coincided with a major seminar in nursing entitled 'Professional Development in Clinical Nursing - the 1980s', convened by the Chief Nursing Officer of the DHSS (DHSS, 1982a). The aim was to consider such objectives as improvement in standards of nursing care and enhanced career prospects and, as a 'first step in a series of initiatives', it was proposed that 'newly registered nurses should have a period of professional consolidation and development following registration. This period would consist of supervised and supported practice in a designated training area and would take the form of a "core professional module" - applicable to nurses in any branch of nursing. A small number of experimental schemes are to be evaluated and for these a common framework will be required' (DHSS, 1982b).

The decision was to start with the newly registered nurse rather than other grades of nurse, although research studies (such as by Pembrey, 1980, Farnish, 1983, and Lathlean and Farnish, 1984) were clearly indicating the development and training needs of ward sisters and the key nature of their role. However, the schemes were also aimed, implicitly if not explicitly, at tackling the broader issues of increasing standards, the better use of resources and the retention of trained nursing staff, as well as the development of individuals.

Although the ward sister role has been the subject of much research, very few studies have concentrated on the role of the staff nurse immediately post-registration. One notable exception is the work of Vaughan who, in a small-scale study, examined the factors affecting the transition between student and staff nurse status (Vaughan, 1980). She concluded that the greatest areas of difficulty were found in relationships with other staff and in management tasks. More recently, and again in a very small study, Shand (1986) has focused specifically on the role and educational needs of the newly qualified staff nurse in an acute services unit, and another study (Humphries, 1987) has sought in part to replicate that of Vaughan, with very similar results. Nevertheless, it remains an area in which information is largely anecdotal or locally based.

THE RATIONALE FOR AN EVALUATIVE STUDY

Having recommended the establishment of programmes for the professional development of newly registered nurses, the DHSS saw merit in the evaluation of a small number of pilot schemes. It was hoped that this could pave the way for a much larger number of similar initiatives, or at least provide substantial research-based indication of the best way forward.

The evaluation of an experimental scheme for the training of ward sisters was already underway in the Nursing Education Research Unit (see chapter 18). It seemed appropriate to locate there also this related project – an evaluation of the effectiveness of three professional development programmes for post-registration nurses – and to adopt a similar research approach, that of action research.

The effect of this was both to consolidate and to expand the area of the unit's work concerned with continuing education and the role of trained nursing staff. It also gave opportunity for the further development of action research and evaluation techniques. The two projects were envisaged to be highly complementary in terms of their methodology and subject areas, a view that was borne out in reality.

RESEARCH APPROACH

The professional development evaluation project took place over a 3-year period (May 1983 – May 1986) and aimed to:

1. monitor the establishment and conduct of the experimental pilot schemes;
2. assess their effectiveness in providing appropriate professional development for newly registered nurses;
3. assist in the modification and improvement of the schemes;
4. assess the extent to which the schemes would be applicable elsewhere;
5. assess the implications for patient care.

It specifically sought to identify the resources involved in setting up and maintaining the schemes, the outcomes with respect to the knowledge and skills of the newly registered nurses, and the effects of the schemes both on the organisations and on patient care.

The approach chosen was 'in line with current thinking in evaluation research, particularly in education, and [was] set in an action research framework. This approach is informed by a certain view – and one gaining increasing recognition – of what is the appropriate foundation for the study of society and nursing in particular' (Lathlean et al, 1986).

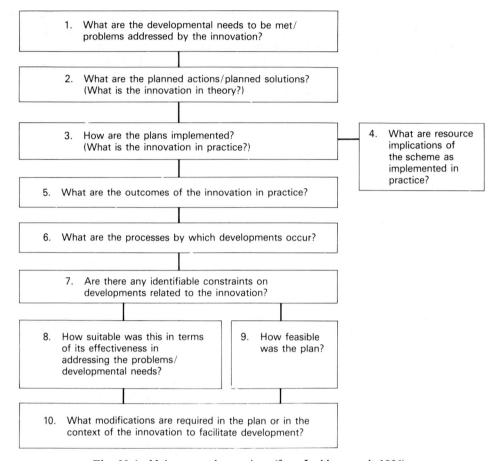

Fig. 20.1 Major research questions (from Lathlean et al, 1986)

The evaluation strategy adopted is one where the emphasis is less on hypothesis testing and more on the discovery of issues and their development into categories for further study and analysis. The research usually proceeds in a series of stages from relatively open-ended enquiry to more structured and focused data collection. The researcher does not seek to demonstrate causal relationships between variables but rather to illuminate and understand the complex processes of, in this instance, individual and organisational change.

Further, an 'intensive' research design (Harré, 1979) was chosen, where the interest is in how a process works in a particular case or small number of cases, rather than in the discovery of the common properties of a whole population (Sayer, 1984). This raises issues of representativeness and generalisability. The researcher does not pretend that the findings of the study are representative of a whole population, nor even typical. Nevertheless, they can be illustrative of possibilities, particularly if the data are presented in such a way that others may judge their relevance to their own situation. Yin (1981) also argues that the merit of case study lies in the attempt 'to examine . . . a contemporary phenomenon in its real-life context [and not] deliberately divorce it from its context' as occurs in an experimental study.

Action research has been described elsewhere, in chapter 18. Its features can vary but, commonly, emphasis is placed on problem solving or the facilitation of development as well as on the advancement of knowledge. Sometimes, the researcher is directly involved in implementing changes in addition to making recommendations for change, based on research data. However, in this project the researchers attempted to provide information on which the practitioners and policy-makers could base their decisions, mainly through collaboration with them and by informal and formal feedback to individuals, groups and committees. Nevertheless, the action component was not such a powerful feature of this project as in the ward sister study.

Table 20.1   Summary of research methods

First phase (May 1983 – December 1984)	Second phase: detailed study (January 1985 – May 1986)
Relatively open-ended interviews (course staff; ward sisters; managers; course members) Observation in various settings (e.g. wards, study days) Attendance at meetings (e.g. district planning teams, project management team, steering group, informal) Analysis of literature and documentation	*Study of cases* Semi-structured interviews of 12 NRNs (6 CMs; 6 non-CMs) plus their sisters, managers, tutors on four occasions Observation of NRNs on own wards, occasional study days Completion of 'formats' by NRNs, WSs and tutors on specific activities undertaken during sample weeks *Questionnaire study* Questionnaires (4) completed by: 1. All NRNs registering at a specific time (96)★ 2. Sisters of these NRNs (86)★ . . . at start of 6-month period 3. Same NRNs as for item 1 (92)★ 4. Same sisters as for item 2 (100)★ . . . at end of 6-month period *Other data collection* Semi-structured interviews of: ● course staff and managers ● steering group members Questionnaires completed by course staff (past and current) Attendance at meetings, e.g. district planning teams, project management team, steering group informal Analysis of literature and documentation

Key
NRN, newly registered nurse; WS, ward sister; CM, course member; non-CM, An NRN not on the course

★Figures in brackets indicate number of responses
(From Lathlean et al, 1986)

DESIGN AND METHODS

The project was in two main phases, each lasting about 18 months. The first phase included a literature review, the development of an historical account of events and the identification of key issues. It led to the production of a series of major research questions (Figure 20.1) and to the clarification of a set of presuppositions or assumptions, which were to underpin the second phase of the study. The clarification of presuppositions was an attempt to answer such questions as, 'What is nursing?', 'What is *good* nursing?' and 'In what ways can the individual nurse, ward or organisation contribute to this?'. They were fundamental to the project because 'they informed the choice of data to be collected in the second stage . . . they provided the categories to be used in the analysis of these data and . . . an indication of the values implicit . . . in the project' (Lathlean et al, 1986).

The second phase comprised a study of cases (12 newly registered nurses and their wards during a 6-month period), a questionnaire study involving newly registered nurses and their ward sisters on two occasions, and other data collection such as interviews with programme organisers, observation and participation in district and national level meetings. (The methods used are summarised in Table 20.1.)

The critical focus was the study of cases (including both those taking part in the course and those not), and the main areas examined were the:

1. characteristics of the newly registered nurse;
2. characteristics of the nurse's ward sister;
3. structure and culture of the ward;
4. learning, development and support needs of the nurse;
5. learning and development opportunities;
6. processes of change;
7. constraints;

at the beginning, end and during a 6-month period.

The questionnaire study enabled the collection of data from a much greater number of people and was used primarily to ascertain the extent to which the cases were illustrative of the whole group.

SELECTED FINDINGS

The range of data gained was considerable and included the needs of the nurses and the organisation, the processes that occurred during the development of the schemes and the outcomes, as well as constraints encountered and the resource requirements. A few of the major factors emerging are highlighted and their implications presented. First the scheme itself is briefly described.

The schemes in practice

Each of the three schemes was based on a common framework provided by the DHSS (DHSS, 1982b). The framework described a programme of 6 months working in a designated training area, with approximately 16 days study leave. The sister in charge of the training area was to be the person with main responsibility for developing and monitoring the individual registered nurses. The course tutor(s) were to be responsible for the theoretical content, with a 'clinically experienced nurse' as facilitator for the course members.

In practice, the schemes were developed slightly differently in each of the three health districts to take account of local resources, needs and preferences. For example, the number of study days varied from 11½ to 18, and the course members comprised between 20 and 30 per cent of the newly registered nurses in each district during the first 18 months (representing 24, 25 and 72 nurses respectively), rising to between 39 per cent and 62 per cent in 1986. Each district had at least two members of staff with major parts to play in the scheme at any one time. All had one or more course tutors, but in two of the districts the tutor and facilitator roles were combined.

The needs of newly registered nurses

Although there were often considerable individual differences, the newly registered nurses were found to have needs for development in all of the following seven aspects of their role:

1. Knowledge and skills required for clinical and managerial aspects, including management of patient care, ward management, clinical skills and knowledge and understanding of the role.
2. Interpersonal skills and knowledge, including communication with patients, relatives and other staff, teaching and expression of ideas and views.
3. Autonomy, including the ability to make decisions and the capacity for self direction and analytical thought.
4. Personal development such as awareness of own needs, strengths and weaknesses, and self-confidence.
5. Attitudes to professional philosophy and issues.
6. Career planning and commitment to staying in nursing.
7. Coping with stress in own role.

There were also issues identified within the wards such as the suitability of some wards as learning environments, the organisation and standards of patient care, and the roles and capacities of other members of the health-care team.

Opportunities for development and support

Opportunities for learning and development during the first few months as a staff nurse came from a number of sources, as shown in Figure 20.2. These were activities, occasions and events where the nurse perceived she had actually learnt something or which provided support. To estimate the quantity and quality of opportunity experienced by the 12 case study nurses, scores were given on a 1-7 scale, where 1 indicated very limited opportunity and 7 indicated considerable opportunity with good learning potential. The scores were aggregated and an average rating for each category of opportunity was gained (Figure 20.2). As expected, course members tended to have more and better opportunities than did those nurses not on the course, but this was not always the case. For example, course members spent less time working with their ward sisters than non-course members, probably because of their greater absence from the wards on study days.

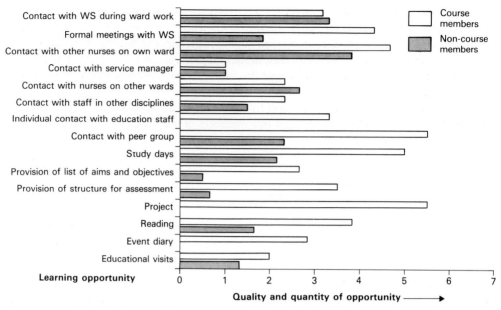

Fig. 20.2   Comparison of average ratings for opportunities for course members and non-course members
(From Lathlean et al, 1986)

Developments in nurses

Just as the needs of the individuals varied (some started off being more knowledgeable, skilled or competent in various aspects), so did their development over the 6 months. But, overall, those on the course tended to show a greater range and depth of development across all the different parts of their role, including technical and interpersonal knowledge and skills, autonomy and personal and professional aspects. When considering the apparent *extent* of change taking place during the 6 months among the 12 case study nurses, five out of the six course members developed more than the non-course members. This was particularly marked in areas such as increased knowledge of research-based information for nursing care, the confident management of a ward (two of the six non-course members developed little and could not be confidently left in charge at the end of the 6 months), and understanding of the role of the registered nurse.

They also tended to change more in respect of their interpersonal skills and knowledge, such as communication with patients and relatives, dealing with distressing situations (where development was *only* apparent among the case study course members), developing an awareness of different ways of teaching and greater ability to work with other staff and delegate appropriately.

Improvement was found among half of the course members, but only in one of the non-course members, in organising and setting priorities. Four course members appeared much better able to make decisions, but the three non-course members of greatest concern developed little if at all. Course members also developed more in terms of thinking analytically, contributing ideas and being critical and questioning. These aspects were referred to as 'autonomy', and this appeared to be a *key* element in that all the newly registered nurses who did not develop in this respect showed a low level of development generally.

The nurses also changed personally, for example in their self-awareness, openness, responsibility and motivation relating to work, response to stress and soundly based confidence. This was always far more pronounced among the group of six course members than the others. In fact, in some aspects, one or two of those not on the course actually deteriorated (for example, in their responsibility and motivation to work, response to stress, and soundly based confidence).

Since course members tended to change and develop more than other nurses in the same period of time, it was important to find out what facilitated these changes. Learning and development seemed to be promoted in three major ways:

1. by general processes such as experience, learning from observing others (role modelling) and individualised learning;
2. by independent learning such as skills practice with feedback, individual study and educational visits;
3. by facilitative and supportive processes such as discussion of experience, feedback on abilities and progress, comparison with peers, expression and justification of own views and discussion of feelings.

The general processes were found to occur to some extent in all nurses, but independent learning was far less common among those not on the programme. This group of nurses also experienced facilitative and supportive processes rarely if ever, and this way of learning seemed to be most beneficial in promoting aspects of autonomy and personal development – the apparent key to success as a newly registered nurse.

In summary, those on the programme tended to develop more rapidly because they experienced certain processes more: for example, they had greater opportunity for learning by self-direction, easier and more continuous access to a facilitator, contact with a peer group, and addition of perspective and educational input from outside the ward.

THE IMPLICATIONS OF THE STUDY

The findings suggest that there is a need for a comprehensive plan for staff development that recognises that all trained staff require continuing education and support. Also there are important aspects in the organisation (such as the way in which care is managed, resources are used and standards achieved) that must be developed as well if individuals are to thrive. Formal learning opportunities such as courses and study days may be part of this, but, if the provision is to be sufficiently flexible to meet both individual and organisational needs, a range of different opportunities should be encouraged. This should include:

1. the joint identification of needs between nurses, their managers and others (such as peers and educators);
2. regular review of progress (incorporating self-assessment, peer and manager review);
3. role-based learning in appropriate clinical/practice settings;
4. opportunity for peer group membership to share knowledge and experience aided by facilitators;
5. support and guidance from outside the clinical setting;
6. time away from the work for discussion and reflection.

The study also reinforced the need for national commitments and policies in relation to continuing education, as well as attempting to assess the quality of continuing education. Both of these areas have received a fair degree of attention since the completion of the study.

CURRENT INTEREST AND FUTURE INITIATIVES

There has been considerable interest shown in continuing professional education at a national level, particularly by the statutory and professional nursing bodies. Both the English National Board (ENB, 1985) and the United Kingdom Central Council for Nursing, Midwifery and Health Visiting (UKCC, 1986) have highlighted its importance. The UKCC has issued a discussion document on mandatory periodic refreshment for nurses and health visitors (UKCC, 1987), a document that embodies – or implies – many of the above mentioned principles. The Department of Health, too, is aware of the value of continuing education, not only in terms of individual development but also to aid career progression and to help in the retention of nurses (Department of Health, 1988).

A national study by Rogers and Lawrence (1987) has indicated the very great variety in the extent of continuing education opportunities across the country. Clearly, there is need for the development of 'explicit philosophy and policies in relation to continuing professional education' (Rogers and Lawrence, 1987) throughout regional and district health authorities, as well as for the expansion of what has often been sparse, or even non-existent, provision.

Attention has also turned to the assessment of standards of nursing education, including performance review and the development of performance indicators, and the English National Board has sponsored a major research project in relation to this.

There is considerable room for further research in this area. First, there would be merit in undertaking follow-up studies of those who have been part of professional development programmes to ascertain the long-term effects of their experience. Although the short-term benefits have been established, little is known about whether these are sustained. For example, does participation in a programme as a newly registered nurse have a positive effect on career plans, attitudes to nursing, retention in the profession and performance over a period of years?

Though district health authority autonomy in the development of continuing education ensures that local needs are met, much can be gained from the collation and cross-fertilisation of approaches and philosophies nationally. More work should be done to bring together information on different programmes so that districts can gain from the experiences of others.

A third important aspect for consideration is that of the role of the newly registered nurse. This has been altering and is likely to do so much more with the implementation of proposals such as UKCC's Project 2000, changes in the structure and organisation of basic training, the expansion of primary nursing, and other developments. Indeed, the examination of the changing nature and function of nursing roles should be a continuing priority in nursing and nursing research since it is a vital prerequisite to the provision of the most effective nursing care.

REFERENCES

Department of Health and Social Security (1982a) *Professional Development in Clinical Nursing – the 1980s*. London: DHSS.

Department of Health and Social Security (1982b) *Framework for Professional Development Programmes for Nurses*. London: DHSS.

Department of Health (1988) *The Way Ahead: Career Pathways for Nurses, Midwives and Health Visiting*. A Report to the NHS Management Board. London: Department of Health.

English National Board for Nursing, Midwifery and Health Visiting (1985) *Professional Education/Training Courses: Consultation Paper*. London: ENB.

Farnish S (1983) *Ward Sister Preparation: a Survey in Three Districts*. NERU Report No. 2. Chelsea College, University of London: Nursing Education Research Unit.

Harré R (1979) *Social Being*. Oxford: Blackwell.

Humphries A (1987) *The Transition from Student to Staff Nurse: a Study of Features Affecting Newly Qualified Nurses*. Unpublished BSc (Health Studies) degree thesis, University of Leicester.

Lathlean J and Farnish S (1984) *The Ward Sister Training Project: an Evaluation of a Training Scheme for Ward Sisters*. NERU Report No. 3. Chelsea College, University of London: Nursing Education Research Unit.

Lathlean J, Smith G and Bradley S (1986) *Post-Registration Development Schemes Evaluation*. NERU Report No. 4. King's College, University of London: Nursing Education Research Unit.

Pembrey S E M (1980) *The Ward Sister: Key to Nursing*. London: Royal College of Nursing.

Rogers J and Lawrence J (1987) *Continuing Professional Education for Qualified Nurses, Midwives and Health Visitors*. Peterborough and London: Ashdale Press and Austen Cornish.

Royal College of Nursing (1979) *Standards of Nursing Care*. London: Royal College of Nursing.

Royal College of Nursing (1981a) *Towards Standards*. London: Royal College of Nursing.

Royal College of Nursing (1981b) *A Structure for Nursing*. London: Royal College of Nursing.

Royal College of Nursing (1983) *Towards a New Professional Structure for Nursing*. London: Royal College of Nursing.

Sayer A (1984) *Method in Social Science: a Realist Approach*. London: Hutchinson.

Shand M J (1986) *Report of the Survey into the Role and Educational Needs of the Newly Qualified Staff Nurse in the Acute Services Unit*. Grampian Health Board, unpublished report.

United Kingdom Central Council for Nursing, Midwifery and Health Visitors (1986) *Project 2000*. London: UKCC.

United Kingdom Central Council for Nursing, Midwifery and Health Visitors (1987) *Mandatory Periodic Refreshment for Nurses and Health Visitors*. Discussion Paper. London: UKCC.

Vaughan B (1980) *The Newly Qualified Staff Nurse: Factors Affecting Transition*. Unpublished master's thesis, University of Manchester.

Yin R (1981) The case study crisis: some answers. *Administrative Science Quarterly*, **26**(1): 58-65.

Chapter 21

Communication Skills Teaching in Nurse Education: A Curriculum Development Project

Jill MacLeod Clark and Anne Tomlinson

BACKGROUND

The teaching of communication skills to nurses in the UK is a relatively new phenomenon. While the topic has been addressed in many psychiatric nursing courses for over two decades, recognition of the need for such teaching in general nurse training did not generally materialise until the late 1970s (Macfarlane, 1980; Faulkner 1985). With hindsight, it is difficult to comprehend why so many generations of nurses have been deprived of educational input in an area that is of such central importance to all nursing practice.

The stimulus for change and for raising the profile of communication skills in nursing is not easy to pinpoint accurately, but at least two factors can be implicated. These are the changes in the philosophy and practice of nursing care and findings from research studies that have demonstrated inadequacies in nurse–patient communication. The dramatic shift in emphasis in the philosophy and practice of nursing over the past decade or so has inevitably influenced the content of nursing curricula. The incorporation of the principles of the nursing process and individualised patient care has highlighted the need for nurses to be skilled communicators.

Assessment of patients' needs and problems, the planning of care with the patient or client and the subsequent evaluation of care are all activities that require specific and effective communication skills.

A further development in nursing, which has focused attention on the need for nurses to develop their communication skills, is the shift in emphasis towards health rather than sickness. This shift has important implications in terms of the skills required both when acting as an effective health educator and when encouraging patients and clients to become more involved in and to take more responsibility for their own care.

The second factor that has undoubtedly increased awareness of the need to help nurses develop their communication skills is the plethora of research findings that have demonstrated inadequacies in communication. For example, a succession of studies has been published, which indicate that patients are more dissatisfied with communication than with any other aspect of their care (Cartwright, 1964; Raphael, 1969; Reynolds, 1978).

Further evidence that communication between nurses and patients is often poor or ineffective has accumulated over the past decade. Researchers have examined nurse–patient interaction in a variety of clinical settings and their findings have been strikingly consistent. For example: deficiencies in nurse–patient communication have been identified in relation to both the quantity and quality of interaction in, among other areas, intensive care units (Ashworth, 1980), medical wards (Faulkner, 1980), radiotherapy wards (Bond, 1983) and surgical wards (Macleod Clark, 1983). In seeking an explanation for their findings, all these researchers postulated a link between poor communication and the lack of appropriate communication skills teaching in nurse education programmes.

This background provided the impetus for a curriculum development project in this area. The overall aim of the project was to explore both the feasibility and the effectiveness of incorporating a structured communication skills input into basic nurse education programmes. Funding and support were provided by the Health Education Council, who were conscious of the need for nurses to possess basic communication skills in order to fulfil a health education role.

The Communication in Nurse Education (CINE) project was initiated in 1980 under the overall direction of Dr Ann Faulkner of the Department of Nursing Studies, University of Manchester. Two project officers were appointed, one of whom (Anne Tomlinson) was based in the Department of Nursing Studies, King's College. The project was designed in three parts:

1. A survey of DNEs' and tutors' perceptions of communication skills teaching.
2. A curriculum development project aimed at evaluating the integration of a communication skills teaching programme into the first 18 months of basic nurse training.
3. A study to investigate the preparation of nurse tutors for communication skills teaching and their subsequent experiences of putting such teaching into practice. The approaches used and the findings for each part of the project are summarised briefly.

PART I: SCHOOLS OF NURSING SURVEY

The purpose of this survey was to establish the extent to which communication skills were currently being taught in schools, the extent to which teachers were prepared for communication skills teaching, and attitudes and beliefs about the place of such teaching in basic nurse education. Questionnaires were initially sent to all Directors of Nurse Education (DNEs) in England, Wales and Northern Ireland. Subsequently, a further batch of questionnaires was sent to each school to be completed by the tutor(s) with responsibility for teaching communication skills.

As part of this survey, schools were also asked to indicate whether they would be interested in participating in the next phases of the project.

Findings

Response rates for both parts of the survey were high – 84 per cent for the DNEs and 75 per cent for the tutors. In general, there was a high level of agreement between the two groups in terms of their perceptions and beliefs about communication skills in the curriculum.

The majority of respondents felt that it was very important that communication should be taught to student nurses. However, almost all respondents reported that less than 5 per cent of curriculum time was devoted to the topic. Communication was both taught as a separate subject and integrated within other sessions in nearly every school. In Scotland almost half the tutors who found themselves teaching this subject did not feel that they had had any preparation for such teaching. In the rest of Britain 73 per cent of the tutors had had some preparation, although overall less than 5 per cent of them felt adequately prepared to teach this subject.

The view of the DNEs was that only 2 per cent of their staff were well prepared for teaching communication skills. The majority of tutors felt that there was inadequate provision of appropriate courses, and frequently commented on the difficulties inherent in teaching the subject. Interestingly, 96 per cent of schools possessed a good range of audio-visual aids and equipment, including tape-recorders, videotape recorders and cameras. However, these resources were often reported to be underutilised. Seventy per cent of the tutors wished to attend a course on teaching communication skills. They identified a lack of information on how to teach the subject, and the majority felt that it was a neglected area in courses for nurse teachers.

Full details of the questionnaires used in the survey and the findings can be found in the report of the survey (Faulkner et al, 1986).

PART II: CURRICULUM DEVELOPMENT PROJECT

The aim of this project was to explore the feasibilities and effects of incorporating structured communication skills teaching input into the first 18 months of an RGN programme. Projects such as this are essentially a form of evaluation research and usually involve a mix of methods encompassing both quantitative and qualitative approaches to data collection.

A quasi experimental design was used in an attempt to measure the impact of the CINE input by comparing groups of students who received the teaching with similar groups who did not. However, the limitations of this approach were recognised. The unique nature of each school of nursing means that the data generated from a curriculum development project need also to be treated as a set of case studies. While important insights can be gained from examining the outcome of a project in terms of increments in students' knowledge and skills, equal weight must be placed on more qualitative data that address the process of developing a curriculum and the context in which curriculum change takes place (Parlett and Hamilton, 1972).

As this was a national study involving six schools of nursing throughout England, two project officers were appointed to act as tutors/facilitators in the schools where the CINE input was being implemented. An independent evaluation officer was appointed with responsibility for the data collection and analysis.

Sample

Four schools, two in the north of England and two in the south, were identified as 'experimental' schools, i.e. where students would receive the CINE teaching input. This yielded a sample of 166 students. Two further schools were identified with similar characteristics to the 'experimental' schools to act as a comparison group. Again, one of these schools was in the north of England and one in the south, and the student sample from these schools was 97.

Method

Teaching input

In each 'experimental' school a link tutor from the staff was nominated to work with the project officer. Curriculum time was negotiated to allow a maximum of 12 2-hour sessions over an approximate 18-month period for two cohorts of students.

Detailed organisation of CINE input varied from school to school, but the overall pattern adhered to involved two introductory sessions related to the importance and relevance of communication in nursing, six communication skills sessions addressing skills such as listening, questioning and reinforcing, and as many sessions (usually two to four) as individual programmes would allow, in which the skills were integrated and applied to specific areas of nursing practice. Full details of the teaching sessions given in each of the schools can be found in the curriculum development report (Faulkner et al, 1988). The emphasis in the teaching was on experiential methods, encouraging participation from the students and maximising opportunities for skills practice.

Evaluation of the impact of CINE input

The aim of this evaluation was to examine the effect of the communication skills teaching input in terms of students' attitudes, knowledge and skills. In a study such as this a great deal of time must go into the development of appropriate measurement tools in order to assess pre- and post-test differences. Indeed, the validity of the findings relies wholly on the appropriateness and reliability of the tools used.

The issue of assessing communication skills and behaviour is particularly complex. Researchers have found it exceedingly difficult to devise reliable and objective measures in this field (Ellis and Whittington, 1981; Neeson et al, 1984). It is perhaps not surprising that the task of devising a behavioural tool for measuring students' communication skills proved to be the most challenging aspect of the project. Details of the process of devising and using the tools can be found in the curriculum development report (Faulkner et al, 1988). Pre- and post-test measures ultimately utilised included the following:

1. Demographic data (pre-test only).
2. Academic achievement.
3. Attitudes towards nursing.
4. Attitudes towards communication.
5. Attitudes towards communication skills teaching.
6. Knowledge about communication skills.
7. Confidence in ability to communicate with patients.
8. Skills and behaviour, based on students' written response to patients' questions or statements and situation, taken from typewritten vignettes or video-recorded stimulus material.
9. Skills and behaviour based on verbal and non-verbal skills displayed during video-recorded role plays of patient assessment interviews.

Pre- and post-test data were collected from all students in the samples from both experimental and comparison schools. Pre-test assessment was undertaken in the students' first week of introductory block and revealed that experimental and comparison groups were very similar in terms of demographic characteristics, academic achievements and pre-test knowledge, attitude and behaviour scores. Post-test assessment took place soon after the completion of the CINE input.

In addition to the pre- and post-test information, a substantial amount of more descriptive qualitative data was collected. This was derived from the evaluation officer's tape-recorded discussions with students and tutors, and written evaluations of the teaching input from students. The CINE tutors also kept comprehensive records and field notes of their observations and experiences during the project in relation to students' and tutors' reactions to the teaching and the curriculum development, the involvement of link tutors and the dynamics within the schools of nursing.

Findings

Post-test measures of attitudes towards communication revealed that students receiving the CINE input were much more likely to believe that communication skills can be learnt and developed than did the comparison group, who tended to believe that the ability to communicate effectively is innate. Students in the comparison group were more likely to attribute the development of communication skills to learning in a 'ward situation', whereas the group receiving the CINE input attributed more learning to the input they received in school. Students in the experimental groups were also more aware of the importance and complexity of communication in nursing than the comparison group. The experimental group also emerged at post-test as feeling less confident of their own ability to communicate well than did the comparison group. This insight would appear to reflect their awareness of the difficulties of putting good communication into practice and the fact that they had confronted their own skills during role-play exercises in the CINE input.

Post-test evaluation of knowledge demonstrated that the students receiving the CINE input had, not surprisingly, much greater increments in their knowledge of components of communication and in their ability to recognise skills and analyse transcripts accurately than students who had not received the input.

The differences between the two groups at post-test in terms of measures of skills and behaviour were particularly interesting. Here the experimental group was more likely to produce an appropriate and more 'skilled' response to vignettes involving complex or potentially threatening situations, while the control group tended to use avoidance strategies. Differences were also demonstrated in the videotaped role-play assessments. Students in the comparison groups showed greater increments in information giving than the experimental group. In contrast, those receiving the CINE input demonstrated greater development in terms of their use of listening and questioning skills and in their ability to recognise and respond to cues.

Data collected from discussions with the students receiving the CINE input and from their written evaluations demonstrated that, overall, students were very positive about the course. Not all students enjoyed the experiential work, especially the role-play. However, after the input, almost every student stated that they could recognise its value and importance. Students also consistently stated the need to continue the communication skills teaching throughout the course and, especially, to help them to apply the skills in their clinical practice.

The CINE tutors' experiences in liaising with the schools and attempting to initiate the curriculum change produced several insights into the practicalities of such teaching. It became clear that small groups were essential for most of the input. They found that 12 students was the maximum number, and this meant that large groups had to be divided and teaching input duplicated in some cases. An ideal number for the experiential teaching was found to be eight. Their experiences with these cohorts of students also illuminated the importance of introducing role-play and feedback slowly. The use of video-tape and transcript stimulus material was consistently effective in generating open-minded discussion and in focusing on specific skills. In addition, audio-taped feedback was often found to be as useful, and more practical, in skill practice exercises than was video-taped feedback.

Interviews with the members of teaching staff in the schools and the CINE tutors' field notes of the impact of the curriculum development provided some valuable descriptive data. In general, most tutors professed enthusiasm for communication skills teaching, although few felt qualified to undertake such teaching. The realities of introducing the CINE input into the curriculum did present several problems, although not all of them were encountered in each of the four experimental schools. The problems could be attributed to several critical areas. These included teaching overload, difficulties in negotiating curriculum changes, space shortages, lack of support from colleagues and superiors, and lack of confidence in integrating experiential teaching approaches into an existing programme.

It is, of course, highly probable that these are all problems and difficulties that could be encountered during any attempt to incorporate a substantial amount of new teaching into any curriculum. However, it was clear at the end of the CINE input that the tutors in schools were not overconfident about their ability to continue the input in their own way and under their own steam. Indeed, three out of four of the experimental schools requested continued input and support from the CINE tutors, and this was provided where possible.

PART III: THE PREPARATION OF NURSE TUTORS FOR COMMUNICATION SKILLS TEACHING AND CASE STUDY EXAMPLES OF THEIR SUBSEQUENT EXPERIENCES

The aim of this aspect of the project was to investigate the preparation of nurse tutors in terms of communication skills teaching, and to explore the experiences of a small sample of tutors when attempting to put communication skills teaching into practice. Data collected throughout the first two parts of the project drew attention to the fact that many tutors do not feel adequately prepared to use experiential teaching approaches in general, nor to teach communication skills in particular. Discussions with those working in tutor training establishments revealed great awareness of this problem. Each course already contained an element of such teaching, but all course leaders expressed great interest in developing the skills teaching input in these areas further.

Method

Two of the institutions where interest was expressed were selected – one in the north of England and one in the south. The CINE team negotiated to take over part of the existing curriculum in order to update tutors' communication skills, and to give students intensive input in terms of experiential teaching methods and approaches to teaching communication skills.

Forty-two tutor students (21 on each course) took part in classes designed to prepare them for using experiential teaching methods and for teaching communication skills. The CINE input consisted of a 2-day workshop and 10 more half-day sessions. At the end of the courses, 86 per cent of the students on the 'south' course and 100 per cent of those on the 'north' course claimed that they were committed to adopting these approaches when they went back to teach in their schools.

Students were asked to state whether they definitely intended to include communication skills teaching in their role on return to the school and whether they would be willing to be involved in the follow-up study. As a result, 12 students were identified whose experiences would provide case-study material needed to illuminate the process and outcome of their attempts to put the skills they had learnt into practice. CINE tutors would act as resource and support agents and would provide intensive follow-up in the form of regular visits and telephone calls. The remaining 30 tutor students in the sample were to be sent a follow-up questionnaire about their experiences 1 year after their return to their schools of nursing.

Case study data were collected over a period of 1 year in the form of tape-recorded interviews between researchers and tutors, researchers' field notes of telephone conversations and discussions and observation notes of actual teaching sessions run by the tutors being studied.

Findings

Data analysis from this part of the project is still in progress. However, some interesting indicators and trends are emerging. Perhaps not surprisingly the experiences in each of the 12 'case studies' vary greatly. Some have failed to include experimental approaches on communication skills sessions into their teaching. Others have achieved partial success. One or two have achieved what they set out to achieve. All of the tutors have experienced some problems and encountered a few serious constraints. These include difficulties in negotiating time and space, lack of support from colleagues in relation to the organisation of small group work, use of equipment, involvement in teaching and a general undervaluing of the subject matter and approach. These problems have emerged in spite of lip service being given to the importance of communication skills teaching in the curriculum in apparently 'progressive' schools. The tutors in the project also recognise that the difficulties are exacerbated by their own lack of confidence and experience in the area of communication skills teaching. In some cases this is compounded by low morale in the school of nursing and poor staffing levels.

As mentioned previously, some of the tutors in the 12 case studies have succeeded in meeting their objectives. It is hoped that further analysis of the data will illuminate personal and organisational factors that have influenced the relative success or failure of individual tutors in their attempts to include communication skills teaching in their role. Such findings could prove to be immensely valuable in the management of future curriculum developments and changes.

DISCUSSION

Over 6 years the CINE project has succeeded in raising many important questions and has provided some valuable insights. Although there are no answers as such, experience gained during the process of curriculum development has demonstrated that it *is* feasible to integrate a substantial amount of communication skills input into nurse education programmes.

Moreover, students receiving this input appear to gain in terms of their knowledge, skills and understanding of the complexities and challenges of effective communication. It has also become clear that a great deal more teaching, practice and support is needed at basic and post-basic education levels if nurses are to develop their full potential as professional communicators.

The form that the teaching and practice of communication skills should take is far from clear. There is convincing evidence that experiential methods are more appropriate and effective than didactic or 'chalk and talk' approaches (Ellis and Whittington, 1981). Beyond this, issues such as the timing and focus of practice sessions have not been examined rigorously. There is also evidence that communication skills developed and improved in the safe classroom environment must be regularly practised in the real-life situation. This has implications for the teaching of communication skills in nursing, where the question of the effectiveness of practice and feedback in the clinical situation needs to be examined closely.

The problems inherent in attempts to assess an individual's skills have been discussed previously. As communication skills teaching gains momentum in nursing, the greater will be the need to develop appropriate and acceptable methods of assessing the impact of this teaching. The approach devised for use in Part II of this project has potential for further development, but it, like many other approaches, is far from perfect. It is also unrealistic to imagine that one simple rating scale could ever be sensitive enough to evaluate a set of skills and behaviours as complex as those encompassed by the term 'communication'.

If communication skills teaching is to gain its rightful place as the core of nurse education programmes, the issues of how it is best taught and best assessed *must* be addressed urgently.

The final part of the project focused on the process of preparing tutors to fulfil a communication skills teaching role. This again has proved to be a problematic area and many questions have arisen, which need to be examined carefully. In particular, the impact that such teaching can have on the dynamics within a school could usefully be addressed. More pragmatically, the question of who should teach communication skills requires exploration. The methods and approaches used in such teaching demand different strengths, qualities and motivations perhaps to those required when a 'chalk and talk' approach is employed.

Since work on the project commenced, many changes have taken place within the profession. There now appears to be a general acceptance of the need for communication skills to be included in all nurse education programmes. However, findings from the project suggest that in some cases the acceptance is at the level of lip service rather than true commitment.

There are still vast numbers of practising qualified nurses who have not had access to any formal communication skills training during their career. Moreover, only a small minority of student nurses are given adequate preparation in current education programmes. It is essential that the profession demonstrates true commitment by providing genuine support and resources for educational updating and research.

As patients and clients become more involved with their care, and as health promotion and preventive care aspects of the nurse's role expand, greater demands will be made on nurses' communication skills. It would be immoral and shortsighted to fail to provide the education and support that nurses will need to meet the challenges of their changing roles.

REFERENCES

Ashworth P (1980) *Care to Communicate.* London: Royal College of Nursing.

Bond S (1983) Nurses' communication with cancer patients. In: *Nursing Research. Ten Studies in Patient Care,* ed. Wilson-Barnett J. Chichester: John Wiley.

Cartwright A (1964) *Human Relations and Hospital Care.* London: Routledge and Kegan Paul.

Ellis R and Whittington D (1981) *A Guide to Social Skill Training.* London: Croom Helm.

Faulkner A (1980) *The Nurse's Role in Giving Information to Patients.* Unpublished MLitt thesis, University of Aberdeen.

Faulkner A (1985) The organisational context of interpersonal skills. In: *Interpersonal Skills in Nursing: Research and Applications,* ed. Kagan C. London: Croom Helm.

Faulkner A et al (1986) *Communication in Nurse Education - Survey of Schools of Nursing Project Report.* London: Health Education Council.

Faulkner A et al (1988) *Communication in Nurse Education, Curriculum Development Report.* London: Health Education Authority.

Macfarlane E A (1980) Nursing theory: the comparison of four theoretical proposals. *Journal of Advanced Nursing,* **5**: 3-19.

Macleod Clark (1983) Nurse patient communication in surgical wards. In: *Nursing Research. Ten Studies in Patient Care,* ed. Wilson-Barnett J. Chichester: John Wiley.

Neeson B et al (1984) Teaching communication skills to nurses - evaluating the development of skills. *Nurse Education Today,* **4**(3): 54-58.

Parlett M and Hamilton D (1972) *Evaluation as Illumination; a New Approach to the Study of 'Innovatory Programmes'.* Occasional Paper 9. University of Edinburgh: Centre for Research in the Educational Sciences.

Raphael W (1969) *Patients and their Hospitals.* London: King Edward's Hospital Fund for London.

Reynolds M (1978) No news is bad news: patients' views about communications in hospital. *British Medical Journal* **1**: 1673-1676.

Chapter 22

Communication and Health Education in Nursing: Exploring the Nurse's Role in Helping Patients and Clients to Give up Smoking

Jill Macleod Clark, Sheila Haverty and Sally Kendall

BACKGROUND

In recent years, increasing emphasis has been placed on the need to exploit the potential of nurses 'to act as promoters of health as well as carers of the sick' (WHO, 1978). Recognition of the extent to which certain diseases are preventable has focused attention on the need to help nurses develop their health education role.

There are innumerable areas in which nurses and other health professions can attempt to influence their patients and clients. These include diet, stress, alcohol, drugs and smoking. Of these, smoking is the one that has received perhaps the greatest attention in the last decade. Smoking is an aspect of health education that has been continuously debated. However, it is also an area where there can be no doubt about the need to inform the public about the dangers and health risks associated with the habit. It is estimated that one-sixth of all deaths occurring in Britain can be related to smoking (Royal College of Physicians, 1983).

In the UK, recent figures show that approximately 34 per cent of the population are regular smokers (OPCS, 1984). There is clearly a great deal of scope for nurses to play an effective role in terms of encouraging patients and clients to stop smoking, since at any one time approximately one-third of those they come in contact with are likely to be smokers. However, in order to act as effective health educators it is essential that nurses are equipped with the appropriate attitudes, knowledge and skills. Research into the role of the nurse as a health educator in relation to smoking cessation has produced contradictory findings. For example, a study conducted by Burt et al (1974), yielded a 62 per cent cessation rate among patients who were visited at home by health visitors following a myocardial infarction. A large community project in Finland involving nurses and other health professionals has also reported high levels of success in terms of helping patients and clients to stop smoking (Vartianen et al, 1986).

On the other hand, several researchers have highlighted nurses' lack of skills and knowledge in relation to their health education role. Syred (1981) found that nurses in hospitals avoid fulfilling a health education role, and a study of nurses' health education skills in relation to smoking (Faulkner and Ward, 1983) suggested that nurses lack the skills and knowledge required to fulfil this role effectively. These deficits are not confined to the UK. In 1983, Swenson and Dalton described the knowledge of and attitudes towards smoking of a sample of American nurses. They found that nearly a third of the nurses were unable to correctly identify three adverse consequences of smoking.

There must, clearly, be a relationship between nurses' knowledge in specific areas and the educational input they have received. Until recently the preparation of nurses for their health education role has not been seriously addressed in most nurse education programmes (Randell, 1980, 1982). This fact is exemplified by the findings of a small study by Ward and Faulkner (1983) in which the limitations of nurse tutors' knowledge about smoking were illuminated.

In response to a growing awareness of the need to address this gap in nursing communication, the Health Education Council (HEC) initiated the development of resource materials in this area. In 1983, the HEC produced smoking packs designed to give guidance and support to nurses who wished to encourage their patients and clients to give up smoking. The packs contained practical information about how to help people to stop smoking and some literature to pass on to those who were thinking about giving up.

The impact of these packs was evaluated in terms of acceptability and their effect on nurses' knowledge levels. Aspects of this evaluation study form the first part of the research reported in this chapter. Findings from the evaluation confirmed those of the previous studies of nurses' knowledge about the effects of smoking (Swenson and Dalton, 1983).

Moreover, although motivated to undertake an active health education role, nurses felt acutely aware of their limitations in terms of both knowledge and skills. A second study was, therefore, undertaken, in which a group of nurses attended workshops designed to enhance their knowledge and skills in relation to helping people stop smoking. The process and outcomes of their interventions with patients and clients were subsequently examined. This study forms the second part of the research reported in this chapter.

PART I: AN EVALUATION OF NURSES' KNOWLEDGE AND SKILLS IN RELATION TO SMOKING

In 1983, the HEC published two versions of a resource pack designed to help nurses fulfil a health education role in relation to helping people stop smoking. One version was produced for nurses working in hospitals and the other for nurses working in the community. The impact of these packs was comprehensively evaluated in terms of use and acceptability, their effect on nurses' knowledge levels, and patterns of distribution and uptake. Full details of the research can be found in a series of project reports (Macleod Clark et al, 1985). The research described in these reports concentrated on the part of the project concerned with assessing the impact of the packs on nurses' knowledge and perceptions of their health education skills.

Prior to publication of the packs, three health districts were identified that were able and willing to offer access to large numbers of hospital and community nurses and that expressed interest in the research. One of these districts was situated in the north of England, one in the south and one in central London. In each of these selected districts, permission was obtained from the relevant district nursing officers and directors of nurse education for the researchers to contact nurses employed in their district.

A quota-sample framework was drawn up to ensure that the main categories of personnel for whom the packs had been produced were adequately represented. These included health visitors, district nurses, registered and enrolled nurses and second- and third-year student nurses.

Before publication of the packs a total of 431 nurses completed a comprehensive questionnaire designed to assess their knowledge about smoking and their attitudes and skills in relation to the nurse's role in smoking cessation. Nurses' knowledge about smoking was tested using a self-completion questionnaire based on information contained in the resource packs. The areas covered included current statistical information about smoking, physiological and pathological effects of smoking, and the nurse's approach to and skills in educating patients and clients about smoking. After completing the pre-test the respondents were asked if they would allow the researcher to contact them again, and they were then each sent a copy of the relevant resource pack.

Approximately 3 months after receiving the packs, each respondent was contacted again and asked if he or she would complete a much shorter version of the pre-test questionnaire. At the same time, the respondents were asked to answer questions related to their opinions of the packs and the extent to which they had used the information with patients *or* clients. A series of questions was also asked concerning the respondent's own smoking behaviour. A total of 330 post-test questionnaires was obtained, representing 76.6 per cent of the pre-test sample.

Findings

The comprehensive nature of the questionnaire and the answers given by the respondents provided a good database on their knowledge in terms of the prevalence of smoking, physiological and pathological effects and approaches to health education interventions.

In the pre-test, several questions were asked about the incidence of smoking in the population. Answers to these questions were generally inaccurate. For example, in the pre-test only 3.3 per cent gave an adequate answer to a question about the number of ex-smokers in Britain. At post-test, after receiving the resources pack, the number of respondents giving an appropriate answer to this question increased to 12.7 per cent. This was a statistically significant difference ($p = < 0.001$). Other questions addressed the potential effects of smoking on body systems. Again pre- and post-test differences in knowledge were demonstrated. For example, at pre-test 41 per cent of respondents were able to identify the potential effects on the gastrointestinal system. In the post-test 53 per cent identified this effect – a statistically significant increase ($p = < 0.05$). Scores on other areas of knowledge such as the effect of cigarette smoking on non-smokers did not change between pre- and post-tests.

Four questions in the pre-test questionnaire asked for responses to situations that could arise when talking to a patient or client about smoking. For example, one situation required the respondent to state how she would respond to someone who said: 'I'm a woman – it's only men who die from smoking'. As reflected in the answers to the factual questions, nurses were unable to provide appropriate background information in this situation. Responses almost all centred around questions such as, 'Do you want to give up smoking?'. Only 11 per cent mentioned that they would attempt to educate the patient or client, and almost 25 per cent referred to 'luck playing a part in the disease' in their responses. Very little difference was demonstrated in these responses at post-test. A large proportion of the respondents spontaneously articulated concern about their lack of knowledge and skills in this area, as well as in other areas of health education such as diet and alcohol.

Overall, the analysis of the data from this study endorsed findings from previous research and illustrated the fragmentary and inadequate nature of nurses' knowledge and skills in the field of smoking education. However, pre- and post-test differences suggest that nurses are able to improve their knowledge in certain areas, such as understanding of disease processes, when provided with useful and accessible information. On the other hand, little change occurred in relation to knowledge of the physiological effects of smoking and specific health education skills. The findings thus demonstrated that although nurses believe they have a role in smoking cessation, written materials alone are not sufficient to equip them with the skills necessary to be confident and effective.

This supports the view that there is a need to increase the amount of curriculum time devoted to the acquisition of health-related knowledge and skills in areas such as smoking in all programmes of nurse education.

In response to these findings, a further research project was undertaken to develop and evaluate a training programme designed to equip nurses with the appropriate knowledge and skills to fulfil a health education role in relation to smoking cessation.

PART II: HELPING PATIENTS AND CLIENTS TO STOP SMOKING – DEVELOPING AND ASSESSING THE EFFECTIVENESS OF THE NURSE'S ROLE

The second phase of the research was designed to meet the following aims:

1. To identify and develop an appropriate model for helping nurses to acquire and enhance their health education skills.
2. To explore the content and process of nurses' health education interventions in relation to smoking cessation.
3. To assess the effectiveness of nurses' health education interventions in relation to smoking cessation.

Method

A case study approach was taken to meeting these aims, in which a small cohort of trained nurses, midwives and health visitors took part in a short training programme and were subsequently followed up. Full details of this research can be found in the Project Report (Macleod Clark et al, 1987). A summary of the approach taken and the main findings are presented here.

A training programme consisting of two 1-day workshops was developed, which would build on the cohort's existing abilities and equip them with the additional knowledge and skills they would need to undertake an effective health education role in relation to smoking cessation.

Twenty people were recruited to the training programme, all of whom had expressed an interest in helping smokers to give up the habit. They included hospital nurses, health visitors and midwives. The teaching input was spread over two study days, the main aims of which were as follows:

1. To provide a sound knowledge base on which nurses could base their health education input related to smoking cessation.
2. To suggest a framework around which nurses could base their interventions.
3. To help nurses develop the communication skills required to be effective health educators.

The first study day essentially consisted of lectures, which were intended to expand the nurses' knowledge in the area. These were preceded by a knowledge quiz, which gave the researchers an indication of the existing baseline knowledge and also served to raise the nurses' awareness of their own lack of knowledge. The earlier research reported in this chapter had highlighted a particular knowledge deficit among nurses related to morbidity and mortality statistics and the physiological and pathological effects of smoking. This was replicated by the quiz. Lectures were, therefore, given on the physiological and pathological effects of smoking, statistics and cessation strategies. Each session was followed by discussion. There was also some discussion about the usefulness of theories and models of health education, and feelings about non-smoking policies in health service premises were explored.

There was a 2-week gap between the two study days, and during this period the participants were asked to audio-record themselves talking to someone who wanted to give up smoking. The aim was to provide baseline data on a health education intervention before any skills training had been given.

The second study day was mainly concerned with the framework for health education and communication skills in theory and practice.

The framework

The research team felt strongly that nurses need a framework on which to base their health education, and this was supported by findings from researchers such as Syred (1981). The framework was devised by the researchers and was based partly on the health belief model (Becker 1974) and partly on the nursing process. It was felt to be important that the nursing process was used as a basis as many nurses are already familiar with its principles and the individualised approach is essential to effective health education.

Many different strategies have been applied to the task of helping people give up smoking. The strategies of choice must be compatible with demands and constraints of the health professionals' work and must meet the needs of the patients and clients concerned. The strategy therefore proposed for use as the basis of nurses' interventions with smoking patients and clients was derived from the minimum intervention model used by general practitioners (Russell, 1979). However, the approach developed differs substantially from this minimum intervention strategy in one important respect. The difference in our approach is that a heavy emphasis is placed on the assessment of each individual's motivation, knowledge and needs.

The stages of the suggested approved framework can be seen below.

Framework for interventions

Assessment

Assess the smoker in terms of motivation to give up, health beliefs and fears or worries about continuing to smoke or giving up. Information should relate to the individual's health beliefs.

Planning

Plan a course of action to stop smoking *with* the smoker, not *for* him or her. Utilise knowledge of cessation techniques and outside agencies, such as smokers' clinics, constructively. Suggest coping strategies.

Implementation

The client implements the plan; the nurse's role is one of support and encouragement. The nurse can act as referral agent if support is impractical, e.g. on a short stay ward.

Evaluation

Evaluate the intervention in terms of client attitude and behaviour and your own approach. If the plan has failed, look at where it went wrong and start again. Reinforce positive changes in smoking behaviour.

Putting such a framework into action demands certain communication skills from the participants. These skills were first explored in theory and then in practice using role-play and analysis of the baseline audiotapes. Although the importance of non-verbal skills was acknowledged, verbal skills were the focus of the training. The particular skills needed to carry out each stage of the framework were identified and practised.

A particularly useful technique in the exploration of these communication skills is to record the baseline intervention on audiotape. The participants analysed their own interventions, identifying the positive use of skills and also where communication was not effective. Not surprisingly, at this stage there were many examples of ineffective communication in the baseline interventions. These included an inability to listen, the use of more closed or leading questions than open questions and a lack of structure within the interventions.

Following the two study days the participants were asked to talk to up to five patients or clients about giving up smoking. A tape-recording was made of each intervention, and data were collected from all the patients and clients involved. The informed consent of these patients and clients was obtained at the outset.

Regarding selection of patients and clients, the researchers had already applied for and obtained ethical clearance from three health authorities, which enabled patients and clients to be approached.

As the nature of data collection (audio-recording) required a high level of motivation and commitment from the participants, it was felt to be most satisfactory if they selected their own patients/clients for the purposes of the research.

They were asked to select patients/clients on the basis of the following criteria: they smoked regularly, they were motivated to give up smoking (it was suggested that a check-list could be used to establish the level of motivation if this was not obvious) and they were aged between 16–60 years. Children were not included as this requires a different kind of intervention, more concerned with primary prevention. Similarly, the very elderly smoking population are more likely to be at a stage where tertiary prevention is more appropriate. However, in practice, one or two patients/clients aged over 60 years were included because they had a high level of motivation to stop smoking.

Sex and socioeconomic group were not specified, but it was expected that more women than men would be involved because of the areas of work from which the health professionals came.

Data were collected from a total of 68 patients and clients. Of the 20 participants attending the study days, 16 contributed to the data collection process. They comprised three ward nurses, seven health visitors and six midwives.

Data from the study were collected and analysed under the following headings:

1. Demographic data from patients and clients.
2. Patients' and clients' smoking history.
3. Patients' and clients' motivation to stop smoking.
4. Patients' and clients' beliefs and worries related to smoking and giving up smoking.
5. Expired carbon monoxide measurements.
6. Outcomes of interventions in terms of change in smoking behaviour, motivation, beliefs and worries at 6-month and 1-year follow-ups.
7. Analysis of audiotape-recorded interventions.
8. Relationship between process of health education interventions and outcomes.
9. Patients' and clients' perceptions of nurses', midwives' and health visitors' interventions.
10. Nurses', midwives' and health visitors' perceptions of their involvement in study days and project.

Of the 68 participants in the study, 54 (80 per cent) were followed up at 6 months and 42 (62 per cent) were followed up 1 year after the interventions. Those not followed up could not be contacted due to moving away, and moving abroad, and two were unwilling to continue the study for personal reasons. Each of the 42 remaining in the study was visited by one of the project officers.

Findings

A comprehensive account of the analysis and findings can be found in the Project Report (Macleod Clark et al, 1987). A brief summary of the results is presented here.

Smoking behaviour

All patients and clients were again asked if they had changed their smoking behaviour since the initial interview. As can be seen in Table 22.1, seven were still non-smokers, five claimed to have cut down substantially, 13 had made at least one attempt to stop, and 17 had not changed their behaviour in any way.

Expired carbon monoxide measurements were repeated and, in order to validate any claims either to have stopped or to have substantially cut down smoking, urine samples were collected for urinary cotinine measurement.

Table 22.1 Outcomes of health professionals' interventions in terms of change in smoking behaviour at 1 year follow-up (*N*=42)

Smoking behaviour	*n*	%
Stopped smoking	7	17
Cut down substantially	5	12
Made at least one attempt to give up	13	31
No change in behaviour	17	40

Analysis of audiotape-recorded interventions

Analysis of the tape-recorded interventions was carried out using a skill-based analysis. This was also closely linked to the intervention framework, in order adequately to measure first the use of the communication skills learned at the study days, and second, the participants' use of the intervention framework in practice.

The participants were generally able to make a detailed assessment of the clients through their use of open and closed questions about smoking history, daily smoking pattern and clients' everyday lives. The hospital nurses were less able to do this as they often had only just met the patient/client, whereas the health visitors and midwives often knew their clients quite well.

The participants were able to assess their clients' desire to be healthier, but sometimes did not find out a great deal about their true level of motivation to stop smoking. However, some tape transcripts show clearly that talking with the health professional was influential in raising the client's level of motivation, and this was borne out by the smoking cessation rate from this study.

The participants were asked to plan with the client how to go about stopping smoking. They were helped in this by the information about cessation strategies and ways of coping with stopping smoking (which had been discussed in detail at the first study day). In practice, however, they found this part of the framework quite difficult. One or two clients with strong motivation to stop smoking participated to some extent in working out a cessation strategy. In general though, the study participants tended to fall back on prescriptive advice, telling the clients what was 'best', and not focusing on the client's needs or allowing the client to think about what would work best for them.

The health visitors and midwives found it easier to offer support and follow-up as they would have the opportunity to see the client again. The hospital nurses found this more difficult, although one of them telephoned the patients a week or so after they had left hospital to see how they were getting on. Clients were often not actually referred to other agencies, for example a smokers' clinic, or to see a health visitor after leaving hospital.

Relationship between process of health education interventions and outcomes

Very few previous studies have attempted to demonstrate any relationship between outcome following an intervention and what is actually said during the intervention. Since in this study audiotape-recordings were collected of every health education intervention as it occurred, it was possible to explore the relationship between interventions and outcomes.

Given the limitations in terms of sample size, only tentative conclusions can be drawn. However, there did appear to be some relationship between the use of specific skills, such as the use of open questions, listening and positive response to cues, and successful outcomes in terms of smoking cessation. Moreover, successful interventions were also characterised by clear evidence of patient/client involvement in the planning process and, most markedly, a high ratio of patient/client talk to health professional talk. In other words the patient or client fully participated in the interaction. This is clearly an area that requires further investigation.

Patients' and clients' perceptions of interventions

Each patient and client was followed up in order to ascertain any changes in smoking behaviour or motivation to stop smoking. These outcome measures have been discussed above. At these interviews, the respondents were also asked to evaluate the intervention by saying how helpful (or not) it had been to talk to the nurse, midwife or health visitor, what other factors had influenced them, and whether or not they felt that the intervention itself had affected their subsequent smoking behaviour.

Fifty per cent felt that the intervention had been helpful. Some said simply that it had been 'very helpful' while others gave fuller responses such as 'she was the reason that I stopped' or 'it helped because she (the nurse, midwife or health visitor) was trying to give up too' and 'I didn't give the help I got a fair chance'. Less than one-third (29 per cent) felt that the intervention had not been helpful. Comments included 'She didn't tell me anything new' and 'It's easy for a non smoker to preach'. It is important to remember when looking at these comments that discussing their smoking behaviour at length was as new to the patients and clients in the study as it was to the health professionals. Indeed, it was apparent from some of the tapes that many of the respondents had never before been asked to talk about themselves in relation to smoking, and they welcomed the chance to do so.

When asked what else might have been helpful, one-third were completely satisfied with the help they received. Six people (11 per cent) would have liked more support and encouragement. Other areas mentioned were more shocking and frightening information, more on the benefits of stopping smoking and more information on other available help, such as hypnosis.

Asked what they recalled from the interventions, two-thirds were able to recall some aspects of the conversation. Since the follow-up was 6 months after the intervention, this demonstrates that, for many respondents, what was said had considerable impact. About 13 per cent particularly remembered 'passive smoking' being talked about, which was encouraging as the majority of respondents were young women with children. Four people particularly remembered the carbon monoxide monitor, and, incidental to this, the majority of people who had changed their smoking behaviour were keen to repeat the carbon monoxide measurement, which gave the impression that it has a strong motivating effect. This impression is supported by evidence from Jamrozik et al (1984) that the carbon monoxide monitor can be used to enhance motivation to give up smoking, especially in socioeconomic groups III – V. Other aspects of the intervention that respondents recalled were mainly related to specific diseases. These included lung cancer, stomach ulcers, emphysema, heart disease and hypertension. In some cases the disease processes recalled correlated with the beliefs and worries expressed in the motivation check-list, indicating that the nurses, midwives and health visitors were recognising cues given by the patient or client and were attempting to discuss their beliefs and worries with them.

Participants' perceptions of their involvement in study days and project

Following completion of data collection, the nurses, midwives and health visitors participating in the study were invited to attend an evaluation session.

They were asked to evaluate the study days and to assess the impact the training had had on their practice. Most of the comments were favourable. Prior to the study days, many had limited involvement with smoking education. When asked about their involvement they made comments such as, 'I wasn't very interested or motivated' and 'very little involvement – I thought I was doing it but I wasn't' or 'I discussed it briefly in passing'.

Following participation in the study, one participant commented, 'I'm more aware of the need to help smokers, and how to be more sensitive in listening', and another said, 'It makes me think more about the way in which I approach individuals in conversations about smoking'. A midwife said that she discussed smoking more readily and encouraged her clients to give up, and overall there was a noticeable change from comments made prior to the study days.

Similarly, when asked how they intended to develop their future practice as health educators in relation to smoking cessation, the majority of the comments were favourable, along the lines of the health visitors who said, 'I will continue to improve my skills' and 'Discussion of smoking will be part of my routine visiting'. A midwife thought that she would 'take an active role in running stop-smoking groups'.

Suggested changes in the content of the study days included more role-play and self-analysis of tape recordings, and more advice on how to select clients who would respond to an intervention and how to assess someone's real motivation to stop smoking.

DISCUSSION

The very positive findings from this study of health professionals' attempts to help their patients and clients to give up smoking have important implications for nursing education and practice.

The case study approach taken in this research project enabled us to build a rich and detailed picture of the group of patients and clients involved. The individuals in the sample were predominantly female and ranged in age from 16 to 76 years, and the majority were classified as socioeconomic groups III and IV. Most had been smokers for between 10 and 20 years, and the majority smoked between 20 and 30 cigarettes a day. In general, the sample was relatively well informed about the effects of smoking. Half admitted that they were worried about the effects of smoking on the health of their babies and family and the effects of smoking on their own health in terms of breathlessness, lung cancer and heart disease. When asked to predict how they thought they would feel if they were able to give up smoking, the majority felt that they would enjoy better physical health as a consequence. Just over half anticipated that giving up would result in extra stress. Interestingly, over two-thirds believed that they would put on weight. These findings have important implications for the way in which health professionals may need to tackle the issue of smoking cessation with their clients. Attempts to help people give up smoking are unlikely to be successful unless the individual's very real concerns about the negative effects of cessation are addressed. Conversely, some statistically significant correlations were demonstrated between individuals' motivation to stop smoking and the degree to which they were afraid of the effects of smoking, and their belief that giving up smoking would make them feel healthier. Thus, it is essential to harness and exploit these concerns and motivations when attempting to help people to stop smoking. Seventeen per cent of the sample who were followed up after 1 year had successfully given up smoking. These figures compare very well with previous studies carried out in the UK, which have primarily concentrated on the general practitioner's influence on smoking cessation. For example, a study by Russell et al (1979) used minimum intervention and achieved a cessation rate of 5 per cent. Later work, which included nicotine chewing gum as part of the intervention, increased the cessation rate to 9 per cent (Russell et al, 1980) and 15 per cent (Jamrozik et al, 1984).

In this study of health professionals' interventions there was, perhaps predictably, a significant relationship between being confident and motivated to give up and subsequent success. Again, this emphasises the wisdom of concentrating attempts to help people give up smoking on those who are truly motivated to succeed. Regarding individuals not yet motivated to stop smoking, energies could more profitably be directed towards increasing motivation to stop rather than the stopping process per se. Analysis of the tape-recorded conversations in this study revealed the importance of assessment in health education interactions. With hindsight, it is clear that many patients and clients were not really strongly motivated to give up, although, at the outset of the intervention, they had claimed to be so. Using a nursing process framework, the assessment would lead to a plan of intervention that could initially lead to increased motivation rather than to the facilitation of smoking cessation.

Moreover, success in smoking education interventions need not be judged solely in terms of smoking cessation figures. As was discussed previously, many of the patients and clients in the study attempted to change their smoking behaviour subsequent to the health professionals' interaction with them. Forty-three per cent of them made at least one serious attempt to give up smoking and a further 12 per cent reduced the amount they smoked substantially. This means that 60 per cent of the sample may have been influenced in some way by the health professional's attempts to help them stop smoking. These influences were particularly apparent in the health visitors' and midwives' interventions with their clients. Two-thirds of the clients seen by health visitors subsequently changed their behaviour. Four clients gave up smoking, and a further 12 reduced their cigarette consumption or made an effort to stop. Similarly, nearly half of the pregnant women seen by midwives subsequently made an attempt to stop smoking. These findings suggest that if contacts and support were increased by these groups of health professionals, higher smoking cessation rates may result.

Further research is needed in two main areas. First, it is important to investigate and encourage the potential of health visitors and midwives to influence the smoking behaviour, and indeed other health-related behaviour, of their young female clients. Second, in the research described in this report it was only possible to undertake a limited analysis of the link between the process of health education and the outcome in terms of behaviour change. We believe that there may be important relationships between the use of certain approaches and subsequent outcomes. Tentative links have already been established between the extent of involvement by patients and clients in an interaction and outcome in terms of smoking cessation. However, these are speculative given the limited sample size, but this is an area that needs further investigation and which is relevant to all health education interactions, not just to those initiated by nurses, midwives or health visitors.

Through this analysis of over 60 case studies of health professionals' attempts to help their clients and patients to stop smoking, we have gained considerable insight into their potential as health educators. At a simple outcome level it is clear that they can be highly effective in helping and supporting their patients to stop smoking. The proportion of patients and clients who changed their smoking behaviour following the nurses', midwives' and health visitors' intervention compares very favourably with the results of studies using other groups of health professionals, such as general practitioners.

This research project has illuminated the fact that the nurse–patient/client relationship provides an ideal basis from which to develop a health-promoting approach to care. However, it is also quite clear that such an approach differs radically from the ones that nurses, and indeed other health professionals such as doctors, are trained to adopt. A certain amount of 'unlearning' must, therefore, take place, and it would be naive to expect nurses, midwives or health visitors to become effective in their new role without appropriate training.

The participants in this study were given a 2-day 'training programme' to introduce them to the principles of a health promotion approach to care, and prepare them to help patients and clients stop smoking. This short training programme also incorporated student-directed learning activities in the student's own time. The participants' evaluations of the training workshops and our own perceptions of them were closely aligned. The 2-day programme was felt by all to be the bare minimum to allow for knowledge and skills increments and attitude shifts.

In an ideal world much more time would need to be allocated for trained staff who have not been exposed to this kind of input in their initial nurse training. This last point is important because the vast majority of practising nurses, and indeed doctors, have not been subjected to a 'health' orientated approach in their basic education programme. Hopefully, if Project 2000 (UKCC, 1986) is implemented, future generations of nurses will be encouraged to develop the knowledge and skills necessary for fulfilling a health education role from the beginning of their training. However, the reality is that thousands of trained health professionals are in need of continuous education and updating in the principles and practice of health promotion. While there is no doubt from the results of this study that nurses require an input of knowledge related to smoking, their greatest deficit, as perceived by themselves, lies in the attitudes and skills required to put health promotion into practice. Training programmes designed to meet these needs must therefore be developed.

A particular problem that emerged from the analysis of the tape-recordings was the difficulty that participants found in moving away from a prescriptive approach towards an approach that involved patient and client participation in decision-making. The training programme used in this study was effective as a stimulus to change in attitudes and skills, and facilitated the acquisition of new knowledge. However, it became clear from the analysis of the tapes that the participants had only made limited changes in terms of their actual practice, particularly in their use of the framework where almost all those taking part found difficulty in encouraging patient and client participation in the planning of a strategy for giving up smoking. Such a shift in approach requires radical rethinking of the principles, philosophy and practice of nursing and is unlikely to take place quickly. Again, this difficulty is unlikely to be exclusive to nursing but will have to be faced by doctors and other health professionals where 'prescription' and the medical model have been accepted for decades.

This research, therefore, has illuminated the need critically to review existing basic and post-basic education programmes in nursing, midwifery and health visiting, particularly in the light of the many changes currently under consideration. If nurses, midwives and health visitors are to fulfil their potential as health educators and promoters of health, the emphasis in their education must become that of health rather than illness. This does not mean that the equally important role of caring for the sick should be undermined, merely that it should be put into perspective.

REFERENCES

Becker M (1974) The health belief model. *Health Education Monographs*, **2**: 409-419.

Burt A et al (1974) Stopping smoking after myocardial infarction. *Lancet*, **i**: 304-306.

Faulkner A and Ward L (1983) Nurses as health educators in relation to smoking. *Nursing Times*, **79**(15): 47-48.

Jamrozik K et al (1984) Controlled trial of three different anti-smoking interventions in general practice. *British Medical Journal*, **289**: 1499-1515.

Macleod Clark J et al (1985) *Helping Patients and Clients to Stop Smoking - the Nurse's Role*. Phase 1 Reports ABC and Summary Report. London: Health Education Council.

Macleod Clark et al (1987) *Helping Patients and Clients to Stop Smoking. Assessing the Effectiveness of the Nurses' Role*. Research Report No.19. London: Health Education Council.

OPCS (1984) *General Household Survey*. London: HMSO.

Randell J (1980) *Health Education in Nursing - a Survey of England, Wales and Northern Ireland*. London: Health Education Council.

Randell J (1982) *Nurse Tutors, Health Education and the Curriculum*. London: Health Education Council.

Royal College of Physicians (1983) *Health or Smoking?* London: Pitman.

Russell M et al (1979) The effect of general practitioners' advice against smoking. *British Medical Journal*, **2**: 231-235.

Russell M et al (1980) The clinical use of nicotine chewing gum. *British Medical Journal*, **280**: 1599.

Swenson I and Dalton J (1983) A comparison of knowledge and attitudes about smoking among nurses. *International Journal of Nursing Studies*, **20**(3): 163-170.

Syred M (1981) The abdication of the role of health education by hospital nurses. *Journal of Advanced Nursing*, **6**: 27-33.

UKCC (1986) *Project 2000*. London: UKCC.

Vartianinen E et al (1986) Ten year results of a community based anti-smoking programme. *Health Education Research*, **1**(3): 175-184.

Ward L and Faulkner A (1983) Tutors as health educators. *Nursing Times* Occasional Paper, **79**(40): 66-67.

World Health Organisation (1978) *Report on the International Conference on Primary Health Care, Alma Ata, USSR*. Geneva: WHO.

Chapter 23

Health Education in Basic Nurse Training

Julienne E Meyer

During the last century the pattern of disease in western society has changed. Statistics of disease and of changes in our social and physical environment indicate that four main health problems exist: those concerned with the ageing population, with unhealthy lifestyle, with mental health and with environmental hazards (DHSS, 1976). Medical and nursing activities have failed to deal with those problems that require a health education approach aimed at prevention.

The importance of health education in nursing has, however, long been recognised (Magowan, 1985), and recent reports in nurse education (UKCC, 1986) and nursing practice (Cumberlege, 1986) have re-emphasised the nurse's role in this respect. Currently nurse educationalists are reviewing nursing curricula in the light of these reports. This chapter gives a brief overview of an exploratory study that investigated the process and impact of introducing a new health education component into a basic nurse training curriculum. A full and more detailed account of the study can be found in Meyer (1986). Health education is a rapidly changing field and current approaches to this discipline must be considered in the context of its historical background.

CHANGES IN HEALTH EDUCATION PHILOSOPHY

A historical review of the development of health education reveals a recent change in philosophy. In an analysis of the state and development of health education, Vuori (1980) argued that, since the scientific revolution, health education has become dominated by medicine.

It took some 200 years for medicine to establish its supremacy over health education, with advances in effective prevention (immunisation, antisepsis and asepsis) and curative (serum therapy antibiotics) measures. For a major part of the twentieth century it was widely believed that medical science would cure all ills and ensure the health of the population. However, since the late 1970s, there has been a general realisation that the complex and costly health-care systems have not actually had an impact on promoting health. Illich (1974) and Mahler (1975), therefore, called for the demystification of medicine and the demedicalisation of health. These sentiments were endorsed by the Declaration of Alma Ata in 1978 (WHO, 1978).

Following Alma Ata, the European region of the World Health Organisation attempted to reconceptualise its orientation to health education within a framework of health promotion (WHO, 1980). Kickbusch (1981) identified four conceptual reorientations:

1. From health prescription to health promotion.
2. From individualistic behaviour modification to a systematic public health approach.
3. From medical orientation to recognition of lay competence.
4. From authoritarian health education to supportive health education.

Literature searches have revealed considerable confusion as to what is meant by health promotion (Anderson, 1984; Baric, 1985; Tones, 1985). Baric (1985) made the following distinction between 'health education' and 'health promotion':

> 'Health promotion is concerned with the creation of a social, political and economic environment conducive to healthy lifestyles, and health education is concerned with raising individual competence and knowledge about health and illness, about the body functions, about prevention and coping; with raising competence and knowledge to use the health care system and to understand its functions; and with raising awareness about social and political and environmental factors that influence health. The main difference, therefore, being not so much in the aims and objectives, but in the levels on which these are carried out.'

From the above it can be seen that there has been a reorientation of philosophy within health education, which nurses must take into account when reviewing their curricula.

THE NURSE'S HEALTH EDUCATION ROLE

It has been argued that nurses have an important role to play in health education. Smith (1979) suggested that nurses are in a unique position to carry out all levels of health education; they are the largest group of health workers and have the most constant contact with patients, so their influence could be very great. Smith saw health education as part and parcel of the nursing process, and the move towards greater involvement of nurses in health education as a logical and rational extension of their role.

There can be little doubt about the professional commitment to health education in nursing. The current interest, reflected in the First International Conference on Health Education in Nursing, Midwifery and Health Visiting at Harrogate in May 1985, may have arisen from the WHO's recommendations that nurses should be trained for primary health care (WHO, 1978) and from the endorsement of this by the English National Board's Statutory Rules Approval Order (ENB, 1983). These state that all nurses should:

> '(18.1a) Advise on the promotion of health and prevention of illness, and
> (18.1b) Recognise situations that may be detrimental to the health and wellbeing of the individual.'

However, despite professional commitment to the concept, research has shown that nurses have not adequately fulfilled their health education role (Faulkner, 1980; Macleod Clark, 1983). Faulkner identified several reasons for nurses' lack of health education skills. One principal reason was thought to be a poor knowledge base, and other factors included nurses' lack of ability in teaching and communication skills. These, together with a lack both of nurses' motivation to teach and of patients' expectation to be taught, led to a behaviour set that excluded health education. A health education role for nurses has been seen to be in direct conflict with medical role expectations (Faulkner, 1980). Macleod Clark et al (1987, and chapter 22) demonstrated that while it has been possible for nurses to acquire a formal knowledge (about smoking), knowledge alone has been insufficient, since nurses also lacked skills and confidence to practise as health educators (about smoking).

In discussing the abdication of the health education role by nurses, Syred (1981) suggested that the problem was to do with education. Randell (1982) found that preparation for a health education role had not been integrated into nurse education programmes. Few schools had a working definition of health education, and there tended to be an approach more towards illness and rehabilitation than towards positive health. Ward staff and clinical tutors have rarely been cited as being involved in its teaching (Randell, 1980). Another study likewise showed that little teaching time has been given to health education in nurse education programmes, and it highlighted the teachers' inability to teach the subject (Ward and Faulkner, 1983). While evidence has suggested that nurses have not been adequately fulfilling their health education role, there is other evidence to suggest that health education in nursing practice has been effective (Carpenter et al, 1983; Wilson-Barnett and Oborne, 1983).

In recent years a variety of initiatives aimed at integrating health education in nursing has been taken (Meyer, 1986), and it is important that these developments are monitored and carefully evaluated. An example of one such attempt to introduce and evaluate a new health education component in a basic nurse training programme is now described.

AIM AND METHODS OF INVESTIGATION

The aim of this project was to describe the process and impact of introducing a health education component into a basic nursing curriculum.

The objectives were:

1. To describe the students' response to the teaching of health education.
2. To describe the effect of introducing a curriculum innovation within a school of nursing.
3. To identify some of the conflicts that may arise through the teaching and practice of health education.

Methods

A qualitative approach, described as 'illuminative evaluation' by Parlett and Hamilton (1977) was chosen for this study, an approach that has been used before in research into nurse education. Lathlean and Farnish (1984), for example, effectively used this method to evaluate experimental training schemes for ward sisters (see chapter 18). Evaluation strategies were used to assess the degree of success of the innovation, the problems encountered and the processes involved. By giving a sufficiently detailed and illuminating description of the facts, problems, issues, experiences and perceptions, it was thought that others might be in a position to judge its application to their own situation. It was hoped that the project might help to direct others interested in integrating health education into their curriculum by suggesting methods of evaluating such an innovation and outlining possible curriculum content.

Research participants

The evaluation was confined to one group of learners (n = 19) preparing for Part 1 of the register in one school of nursing during the first 16 weeks of training. The first 16 weeks of training comprised an 8-week teaching component followed by an 8-week clinical allocation. One learner left after 2 weeks of the introductory course and another during the clinical allocation (both on account of sickness). Data were also gathered from other nurses/health educators interested in introducing health education in nursing (n = 56) and from teachers in the school of nursing (n = 26).

Data collection and analysis

A variety of methods was used to gather the data, including written questionnaires, taped guided interviews, non-participant observation, incident books and diary. A full account of the methods used can be found in Meyer (1986).

Pilot work began in October 1985 and was followed by the main data collection which began in February 1986 and continued until June 1986. The study was divided into two parts – a local review and a national review. The local review gathered data from those directly involved in the innovation and the national review circulated details of the curriculum to experts for comment. Latent content analysis, as described by Fox (1982), was used first to code the data gathered, and then descriptive statistics were used to enumerate the number of times specific concepts were discussed.

The innovation

The health education curriculum was designed by the author in her role as tutor and member of the sub-planning group for health education and communication skills, in conjunction with a senior health education officer. The curriculum was divided into two phases. Phase 1 dealt with the concepts, principles and philosophies of health education, which were taught during the first 8 weeks of the introductory course, and was the focus of attention for this study. Phase 2 was concerned with the application of themes developed in phase 1 to specific clinical areas under study in later modules. The curriculum combined theory and practice (where possible drawing upon local initiatives and ward experiences) and was threaded throughout the 3-year training programme.

Fundamental to the course was the encouragement of students to examine their own health beliefs and attitudes as well as the social, environmental and individual factors affecting health behaviour. A broad understanding of health education was facilitated through an appreciation of the different and varied approaches used by health educators. It was hoped that by enabling the students to appreciate a deeper understanding of the complexities of issues involved, their health education practice would be more appropriate and effective in meeting the needs of individual clients. Informal teaching with class participation was considered to be the most suitable method of teaching this complex subject. Health education was linked with the teaching of sociology and psychology (Table 23.1) and was taught alongside communication skills. Communication skills training was thought to be essential to the practice of health education and followed the format outlined in the communication in nurse education project (Tomlinson, 1984, and chapter 21). Attempts were made to link theory and practice by asking learners to note 'incidents' of health education activity or missed opportunity while working on the wards. These incidents were recorded in books and formed the basis for discussion in clinical tutorials.

Table 23.1   Phase 1 – introductory course

Sessions	Sociology	Health education	Psychology

1	Introduction to sociology:
	  What it is
	  How it developed
	  Relevance to health
		Introduction to health education – nurses' responsibility	Introduction to psychology – different schools of thought

2	Inequalities in health care:
	  Employment/
	    unemployment
	  Poverty
	  Class
	  Race
	  Gender
		Concepts and determinants of health	Perceptual processes

3	Sociology of community:
	  What it is
	  How it is defined
	  How people fit into it
	    as individuals, group
	    members, families
		Health education – the local community	Study of personality

4	Attitude formation and change	Principles of health education	Human motivation
5	Power and authority status and role. Patient, nurse, doctor relationships	Different approaches to health education	Reaction to illness by patient and family
6	Medicine as an agent of social control. Social order	Ethical aspects of education	Conflicts and anxiety
7	Illness behaviour, deviancy and illness	Helping people to make health choices	Intelligence
8	Education: opportunities, inequalities Health service: origins, welfare state, organisation, bureaucracy, institutionalisation	Teaching and instructing health education	Learning theory

Response

National review

Findings of the national review must be viewed with caution since the analysis was only based on 30 replies, which represented a response rate of 54 per cent. However, it was felt that some useful information had been obtained from the national review, which reflected current thinking on health education in nursing.

Local review

Response rates from teachers and learners within the school were high and may be one of the advantages of institutional self-evaluation. The researcher, by working on site, could easily rearrange interviews and the collection of questionnaires to suit the convenience of respondents. The 'subjective' nature of illuminative evaluation is frequently questioned. In this particular study criticism may be directed towards the fact that the teacher was also the researcher. Smeaton (1982) argued the need for illuminative evaluation in nurse education and suggested that teacher-researchers need to become an established reality, as in the case of general education. He suggested that illuminative evaluation had already achieved the status of other more traditional research methods in general education, and that there were sufficient case studies to form guidelines and principles for its use in nursing. The need for teacher-researchers was supported by Simons (1981); she argued that decisions as to who is the most legitimate person(s) to initiate and/or conduct school self-evaluation should be determined on the basis of local knowledge of the context and relationships. In this particular study, working both as teacher and researcher proved to be an asset. In the role of teacher working within the hospitals under study, 'informants' arose informally and volunteered feedback on the innovation. This information was recorded in the researcher's diary. An 'outsider' may not have had such easy access to this type of information.

FINDINGS FROM THE NATIONAL REVIEW

Comments on curriculum outline

Overall there was general approval for the curriculum outline in the national review. The curriculum was thought to be in line with the English National Board's guidelines for curriculum revision (ENB, 1985).

Consensus of opinion

There appeared to be a consensus of opinion as to how health education should be developed in basic nurse training. The national review highlighted that health education should be threaded throughout training and integrated with other subjects. It was also felt that students should explore wider social and political issues and acknowledge the importance of the community. The need to allow students to explore their own values and attitudes was thought to be vital before encouraging client interaction, and the importance of informal teaching methods was also noted. It is interesting that many of the suggestions from the national review were included in the curriculum outline but in practice gave rise to some important issues to be discussed in the local review.

However, despite this general consensus of opinion, there appeared to be a wide variety of approaches to the inclusion of health education within basic nurse training and, therefore, a great need to share ideas/experiences. Similar conclusions were drawn from the Basic Curriculum Project (Scottish Health Education Group, 1986).

Negative comments

The national review highlighted possible problems in the evaluation strategy to be used in the research. In particular, it was suggested that learners and teachers might feel 'swamped' by the data collection. Teachers did not express these feelings, but learners were certainly overloaded.

The curriculum outline was criticised for not stating clearer aims and objectives and also for being too ambitious for an introductory course. Furthermore, it was suggested that there was a need to include more health education resources in the curriculum outline.

Comments were made about the difficulty of putting theory into practice in view of the current constraints on manpower and resources.

FINDINGS FROM THE LOCAL REVIEW

The findings of this study cannot be generalised, as they represent a case study of one instance. However, the research raised some problems and issues that may be of relevance to others interested in developing health education in basic nurse training, and confirmed many of the findings from previous studies.

Positive in theory – reservations in practice

Learners and teachers within the school environment felt positive towards the concept of health education and wanted it to be threaded throughout nurse training. Teachers acknowledged that the need to change was long overdue and suggested that, in the past, health education had tended to be linked with teaching about disease and, where taught separately, had been undertaken by health education officers, with limited time available. This confirmed the findings of a survey carried out by the then Health Education Council in 1980 (HEC, 1980).

While teachers felt positive towards the concept of health education, some reservations were held as regards its implementation. The major area of concern was the amount of time to be spent on its teaching. An already overcrowded curriculum was often referred to and fears expressed that health education would be taught in preference to basic nursing skills. The study found that it was possible to incorporate teaching time for health education, psychology, sociology and communication skills within the introductory course programme. However, it must be noted that the clinical teachers involved felt that this was done at the expense of teaching on practical skills. It was interesting that no feedback from learners indicated this to be a problem. This issue would certainly need to be addressed in a longitudinal study.

Total curriculum review and in-service training

The introduction of health education as a new subject within the curriculum has implications not only for timetable planning but also for the teaching of all other subjects within the curriculum. For 'health' to be placed as a central concept, a reorientation of thinking away from the medical model is needed. For true integration of health education within the curriculum, teachers need to share health-orientated philosophies and approaches to their work. This leads to another issue highlighted in the study – inadequate preparation of teachers to promote the concept of health education. Similarly, Ward and Faulkner (1983) identified teachers' lack of knowledge and skills in health education. Within the school environment it was not thought that all teachers would be prepared to change their thinking towards health.

Change was seen as a threat to some individuals and involved too much work for some teachers who were already overcommitted timewise and unable to take on any further projects.

Need for specialist teachers

While learners enjoyed the communication skills teaching and appreciated its relevance to the health education input, the links between health education and sociology and psychology were not always recognised. Teachers who taught sociology and psychology felt that they had worked in isolation and that the innovation would have benefited from an involvement by them at the planning stage. The fact that teachers felt they were working in isolation perhaps suggested that they were not sufficiently aware of the links to be made with the health education input, and this supported the need for in-service education. Findings also indicated that there may be a need to look outside nurse education for experts to teach specialist subjects. It is interesting that a senior tutor who was studying for an MSc in sociology was unable to teach this subject due to other work commitments.

Another possible reason for the inability of learners to perceive the relevant links between subjects may have been that insufficient time was allocated to teach the content outlined in the curriculum. Both learners and teachers made comments to this effect. It would now seem appropriate either to increase the time commitment to these subjects or decrease the content.

Relevance of health education in the introductory course

Teachers questioned whether learners would appreciate the relevance of health education in the introductory course. In fact, learners realised the importance of health education in the introductory course and wanted it to be taught in future modules. However, some did comment that its relevance became far more apparent once working on the wards.

Problems of content with multi-ability groups

While the teaching of health education was rated highly by learners, a difference in opinion was expressed about some of the content. Teachers had questioned whether the content was too theoretical, and some learners commented that they would have preferred more content related to practical nursing. It is, therefore, not surprising that the lesson most highly rated included the use of a practical role-play (session 7), whereas the lesson that caused confusion looked at the theoretical approaches to health education (session 5). Despite this, some learners commented that they would have preferred more content and depth, and this highlighted the issue of balancing education to suit the needs of large numbers of learners within the context of a classroom.

Need for sensitive teaching methods and support for learners

The national review identified the need for learners to explore their own values and attitudes towards health, but in practice this highlighted some difficulties. While learners enjoyed the opportunity of exploring their own health and suggested that it had helped them to make friends with one another, a few found the experience painful. This collaborated the findings of Mayhew (1986) and raised some important issues, particularly as to what help has been available to support learners with health problems. Few hospitals have had the luxury of full-time counsellors, and the ethics of learners exploring their own health without the necessary support systems must be questioned. In particular, some learners found the issue of smoking especially threatening, and this indicated a need for sensitive teaching methods. Booth (1985) drew similar conclusions.

The national review recognised the importance of informal teaching methods in health education. Learners especially enjoyed the informal relaxed atmosphere and felt that they had learnt more through discussion and exchange of ideas than they could have learnt by traditional teaching methods. Similar findings were highlighted in the CINE project (Tomlinson, 1984 and chapter 21).

Lack of support for health education on the wards

A major issue identified by the study was the lack of support for health education on the wards and the need for practising role models. Some learners found that health education was actively inhibited, depending on the attitude of ward staff.

Learners commented that there was a lack of time for health education on the wards and that it tended to be taught by specialist staff, e.g. diabetic sisters. This raised the question of whether general nurses have a role to play in health education. While it has been suggested that nurses are perceived as credible sources of advice (Syred, 1981), support must be given to nurses to function in that role.

Lack of support for health education was also shown in the reluctance of ward staff to release learners to attend tutorials to relate theory to practice. Tutorials were poorly attended, but those learners who were able to attend found them helpful.

CONCLUSION

In conclusion, the research raised some problems and issues that might be of interest to others involved in developing health education in basic nurse training.

While there appeared to be a consensus of opinion as to how health education should be included in basic nurse training, doubts existed as to how this could be achieved in the current nurse education system.

For 'health' to be placed as a central concept in nursing, a reorientation of thinking away from the medical model was identified. Findings showed a need for total curriculum review and in-service training of both tutorial and ward staff.

The implications for introducing health education were far reaching, and the study highlighted the need for support systems for nurses addressing their own health beliefs, values and behaviours. Sensitive teaching methods involving class participation were likewise indicated.

For true integration of health education in nursing it would appear that commitment is required on all levels: managerial, educational and clinical. The nurse's role in health education needs to be established and supported in practice through multidisciplinary teamwork. It is imperative that nurses should be prepared for this new role and guidelines drawn to direct future initiatives.

ACKNOWLEDGEMENT

The above study (Meyer, 1986) was undertaken with the support of a DHSS Nursing Studentship, in part fulfilment of an MSc in Nursing, while the author was working as nurse tutor.

REFERENCES

Anderson R (1984) Health promotion: state of the art. In: WHO, *Health Promotion: Concepts and Principles*, pp. 12-17. A selection of papers presented at the Working Group on Concepts and Principles, Copenhagen 9-13 July 1984. WHO Regional Office for Europe 1984.

Baric L (1985) The meaning of words: health promotion. *Journal of the Institute of Health Education* (special issue - Health Education and Promotion), **23**(1): 10-15.

Booth C (1985) *Giving up Smoking: an Exploration of Support Systems for Nurses.* Unpublished MSc dissertation, University of Manchester.

Carpenter R G, Gardner A, Jepson M, Taylor E M, Salvin A, Sunderland R, Emery J L, Pursall E and Roe J (1983) Prevention of unexpected infant death. *Lancet*, **i**: 723-727.

Cumberlege J (1986) *Neighbourhood Nursing - a Focus for Care.* Report of the Community Nursing Review, DHSS. London: HMSO.

DHSS (1976) *Prevention and Health: Everybody's Business. A Reassessment of Public and Personal Health.* London: HMSO.

English National Board (1983) *Statutory Rules Approval Order.* Statutory Instrument No. 873.

English National Board (1985) *The Syllabus and Examinations for Courses in General Nursing Leading to Registration in Part 1 of the Register*, (19) ERDB, April.

Faulkner A (1980) Communication and the nurse. *Nursing Times*, **76**(21): 93-95.

Fox D J (1982) *Fundamentals of Research in Nursing*, 4th edn, pp. 391-409. Norwalk, New Jersey: Appleton-Century-Crofts.

Health Education Council (1980) HE in nursing, a survey of nursing in England, Wales and Northern Ireland. London: HEC.

Illich I (1974) Medical nemesis: the expropriation of health. London: Calder and Boyars.

Kickbusch I (1981) Involvement in health: a social concept of health education. *International Journal of Health Education* supp. October-December, XXIV: 4.

Lathlean J and Farnish S (1984) *The Ward Sister Training Project.* NERU Report No. 3. Chelsea College, University of London: Nursing Education Research Unit.

Macleod Clark J (1983) Nurse-patient communication in surgical wards. In: *Nursing Research*, ed. Wilson-Barnett J. Chichester: John Wiley.

Macleod Clark J, Kendall S and Haverty S (1987) Helping nurses develop their health education role: a framework for training. *Nurse Education Today*, **7**: 63-68.

Magowan R (1985) *Health Education - a Midas Touch for Nursing.* Unpublished paper presented at the 1st International Conference of Health Education in Nursing, Harrogate.

Mahler H (1975) Health - a demystification of technology. *Lancet*, **ii**: 829-833.

Mayhew A (1986) Education for health. *Senior Nurse*, **5**(1): 24-25.

Meyer J (1986) *An exploratory study to describe the process and impact of introducing a new health education component into a basic nurse training curriculum.* Unpublished MSc dissertation, University of London.

Parlett M and Hamilton D (1977) Evaluation as illumination: a new approach to the study of innovatory programmes. In: *Beyond The Numbers Game*, eds. Hamilton D et al. London: Macmillan Education.

Randell J (1980) *Health Education in Nursing.* Unpublished report on a Survey of Nursing in England, Wales and Northern Ireland. London: HEC.

Randell J (1982) *Health Education in Nursing.* Unpublished report of a workshop. London: HEC.

Scottish Health Education Group (1986) A Report on Health Education Development in Nursing Curriculum in Three Scottish Colleges 1982-1986. Edinburgh: SHEG.

Simons H (1981) *Against the Rules: Procedural Problems in Institutional Self Evaluation.* Unpublished paper, Curriculum Studies Department, University of London Institute of Education.

Smeaton W (1982) The nurse tutor as researcher. *Nurse Education Today*, **2**(5): 8-9.

Smith J P (1979) The challenge of health education for nurses in the 1980s. *Journal of Advanced Nursing*, **4**: 531-543.

Syred M E J (1981) The abdication of the role of Health Education by hospital nurses. *Journal of Advanced Nursing*, **6**: 27-33.

Tomlinson A (1984) *The Analysis of Qualitative Data from a Curriculum Development Project*. Unpublished paper presented to RCN Research Society Conference, April 1984.

Tones B K (1985) Health Education: A new panacea. *Journal of Institute of Health Education*, **23**(1): 16-21.

United Kingdom Central Council for Nursing, Midwifery and Health Visiting (1986) *Project 2000: a new preparation for practice*. London: UKCC.

Vuori H (1980) The medical model and the objectives of health education. *International Journal of Health Education*, **23**(2): 12-19.

Ward L and Faulkner A (1983) Tutors as health educators. *Nursing Times* (October 5): 66-67.

WHO (1978) *Primary Health Care Report of the International Conference on Primary Health Care*. Alma Ata USSR, 6-12 September 1978. Geneva: WHO.

WHO (1980) *Regional Strategy for Attaining Health for All by the Year 2000*. Copenhagen: Thirtieth Session of the Regional Committee for Europe EUR/RC30/8, WHO.

WHO (1984) *Health Promotion: Concepts and Principles*. A selection of papers presented at the Working Group on Concepts and Principles, Copenhagen 9-13 July 1984. WHO Regional Office for Europe.

Wilson-Barnett J and Oborne J (1983) Studies evaluating patient teaching: implications for practice. *International Journal of Nursing Studies*, **20**(1): 33-34.

Chapter 24

Evaluation of a Ward-based Teaching Programme for Nurses Caring for Patients with a Tracheal Stoma

Brenda De Carle and Jenifer Wilson-Barnett

The overall aim of this study is to evaluate a ward-based teaching programme for nurses who are caring for patients with a tracheal stoma. (Tracheal stoma is used as a broad term to cover both patients who have undergone tracheostomy formation as well as those who have had their larynx removed, usually because of cancer.) The study has been funded by the DHSS and is in the final stage of analysis.

This chapter provides the background to the study, describes the research design and the teaching programme devised. An analysis was not complete at the time of writing, but some preliminary findings are included.

BACKGROUND TO THE STUDY

There has been very little research into the nursing care of patients with a tracheal stoma, although some small-scale studies on certain aspects of physical care have been conducted. For example, Grossbach-Landis (1979) studied the suction techniques of 30 nurses and concluded (p. 237) that 'tracheal suctioning is performed with considerable variation and frequently with questionable regard for sterile technique'. More recently Harris (1984) investigated the prevalence of clean versus sterile suctioning techniques in 142 hospitals in America. She concluded that the technique practised was on the whole a 'clean' technique, regardless of what it was called. Oermann et al (1983) described sensations experienced by 34 patients during tracheostomy care, suggesting that if such information was included in the preoperative preparation, emotional distress would be reduced and coping facilitated.

The psychological and social care of patients who have undergone tracheal stoma formation is an area in which even less research is available (De Carle, 1985). Communication may be extremely difficult in the early postoperative days as patients may be unable to speak.

231

Lauder (1975) identified the nurse as the key figure who must enable the patient to communicate effectively by other means such as deciphering writing and providing appropriate aids such as picture cards, etc. In a descriptive study of 24 patients' experiences after laryngectomy, Beilby (1983) reported that there are still problems with adequate rehabilitation after discharge.

The nursing management of tracheostomy patients in three hospitals was investigated by De Carle (1985). The findings gave a picture of variety in practice and of misunderstanding by nurses. The purpose of the study described in this chapter is a development of his initial work, and comprises an evaluation of an educational programme designed to improve the nursing care of patients with a tracheal stoma.

EDUCATIONAL STRATEGIES

Studies evaluating strategies for integrating principles with practice have identified several problems, such as the difficulty of transferring knowledge learnt in the classroom to other situations and the lack of representation of reality of the practical situation in teaching. Solutions offered have suggested that those who teach nursing should be more directly involved with the actual practice of nursing.

Work by Alexander (1980) is of direct relevance to this concept of planned teaching as her research aimed to facilitate the integration of theory and practice. A planned programme of concurrent theory and directly relevant and supervised practice of nursing (i.e. of college and ward-based instruction) was experienced by student nurses randomly allocated to an experimental group. Their peers in the control group received teaching by entirely college-based methods, as was the norm. Students in the experimental group were thus helped to learn how to learn from their daily work with patients, and to learn from practice rather than from classroom teaching only. Students, teachers and trained ward staff gave a very positive evaluation of the method. Three of Alexander's four recommendations have been incorporated in the present study:

1. That nursing should be taught where nursing is carried out.
2. That teaching methods actively involve the students.
3. That attention is given to teaching ward staff and students how to teach.

PATIENT TEACHING

This is an area of key importance if patients with a tracheal stoma are going to be able to cope successfully. In a review of the literature on patient teaching and its implications for practice, Wilson-Barnett and Oborne (1983) found that, generally, studies indicate that patients do gain from and appreciate more information, resulting in 'less anxiety, more participation and an increased feeling of control over their lives'. However, the type of information and its presentation is important if the patient is going to assimilate it (Redman, 1981). Redman suggests that understanding of new material is possible if the recipient is motivated and the information is clearly presented in small 'doses' and is seen to be relevant. Pagana (1978) describes some information that should be available to patients with a tracheostomy before discharge.

AIMS AND DESIGN OF THE RESEARCH

From reviewing all the available literature and after much discussion with many experts in the field, a teaching programme for nurses was devised.

The aims of the research are as follows:

1. To assess nurses' level of knowledge, understanding and practical skills when caring for patients with a tracheal stoma.
2. To evaluate the effectiveness of the teaching programme, which was designed to enhance nurses' knowledge, understanding and practical skills and to enable them to care more competently and confidently for the physical, psychological and social needs of patients with a tracheal stoma.
3. To describe patients' experiences and their physical, psychological and social adjustment to having a tracheal stoma.
4. To evaluate patients' physical, psychological and social adjustment to having a tracheal stoma when cared for by nurses who have or have not participated in the teaching programme.

Design of the study

This study is an adaptation of the clinical experimental design by Levine (1960). There are two researchers: the first is responsible for data collection from both nurses and patients; the second is responsible for the experimental intervention, i.e. the teaching programme.

The main study design is viewed in two parts with two pairs of wards. After a 6-month time period the whole procedure is then duplicated in two more hospitals with two more wards.

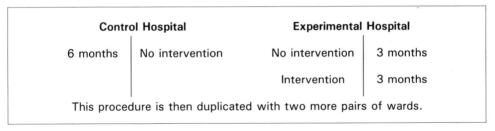

Fig. 24.1 Outline of main study design

In the control hospital no intervention takes place, only data collection. In the experimental hospital data collection also takes place, but, after a 3-month time period, the teaching programme is introduced for a further 3-month time period.

The nurses

All trained and learner nurses allocated to the ear, nose and throat (ENT) wards during the time period of the study are asked to participate. Once consent is obtained they are asked to complete the following:

1. An *interview schedule* to collect biographical details and other items, such as expectations about and feelings towards patients with a tracheal stoma.
2. A *multiple-choice questionnaire* concerning ideal practice in terms of procedures and psychological care. Questions are divided into two parts – the stem and the response. There are 20 questions, the respondents having to choose one out of four answers for each and filling in an answer sheet.
3. *Observation check-lists.* After a period of acclimatisation, nurses are observed performing three practical procedures of tracheal stoma care, namely:
    i   suctioning the airway;
    ii stoma care;
    iii stoma care with the tapes being changed.
   (Observations are only carried out if both the patient and the nurse consent for a specific occasion.)

Trained staff complete the interview and questionnaire and are observed initially and then at 3- and 6-month time intervals in the study. The same process is undertaken with student nurses at the start and end of their ward placements, which are estimated to last on average for 8–10 weeks.

This data collection from the nurses is represented diagrammatically in Figure 24.2.

The patients

All patients undergoing tracheal stoma formation on the ENT wards during the time period of the study who meet the criteria for admission are approached by the researcher. The study is explained and guarantees of confidentiality given. Once signed consent is obtained the patient is assessed with respect to his mood, satisfaction, confidence in personal health and practical coping skills on a number of occasions, planned to be:

1. preoperatively (unless emergency situations);
2. 3 days postoperatively;
3. 1 week postoperatively;
4. 10 days postoperatively;
5. the day before discharge.

The research tools used in this assessment consist of an interview schedule, mood adjective check-list (Lishman, 1972) and a well-being inventory. A sub-group of patients, consisting of those discharged home with a tracheal stoma, is interviewed 4 weeks after leaving hospital.

Outcome measures

For the *nurses*, measures used to indicate changes in understanding and practical skills (relevant to their competence and confidence after participating in the teaching programme) include scores from multiple choice questionnaires and observation check-lists, plus factors identified at initial and subsequent interviews. Scores are, therefore, compared across groups and within the experimental groups before and after the teaching programme.

For the *patients* who have been cared for by nurses who participated in the teaching programme, the measures used to indicate changed mood, satisfaction, confidence in personal

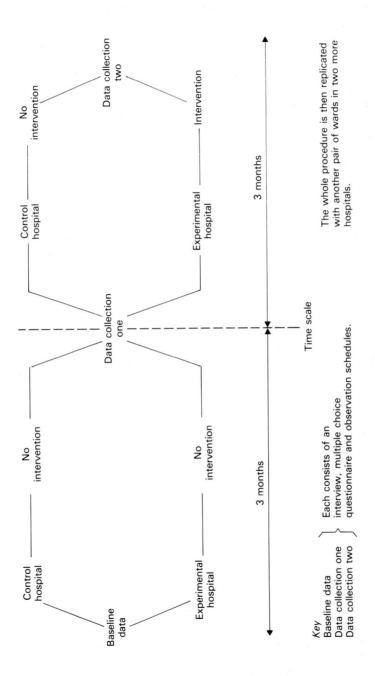

Fig. 24.2 Outline of data collection from nurses

health and practical coping skills include scores from the mood adjective check-list and factors identified in initial and subsequent interviews. Scores are compared for those patients nursed as controls (or before the teaching) with others after this intervention.

The sample

As it was not possible to find two busy ENT wards caring for patients with tracheal stomas in one hospital, two pairs of ENT wards in two different hospitals were used. The wards were matched as far as possible, on factors such as size, layout, numbers of patients and staff complement. It was anticipated that about 100 nurses and 50 patients would be involved in this two-part study. An analysis will be undertaken to ensure that no differences in base-line knowledge and practices exist between groups prior to intervention. Any differences in outcome measures can then be accounted for by the independent variable – the teaching programme.

Outcomes

It is hoped that this study will demonstrate the effectiveness of a teaching programme designed to improve the understanding and practical skills of nurses, enabling them to meet the physical, psychological and social needs of patients with a tracheal stoma more competently and confidently. It is envisaged that patients who have been cared for by nurses participating in the teaching programme will be less anxious or depressed and more satisfied with their care and progress than those cared for by other nurses.

THE TEACHING PROGRAMME

As the independent variable, the teaching programme is being evaluated. This programme is the responsibility of one researcher and is carried out only in the experimental hospital during the intervention phase in the final 3 months of the study (see Figure 24.1).

The teaching programme consists of three main parts:

1. Ward-based tutorials.
2. Working with nurses.
3. Patient teaching cards.

Ward-based tutorials

A continuous series of five ward-based tutorials are held throughout the teaching programme. A record of attendance is maintained to avoid repetition and to ensure that the nurses have the opportunity to attend the full range of sessions. The tutorials usually take place in the afternoon during the cross-over period when both shifts of staff are on duty. They last approximately 20 minutes which, in practice, is the maximum time feasible on a busy surgical ward with operating lists throughout the day, 5 days a week. Tutorials at the weekend are thus particularly helpful and popular, especially among the trained staff. At each session nurses are given copies of the relevant nursing care guidelines devised as the theoretical basis of the study. They outline the nursing actions to be taken, with reasons for this. Each nurse is given a folder so he or she can build up the full series of guidelines for personal use.

The researcher is able to adapt the tutorials to meet the needs of trained staff and learners by altering the approach and emphasis to suit the group. Throughout the series of tutorials, the emphasis is on helping nurses to understand the principles underlying the nursing care. A wide variety of visual aids has been developed and are used as appropriate.

Working with nurses

To help nurses relate information given in the tutorials and outlined in the nursing care guidelines, the researcher actually worked with each nurse caring for a patient with a tracheal stoma. In particular, the researcher tried to ensure that she worked with the nurse at the following times:

1. when the nurse prepared the patient preoperatively for tracheal stoma formation;
2. when the nurse carried out the following three practical procedures:
   i   suctioning the airway;
   ii cleaning the stoma;
   iii changing the tapes;
3. when the nurse discussed psychological and social implications of the tracheal stoma with the patient in preparation for his discharge home.

The researcher aimed to gain rapport with the nurses, caring for patients being seen as a joint effort rather than a 'test' situation. Also, it was important for the researcher to abstain

---

Cleaning the inner tracheostomy tube (plain or speaking)

What to do	*Reason why*
1. Take the inner tube out of the outer tube in your neck and clean it as follows:	Inner tube cannot be cleaned while it is in your neck
a) Hold inner tube under warm (*not* hot), running tap water and clean with stiff brush	Thorough cleaning is important to remove the phlegm that has collected there. Hot water may make tube too hot to handle
b) Rinse inner tube under cool running water, shake and replace inside outer tube in your neck	Inner tube should only be removed for the shortest possible time to prevent blocking of the outer tube
2. Clean the inner tube as often as necessary, usually every 3 hours to begin with	A clean inner tube can make it much easier for you to breathe
3. Between use, your spare inner tube and the stiff brush should be stored dry	There is no need to store them in water, which can sometimes act as a source of infection
4. Do not mix up the spare set of tubes with the tube you are currently using	The inner tubes from one set will not fit properly inside another tracheostomy tube set

Fig. 24.3 Patient teaching card

from extending advice beyond the realms of a nurse with no specific responsibility for the patient. In circumstances when this arose, the researcher encouraged communication and liaison with the ward staff who had a direct responsibility for the patient's well-being.

Patient teaching cards

These cards were designed to be used by nurses when teaching patients to care for their own stoma. They provide a basic outline of the procedure and explain why each step is necessary in very simple language. An example is shown in Figure 24.3 above. They have a very plain format, clearly printed in large type on white card A5 size. Space is available to add specific nursing care points pertinent to a particular patient.

Cards were used rather than a booklet as they could be given to the patient gradually as each new skill was taught. The cards were kept by the patient but were always thoroughly explained and used by any members of the team involved in the teaching of self-care. Cards were invented to cover a wide variety of practical skills including tracheal suction, stoma care, changing the tapes and care of the tube. Some were also devised to form reference cards to give essential details for a patient's discharge.

It is hoped that the three aspects of this teaching programme will enable nurses to care for patients with a tracheal stoma with improved knowledge, understanding and insight into their needs. This will, hopefully, make nurses more confident and competent in their care. As a direct result, it is hoped that patients with a tracheal stoma will be able to learn the skills of self-care to the best of their ability, so that they can live as independently as possible.

CONCLUSION

This chapter has attempted to cover three main aspects of the study set up to evaluate a ward-based teaching programme for nurses caring for patients with a tracheal stoma. By reviewing the background, outlining the study and describing the teaching programme, we hope to provide the justification for this ward-based teaching approach.

As yet, no results are available, but on an impressionistic level the teaching programme has been well received by both nurses and patients. Staff have generally been helpful, interested and willing to learn. Patients have become very involved, using their teaching cards enthusiastically and explaining them to their relatives. Relatives have also commented that they felt much more at ease with the patient, knowing how and why specific care was needed.

However, one has to await the results of the outcome measures to determine whether or not this general impression can be translated into tangible differences in both nurses' confidence and competence and patients' mood and adjustment to their tracheal stoma.

REFERENCES

Alexander M F (1980) *Nurse Education – an Experiment in Integration of Theory and Practice in Nursing.* Unpublished PhD thesis, University of Edinburgh.
Beilby E (1983) *Laryngectomy – an Investigation of Reactions, Requirement and Rehabilitations after Discharge from Hospital.* MSc dissertation, University of Surrey.
De Carle B (1985) Tracheostomy care. *Nursing Times* Occasional Paper, **81**(6): 50–54.

Grossbach-Landis I (1979) Tracheal suctioning: a tool for evaluation and learning needs assessment. *Nursing Research*, **28**: 237-242.

Harris R B (1984) National surgery of aseptic tracheostomy care techniques in hospitals with head and neck/ENT surgical departments. *Cancer Nursing*, **7**: 23-32.

Lauder E (1975) Towards total rehabilitation. *Nursing Digest*, March-April, **3**: 50-51.

Levine E (1960) Experimental design in nursing research. *Nursing Research*, **9**: 203-212.

Lishman W A (1972) Selective factors in memory part 2 - affective disorders. *Psychological Medicine*, **2**: 248-253.

Oermann M H et al (1983) After a tracheostomy - patients describe their sensations. *Cancer Nursing*, **6**: 361-366.

Pagana K D (1978) Teaching your tracheostomy patients to cope at home. *RN*, **41**: 63-66.

Redman B H (1981) *Issues and Concepts in Patient Education*. New York: Appleton-Century-Crofts.

Wilson-Barnett J and Oborne J (1983) Studies evaluating patient teaching; implication for practice. *International Journal of Nursing Studies*, **20**(1): 33-43.

Chapter 25

Nurses' Attitudes towards Cancer: an Educational Evaluation

Jessica Corner and Jenifer Wilson-Barnett

INTRODUCTION

The study described in this chapter is a 3-year Cancer Research Campaign funded project, which commenced in October 1985. The study aimed to look at ways of improving nurses' attitudes, knowledge and confidence in caring for and communicating with cancer patients, using an educational intervention.

The study grew out of a body of research that indicates that the attitudes held by both the general public and health-care professionals are largely negative and stereotyped, so that cancer is seen to be more devastating than other life-threatening diseases. Like no other disease, cancer is associated with fear and inevitable death involving much pain and suffering (Sontag, 1979). There is also evidence to suggest that such attitudes affect the way in which patients present with symptoms, and delay has been a common feature. Among health carers these attitudes have been associated with patterns of poor communication and care for cancer patients.

This study focused on newly qualified nurses, working in general hospitals, who have received no specialist preparation for dealing with cancer patients. Researchers sought to document the attitudes, knowledge and confidence of these nurses in caring for cancer patients, to assess their educational needs, and then to develop a modest educational input that might meet these needs, evaluating the intervention over a 6-month period.

The project also had wider aims, which were broadly educational and methodological. The educational aspect involved examining questions such as 'How best can the continuing educational needs of qualified nurses be met?', 'What sorts of educational experiences do such nurses prefer?' and 'What were the processes by which attitude, knowledge and confidence change occurs?'.

Following a review of previous research in the area of attitudes to cancer, the authors were critical of the rather simplistic approach that many research studies had taken towards such a complex area as attitude and its change. It was decided that some newer, more qualitative approaches to attitude research should be used and combined with more quantitative, established methods, and their relative merits assessed in a triangulation exercise. Thus, the research could take a multi-faceted approach to attitude assessment and educational evaluation.

In this chapter an initial review of previous research in the area is followed by a discussion of the research methods and design of the study, which attempts to highlight the methodological issues involved. Finally, a brief description of some early findings is given, although as yet it is too early to report a full analysis of the data. The project is due to be completed in October 1988.

BACKGROUND TO THE STUDY

Brooks (1979) has summarised the findings of surveys of public attitudes towards cancer as:

1. a tendency for respondents to exaggerate the number of deaths caused by cancer;
2. a tendency to underestimate the numbers cured of cancer;
3. a strong tendency to view cancer as the most worrying of all diseases;
4. a belief that smoking is implicated in lung cancer;
5. a knowledge of other 'causes' for which some scientific evidence exists;
6. a knowledge of some 'early warning signs' of cancer;
7. a tendency to reject early treatment as leading to improved prognosis;
8. a recognition of the non-contagious nature of cancer.

Brooks concludes (p. 457) that 'One is left with the strong impression that cancer is seen to be very threatening, the most dreaded of all diseases, rarely if ever curable and largely unavoidable'.

The research on health-care professionals seems to indicate that the above statement also applies. In an early study, Davison (1965) surveyed 783 health visitors, district nurses and midwives by questionnaire and asked them to predict cure rates for cancers of different sites. Davison interpreted the significant proportion of nurses who greatly underestimated cure rates as 'gross despondency about cancer'. Twenty per cent of the sample also thought that hospital treatment for cancer was 'frequently not worthwhile'. Easson (1967) documented similar pessimism in groups of general practitioners and medical students, the general practitioners scoring less favourably than the students.

In a more recent study by Elkind (1981, 1982), who surveyed 785 nurses, 21 per cent agreed with the statement: 'a patient who has cancer can never really be cured' and two-thirds of the nurses agreed that 'treating cancer patients can do more harm than good'. Forty-four per cent selected cancer of the stomach as the most alarming disease from a list of diseases including: schizophrenia, coronary heart disease, rheumatoid arthritis and chronic bronchitis. As in Davison's study, the nurses failed to predict accurately survival rates for cancers of different sites, with a tendency to underestimate survival. Increasing age and positive experiences with cancer made the nurses more likely to respond positively. However, while training and experience led to a greater understanding of curability, it also gave rise to doubts about the value of treatment for cancer. Elkind concluded that some nurses are likely to find it difficult to pass on anything other than an entirely negative view of the disease.

Haley et al (1968, 1977) developed an attitude scale using an item pool and factor analysis for use with medical students and physicians. This cancer attitude scale (CAS) is based on a Likert-type scale and includes 33 items which examine attitudes to cancer in four different areas:

1. Attitudes towards the patient's inner resources to cope with serious illness such as cancer.
2. Attitudes towards the value of early diagnosis.
3. Attitudes towards the value of aggressive treatment for cancer.
4. Attitudes towards personal immortality and preparation for and acceptance of death.

The CAS has been used in a number of studies and has revealed largely consistent results, although the reliability and validity of the scale are in question. Haley et al's study indicates that as medical students progress through college, they become more positive towards the patient's ability to cope with the knowledge of cancer, but become more doubtful about the value of early diagnosis and aggressive treatment for cancer. These findings are consistent with more recent studies of medical students and with studies of practising physicians (Cohen et al, 1982; Madden and Dornbush, 1986; Raina et al, 1986).

Felton et al (1981) used the CAS to measure nurses' attitudes to cancer. The nurses showed favourable attitudes regarding the value of early diagnosis, the importance of accepting death and patients' inner resources to cope with cancer, but held deep reservations about the value of aggressive treatment. This seems to demonstrate the complexity of nurses' attitudes to cancer; it is not simply an issue of being optimistic or pessimistic about an individual's chances of survival with the disease. Quality of life and value of treatment are also important.

Other studies have demonstrated that health carers assume poorer prognosis for patients with cancer than with other life-threatening diseases. Groszeck (1981) used pairs of vignettes involving patients with cancer and patients with another chronic condition, and found that nurses identified the cancer patient as terminally ill significantly more often than the other patient. Groszeck concluded that nurses continue to perceive cancer as automatically fatal.

The evidence does seem to suggest that the attitudes nurses and other health carers hold towards cancer are negative. It is worrying that there is also evidence in the literature that points to the negative effect that such attitudes have on patient care.

Observational studies by Bond (1978), McIntosh (1977) and Quint (1965) have documented blocking and avoidance behaviours by nurses and doctors in their communications with cancer patients. McIntosh discovered the complexity of communications between doctors, nurses and patients and found that there was often collusion among staff and close relatives not to tell patients the seriousness of their condition. Knight and Field (1981) observed avoidance strategies used by student nurses with terminally ill cancer patients. The students, by the nature of their work, formed deep relationships with these patients, which became difficult if the patient asked questions about their disease. To avoid this, the nurses either suggested by actions that they were too busy to talk, or if they were confronted with a difficult question, used their low status in the ward hierarchy to avoid answering, and referred the patient to the doctor, who was then never summoned. Thus a 'conspiracy of silence' was maintained.

A number of solutions have been offered for the problem and education has been a common theme among them. Hitch and Murgatroyd (1983), in a Delphi study of nursing personnel, examined communication problems with cancer patients. The most important problems were seen as those relating to nurse–patient interaction, particularly in knowing when and how to answer patients' questions. The nurses noted the absence of training opportunities for the development of such communications skills and more education was recommended at every level.

At the University of Rochester School of Nursing and Cancer Control, Craytor and colleagues have undertaken a series of studies since 1972 to determine nurses' perceptions of cancer and cancer patients, and to develop and test an educational intervention to meet educational needs and promote more positive attitudes (Craytor et al, 1978; Craytor and Fass, 1982). As a result of these studies, a teaching package was designed to help nurses to view cancer in a more positive manner and themselves as able to undertake this care. The package was tested with a group of nurse volunteers. After the educational intervention the nurses held less stereotyped perceptions of cancer patients and reported feeling more confident to deal with patients' emotions. These changes endured with time.

The work of Craytor and colleagues became the starting point from which our study developed. Unfortunately, their teaching package had become rather out of date and was not appropriate for use with British nurses, so a new package was developed.

METHODS AND DESIGN OF THE STUDY

Since the study is essentially an educational evaluation, it has attempted to incorporate evaluation within its design. Rather than focusing at one level of evaluation, that is the outcome or product of the intervention, the study attempted to examine parameters of process and context.

Parlett and Hamilton (1977) criticised traditional styles of evaluation which examined the effectiveness of a programme by focusing on achievement of pre-set objectives using different research groups, large numbers and statistical inference. They called for more illuminative evaluation styles that would also take into account the wider contexts in which education programmes function, using description and interpretation rather than measurement and prediction. Stake's (1967) model of evaluation involves three kinds of data: antecedent data (that existing before the programme commences), transactional data (that occurring during the programme between instructor and student) and outcome data (involving data from a wide number of sources, which can take into account programme impact and problems as well as achievements).

Following the work of such authors, the study has attempted to examine the context in which the education occurs, processes of development, appropriateness of different teaching methods, and issues relating to the programme organisation, within a more traditional research design. It was also felt important to incorporate some theory of learning as a basis for the development of the educational package. Among others, Knowles's (1973) theory of adult education and Rogers's (1969) concept of significant learning were considered to be highly relevant, as they highlight the need to involve and utilise individuals' own experiences, their own identified needs for learning and self-direction, and facilitation of learning rather than instruction if meaningful learning is to occur.

The study aimed, therefore, to move in three phases:

1. To collect baseline information on nurses' attitudes, knowledge, confidence and perceived educational needs in relation to cancer care.
2. To develop and pilot an educational package to meet these needs.
3. To evaluate the package with groups of newly registered nurses in two general hospitals.

In the first phase of the study data was collected from 57 newly registered nurses in the two research hospitals. They completed questionnaires including the CAS devised by Haley et al (1968), check-lists of self-competency ratings in caring for cancer patients and perceived educational needs. Group discussions were also held with the nurses to illicit more illuminative data on nurses' experiences, feelings and needs in relation to cancer care.

The majority of these nurses (86 per cent) were caring for cancer patients at least some of the time. Yet they felt ill prepared for this role in two main areas:

1. They felt that they lacked communication/counselling skills to enable them to deal with cancer patients.
2. They also felt that they lacked knowledge of cancer and cancer care.

Feelings of inadequacy in their dealings with cancer patients was a recurrent theme in the group discussions.

An initial analysis of the questionnaires revealed that attitudes among the nurses were negative in relation to the efficacy of active treatment for cancer patients, and that early diagnosis leads to better care for cancer patients and increases the cure rate. There was a general feeling that treatment does more harm than good.

Their perceived educational needs fell into three main areas: communication skills, pain control and early detection and prevention of cancer. These nurses had many worries about looking after cancer patients and felt that the quality of care cancer patients receive from both nursing and medical staff is poor.

The data from this first phase provided useful material for the development of the educational package in the second phase of the study. The package was originally planned to run over eight 2-hour sessions in 4 weeks. Each session focused on a particular topic relating to cancer care, and included references, visual aids and individual and group exercises. This was, in fact, the shape of the package piloted in the second phase of the project. During piloting there were difficulties in nurses being released from wards. Following negotiations with nurse management in the research hospitals, the package was revised into a 3-day workshop, which incorporated the features listed in Table 25.1

The workshop has been evaluated in the third phase of the study using a quasi-experimental research design. All newly qualified staff nurses registering during the data collection period in the two research hospitals were offered some additional education on cancer care and were invited to participate in the research. Three research groups were included in the research design (Figure 25.1) so that the workshop was evaluated against nurses receiving a more

Table 25.1 Features of the workshop

Techniques used
Small group work (10–12 participants optimal)
Experiential learning techniques
Role-play
Discussion
Self-direction
Use of library of resource materials and books
Videos
Case studies
Games
Facilitation of learning
Some more didactic presentations

Topics included
Attitudes to cancer/personal feelings/fears of cancer
Prevention and early detection of cancer
Patient education
Ethical issues
Pain and symptom control
Implications of cancer and its treatment
Reactions to loss and coping with cancer
Communication skills
Orthodox and complementary treatments
Staff, patient and family support
Resources available for cancer patients

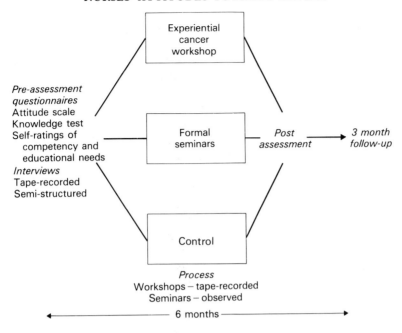

Fig. 25.1 The research design

formal seminar programme covering the same material, but using a predominantly didactic approach, and a third group of nurses who received no education and acted as a control. The participants have all been followed up over a 6-month period. Although random allocation to the research groups was intended, in reality this was not possible and availability for education determined allocation to groups.

The triangulation strategy

As already stated earlier, the study design developed from a feeling of unease about the oversimplistic approach previous research had used in assessing attitudes towards cancer. A strategy of combining quantitative and qualitative methods of data collection was selected, in which triangulation of data from a number of different sources would be undertaken.

A triangulated study combines different theoretical perspectives, different data sources or different methods within a single study in order to overcome the deficiencies and biases that stem from any single method (Mitchell, 1986). The use of triangulation derives from Campbell and Fiske (1959), who developed the idea of using more than one method as a means of validation. Denzin (1978) developed the concept further, distinguishing between different types of triangulation. 'Between (or across) methods' triangulation can be used as evidence of validity when two or more distinct methods yield comparable data. 'Within method' triangulation uses a number of techniques within a particular method. Several scales measuring the same constant in a questionnaire would be an example, and this gives an indication of reliability. Triangulation may also be used to capture a more holistic and complete portrayal of an area of study. In this sense, triangulation may be used not only to examine the same phenomenon from multiple perspectives but also to enrich our understanding by allowing for new and deeper dimensions to emerge (Jick, 1979).

The triangulation strategy adopted for our study involves all three types of triangulation. As can be seen in Figure 25.1, research participants complete a questionnaire and are interviewed before the educational interventions, immediately after it and 3 months later. The questionnaires include Haley's CAS, as described previously; a 15-item self-rating scale relating the subject's perceived competency to care for cancer patients; a 24-item check-list of educational needs; and a 20-item, open-ended knowledge test. These yield quantitative scores for each subject.

The interviews are open-ended, semi-structured and tape-recorded, and yield qualitative data relating to very similar areas to the questionnaires and additional data relating to feelings and experiences of dealing with cancer patients, details of processes involved in any changes identified and evaluation of the educational experiences. Specific questions have been included in the interviews, which relate to the four areas examined by the CAS, and the participants are shown their self-ratings of competency from the questionnaire as a validation of their written response to the self-rating scale.

A further method of triangulation is included in the description of the seminar sessions and tape-recordings of workshops, which yields data relating to process as well as to areas outlined in the questionnaire.

SOME EARLY FINDINGS

One hundred and twenty-seven nurses have been involved in the project, and 42 nurses have attended the five workshops run during the data collection period. Three workshops and concurrent seminar programmes were held at hospital A and two at hospital B. A minority of nurses completed the first questionnaire but declined further involvement, and the remainder are split between the lecture/seminar group and the control group. A full analysis of the data has at the time of writing just commenced.

Anonymous reports evaluating the workshops have all been very good, the most common criticism being that they would have liked the workshop to be longer. Participants welcomed the informality of the sessions and the opportunity to discuss issues and experiences. Participants have all enjoyed and found the experiential learning exercises stimulating. The following are two examples of comments:

'Thank you for treating us as equals and not as we normally are in school . . . the discussion style teaching I found very good, and I think it enabled us to contribute so we could all learn from each other.'

'I think this sort of course would be very valuable *during* nurse training. As a student one has maximum contact with patients, and it is often the student who has to deal with patients' grief, anger, etc. and this can be quite daunting.'

The interview data to date also reveals examples of how nurses recognise that the workshop has improved their confidence and perceived competency to give good care to cancer patients. The following is an excerpt from an interview with one workshop participant:

'*Nurse:* We actually have got a cancer patient here at the moment and really it has just slotted in with this cancer course, because she's on a syringe driver and we talked about that last week . . . she's come in very much out of control . . . as a student it was very easy for me to step back and let everybody else get on with it; now that I'm in charge, if anything happens, I want to know what I'm talking about and to suggest any changes. I just feel a lot happier now.

'*Researcher:* Last time I spoke to you, you said you just didn't know how to approach talking to someone who is dying, do you still feel like that?

'*Nurse:* I think it has made me feel easier about sitting and talking with cancer patients. That I don't have to go in there, and I don't have to say anything. And I suppose it's fear in myself really, about the situation, not really knowing how people are feeling. I don't seem to have that fear and uneasiness that I had a few weeks ago; it just seems to have taken that away.'

These are some examples of nurses' comments, illustrating the kind of qualitative data the research is yielding. A thorough content analysis is at present being undertaken.

The seminars, which were also open to all hospital staff, were poorly attended and motivation for nurses to attend, both those participating in the research and staff generally, seemed to be poor. Data from interviews suggested that this was due more to their organisation than to their content.

Of the control group, most remained pessimistic and felt inadequate to deal with cancer patients. Some gained more confidence through increased experience, but their development appeared to be dependent on their ward environment and support.

IMPLICATIONS OF THE RESEARCH FOR NURSING

While it is obvious that, at the time of writing, the research study is still at an early stage, there are some important implications for nursing practice, education and research that are emerging.

The study is highlighting that the area of cancer care is one that nurses working in the general setting find particularly difficult and feel ill-prepared for. Yet many are caring for such patients regularly. Since the majority of cancer patients in this country will never be referred to a specialist centre, nor be cared for by specially trained nursing or medical staff, this is particularly worrying.

It is anticipated that this study may help to provide some of the solutions to this problem by indicating the kind of educational input that nurses need and how this may be incorporated into continuing education schemes.

By using a triangulation strategy in the research design, the study should produce evidence for relative merits of different research methods in attitude and evaluation research. A comparative analysis of specific quantitative and qualitative methods has long been needed in nursing research to increase our understanding of when and how to select such methods for future research.

REFERENCES

Bond S (1978) *Processes of Communication about Cancer in a Radiotherapy Department*. Unpublished PhD thesis, University of Edinburgh.

Brooks A (1979) Public and professional attitudes towards cancer: a view from Great Britain. *Cancer Nursing*, 2(6): 453–460.

Campbell D T and Fiske D W (1959) Convergent and discriminant validation by multitrait-multimethod matrix. *Psychological Bulletin*, **56**: 81–105.

Cohen R E, Ruckdeschel J C, Blanchard C G, Rohrbaugh N and Horfor J (1982) Attitudes towards cancer. A comparative analysis of cancer patients, medical students, medical residents, physicians and cancer educators. *Cancer*, **50**: 1218-1223.

Craytor J K and Fass M L (1982) Changing nurses' perceptions of cancer and cancer care. *Cancer Nursing*, **5**(1): 43-49.

Craytor J K, Brown J and Morrow G (1978) Assessing learning needs of nurses who care for persons with cancer. *Cancer Nursing*, **1**(3): 211-220.

Davison R L (1965) Opinion of nurses on cancer, its treatment and curability. A survey among nurses in public health service. *British Journal of Preventive and Social Medicine*, **19**: 24-29.

Denzin N K (1978) *The Research Act: A Theoretical Introduction to Sociological Methods*. New York: McGraw-Hill.

Easson E C (1967) Cancer and the Problem of Pessimism. *Journal for Clinicians*, **1**: 7-14.

Elkind A C (1981) The accuracy of nurses' knowledge about survival rates for early cancer in 4 sites. *Journal of Advanced Nursing*, **6**: 35-40.

Elkind A K (1982) Nurses' views about cancer. *Journal of Advanced Nursing*, **7**: 43-50.

Felton G, Reed P and Perla S (1981) Measurement of nursing students' and nurses' attitudes towards cancer. *Western Journal of Nursing Research*, **3**(1): 62-75.

Groszeck D (1981) Nurses' identification of patients as terminally ill. *Oncology Nursing Forum*, **8**(4): 33-37.

Haley H B, Juan I R and Gagan J R (1968) Factor-analytic approach to attitude scale construction. *Journal of Medical Education*, **43**(3): 331-336.

Haley H B, Huynh H, Paira R E A and Juan I R (1977) Students' attitudes towards cancer: changes in medical school. *Journal of Medical Education*, **52**(6): 500-507.

Hitch P J and Murgatroyd J D (1983) Professional communications in cancer care: a Delphi survey of hospital nurses. *Journal of Advanced Nursing*, **8**: 413-422.

Jick T D (1979) Mixing qualitative and quantitative methods: triangulation in action. *Administrative Science Quarterly*, **24**: 602-611.

Knight M and Field D (1981) A silent conspiracy: coping with dying cancer patients on an acute surgical ward. *Journal of Advanced Nursing*, **6**: 221-229.

Knowles N (1973) *The Adult Learner: a Neglected Species*. Houston: Gulf Publishing Company.

McIntosh J (1977) *Communication and Awareness in a Cancer Ward*. New York: Prodist Croom Helm.

Madden R G and Dornbush R L (1986) Attitudes of medical students and faculty towards cancer. *Journal of Cancer Education*, **3**: 177-181.

Mitchell G S (1986) Multiple triangulation: a methodology for nursing science. *Advances in Nursing Science*, **8**(3): 18-26.

Parlett M and Hamilton D (1972) *Evaluation as Illumination: a New Approach to the Study of Innovatory Programmes*. Occasional Papers. Centre for Research in the Educational Sciences, University of Edinburgh.

Quint J C (1965) Institutionalised practices of information control. *Psychiatry*, **28**(2): 119-132.

Raina S, Algere E A, Stolman C, Feverman M and Hill G J (1986) Limitations in testing for attitudes towards cancer. *Journal of Cancer Education*, **1**(3): 153-160.

Rogers C R (1969) *Freedom to Learn*. Columbus Ohio: Charles E. Merrill.

Sontag S (1979) *Illness as Metaphor*. London: Allen Lane.

Stake R (1967) The countenance of educational evaluation. *Teachers College Record*, **68**(7): 523-540.

Chapter 26

Continuing Education in Relation to the Prevention and Management of Violence

Sarah Robinson and Christine Barnes

The research described in this chapter comprises one part of a project that is investigating various aspects of the nurse's role and education in relation to the prevention and management of violence. Commissioned by the DHSS, the project is a response to growing concerns about the level of violence that nurses encounter and the adequacy of their educational preparation for this situation. It has three main components:

1. An analysis of guidelines on the prevention and management of violence produced for nurses by national bodies and district health authorities.
2. A study of continuing educational provision on the subject of violence.
3. An in-depth case study located in the psychiatric facilities of one health district, documenting the views and experiences of learner nurses, tutors, service staff and managers in relation to violence, in terms of both education and practice.

The impetus for the project came from mental health nursing staff, and the case study is, therefore, focusing on education and practice in psychiatric settings. Although guidelines and continuing education courses may be designed specifically for those involved in caring for the mentally ill and handicapped, they are often multispecialty and multidisciplinary in nature. This has increasingly been the case as violence has become a subject of concern in a wider range of settings than hitherto, for example in accident and emergency departments (Winterbottom, 1978; Gosnold, 1978; Cardwell, 1984) and in the community (COHSE, 1977; Dingwall, 1984; Holmes, 1985). The first two parts of the project – the analysis of guidelines and the study of continuing education – are, therefore, concerned with nurses working in all clinical specialties and, in some respects, with nursing auxiliaries as well.

BACKGROUND

Our project was commissioned at a time when little research had focused on nursing practice or education in relation to the prevention and management of violence, although views on many aspects of these topics had been expressed. The late 1960s and 1970s had seen nursing staff working in some of the hospitals involved in enquiries into allegations of patient abuse, stressing their need for advice and guidance as to the degree of restraint they could use without fear of being accused of assault (Martin, 1984). A number of national bodies produced guidelines as to how staff should care for potentially violent patients (National Association for Mental Health, 1971; Royal College of Nursing and Royal College of Psychiatrists, 1972; Department of Health and Social Security, 1976; Confederation of Health Service Employees, 1977), and many individual hospital and health authorities produced guidelines for their own staff. Views on circumstances most likely to lead to the manifestation of violence, signs that may indicate the imminence of an attack, and the way in which such incidents should be handled had been discussed by a number of authors (James, 1972; Frost, 1972; Harrington, 1972; Packham, 1978; Leiba, 1980; Altschul, 1981; Trick and Obcarskas, 1982; Burrows, 1984). The relationship of the ward environment to the incidence of violence had been discussed, and factors such as the nature of the ward regime, staffing levels and admission policies in relation to available nursing resources had all been considered in this respect (Harrington, 1972; Packham, 1978; Martin, 1984).

The view that nurses had become less confident in caring for violent patients had been expressed (Packham, 1978; Altschul, 1981); reasons suggested for this trend included an increasing fear of allegations of assault and changing policies of patient care. It was also suggested that, perhaps, a knowledge and skill base in relation to preventing and managing violence had never been adequately developed, and, with the move away from management by physical restraint and/or chemical sedation, this had become increasingly apparent. Many of the authors cited stressed the need for nursing education at both basic and post-basic level to pay much greater attention to the subject than had previously been the case.

Research into violence in health-care settings had focused primarily on the frequency with which incidents occurred (Fottrell, 1981; Drinkwater and Feldman, 1982; Casseem, 1984; Hodgkinson et al, 1984), and showed that nurses were the grade of staff most likely to be attacked. Studies by Cobb and Gossop (1976) and Campbell and Mawson (1978) had explored the difficulties experienced by nurses in caring for patients in hospitals that had no secure facilities, and papers by Weaver et al (1978a, b) had considered the implementation by nurses of a behavioural modification programme in a locked ward and its effects on the incidence of violence. Research on nursing education in relation to violence was represented by Strong's (1973) study of general student and pupil nurses, in which it was found that 76 per cent of the former group and 61 per cent of the latter were the subject of an attack, and that over half the respondents in both categories said that their training had not prepared them adequately to cope with this event.

The three parts of our project were, therefore, designed to provide information in areas in which little or no research had previously been undertaken. This chapter focuses on the study of continuing education. Following Rogers and Lawrence (1987), continuing education was considered in terms of post-basic courses for which nationally recognised certificates are awarded and in-service courses provided by employing authorities for which nationally recognised certificates are not awarded. At the time that our research was commissioned, the only post-basic course concerned specifically with violence was the English National Board Course 955 – 'Care of the violent or potentially violent individual'. This course was initiated by the Joint Board of Clinical Nursing Studies at the end of the 1970s; it is 15–20 days long and is open to registered and enrolled nurses, midwives and health visitors. The course's overall aim, as stated in the outline curriculum (JBCNS, 1978), is as follows:

'to enable nurses and midwives to gain an increased awareness and understanding of internal and external factors which provoke aggressive and violent responses from patients and relatives, and develop appropriate skills in managing potential and actual violent behaviour.'

Unpublished data, collected by Rogers and Lawrence in their survey of continuing professional education, indicated that some health authorities were providing in-service courses on the subject of violence. Moreover, the exploratory phase of the project described in this chapter indicated that induction courses for nurses and nursing auxiliaries held in some districts included a session on this subject. At the time that the project was initiated, therefore, continuing education in relation to violence comprised:

1. ENB course 955 – 'Care of the violent or potentially violent individual'; and
2. in-service courses of various kinds provided by health authorities, including sessions in induction courses.

AIMS AND METHODS OF THE PROJECT

The overall aim of the research was to document the extent and nature of continuing education opportunities available on the subject of violence, and to identify issues in relation to course membership and content that would be relevant to those responsible for educational provision on this subject in the future. The aims and methods of each part of the project are described separately.

ENB course 955

The aims of this part of the project fell into three main groups.

Course membership

Aims:

1. To obtain information on the course members in terms of clinical specialty, place of work and grade of staff, in order to ascertain whether course membership was biased in particular directions and whether this had changed over time.
2. To ascertain course members' reasons for attending and their expectations of the course.
3. To ascertain the extent to which the course met expectations and whether differences existed between specialties in this respect.

Course details

Aims:

1. To obtain details on the structure and aims of the course at each centre.
2. To examine some aspects of course content in detail, in particular, visits and placements undertaken by course participants and sessions on physical restraint.

Post-course experience

Aims:

1. To determine course members' views on the effect the course had on their confidence.
2. To determine course members' subsequent careers and their perceptions of the usefulness of the course to this career.
3. To identify opportunities for dissemination and feedback to colleagues, and views on opportunities for, and obstacles to, dissemination and use of knowledge and skills gained on the course.

The method selected for achieving the aims of this part of the project was a survey by questionnaire of all those who had attended Course 955 since its inception; the group was too large and too widely dispersed to have considered collecting data by means of interviews. A response rate of 64.5 per cent was achieved, representing 474 of the 735 people known to have attended the course by the end of 1985/beginning of 1986, and it ranged from 53.3 per cent at one centre to 88.2 per cent at another. The tutors responsible for the course were interviewed about their views, experiences and policies in relation to the aims listed in the previous section.

In-service course provision[1]

The aims of this part of the project were:

1. To document the level of provision of in-service courses in 1984 and 1985, and planned for 1986, and to ascertain whether or not sessions on violence were included in induction courses for nurses and nursing auxiliaries in district health authorities in England and Wales.
2. To ascertain details of the courses provided in relation to whom they were available, their length and size.
3. To study views of district personnel on problems in providing courses, such as funding and releasing staff from nursing duties in order to attend courses.

Questionnaires requesting information on these subjects were sent to personnel in each district health authority and in the special hospitals and London postgraduate teaching hospitals (n=212). Following a reminder letter and a second mailing, a response rate of 73 per cent (154) was achieved for this part of the study. A separate questionnaire on induction courses was also sent to each district, special hospital and London postgraduate teaching hospital. Information was sought on whether induction courses were held, and if they were, whether they included a session on violence; a response rate of 65 per cent (137) was achieved.

Data analysis

Questionnaire data were analysed using the SPSS-X package; the main statistical test applied was that for the difference between proportions (Armitage, 1977). Answers to open-ended questions and amplification of closed-item questions were subject to content analysis. Using the categories derived from this analysis, these were then coded to allow for quantification and cross-tabulation.

---

[1]In-service course provision was defined as including courses, seminars, study days and workshops.

FINDINGS AND IMPLICATIONS

Findings presented in this chapter include the following:

1. In relation to Course 955:
   course membership
   reasons and expectations of course attendance
   visits to and placements in other institutions
   teaching physical restraint
   post-course experience
2. In relation to in-service courses:
   extent of provision
   difficulties encountered by some personnel in providing courses

ENB Course 955 membership

At the time the research was undertaken, 10 centres were approved to run the course, and a total of some 80 courses had been held, attended by just over 700 people. Table 26.1 (below) shows that the overwhelming majority (90 per cent) of respondents held hospital posts and that most of them came from the mental health nursing services, particularly mental illness nursing. (In this project mental illness nursing, mental handicap nursing and nursing in secure units or special hospitals were described collectively as mental health nursing.)

This emphasis is no doubt a reflection of the long-standing concern that some mental health nursing staff have had with regard to encountering violence in their work. Although the majority of respondents in this field worked in acute psychiatry, nonetheless a wide range of other psychiatric facilities was also represented, for example rehabilitation, care of the elderly mentally ill and day hospitals. A quarter of the respondents came from general nursing and midwifery in hospital. As anticipated, the largest proportion of this group came from accident and emergency departments, but staff from a wide range of other specialties were also represented among the membership; these included cancer nursing, gynaecology, neurology, burns units and plastic surgery. Only 6.5 per cent of the respondents were community staff, primarily from health visiting. Overall, the composition of the course membership demonstrated a bias towards mental health nursing, but also indicates that, for staff in a very wide range of specialties, violence seems to have been of sufficient concern to motivate attendance on Course 955.

Although analysis of these data by course centre and by year showed some fluctuations, the overall trend remained unchanged.

Just under half of the respondents held ward sister/charge nurse posts, a quarter were staff nurses or midwives and 16 per cent were enrolled nurses. Analysis of these data by year demonstrated a decrease in the proportion of senior staff attending in successive years of the course and a concomitant increase in the proportion of junior staff. Night-duty staff were under-represented in that only 12 per cent of respondents worked solely on nights, with a further fifth doing some night duty work.

Reasons for attending Course 955

From a list of possible reasons for attending the course, respondents were asked to select all those applying in their case. The findings, shown in Table 26.2, indicate that reasons

Table 26.1 Specialty working in immediately prior to taking Course 955

Specialty	Proportion of respondents	
	%	n
Mental health nursing in hospital/unit:		
Mental illness nursing	40.1	190
Mental handicap nursing	10.8	51
Nursing in a regional or interim secure unit	8.0	38
Nursing in a special hospital	5.7	27
Sub-total	64.6	306
General nursing and midwifery in hospital/unit:		
Accident and emergency nursing	12.2	58
General nursing	11.0	52
Accident and emergency with general nursing	1.3	6
Midwifery in hospital	0.8	4
Sub-total	25.3	120
Community care:		
Health visiting	3.2	15
Community nursing	1.5	7
Community psychiatric nursing	1.3	6
Other community posts: community midwifery, school clinic nursing, health visiting with school nursing	0.6	3
Sub-total	6.5	31
Teaching	2.3	11
Other, e.g. nursing in a prison or remand centre	1.3	6
Total	100	474

concerned with responsibilities and interests at the time of course attendance were selected much more frequently than those relating to the future. This finding was reflected by the tutorial staff interviewed, all of whom said that, in their experience, present concerns were the main motivation for course attendance. Differences between specialties, in terms of the frequency with which reasons were cited, were not significant at the 0.05 level.

Expectations of Course 955

Respondents were asked to list their expectations of the course and to indicate whether or not these were met; some interesting differences by specialty emerged in this respect. Content analysis of the expectations listed revealed 12 main categories; these are shown in Table 26.3 (p. 256), as is the proportion of respondents listing expectations in each category. Those concerned with enhancing knowledge and understanding of violence, and learning about management and prevention of violence, were cited most frequently.

Table 26.2   Reasons for deciding to take Course 955

Reason	Proportion of respondents who cited each reason (N = 474)	
	%	n
Responsibilities of post held prior to taking course required an increase in respondents' knowledge and skills in the management of violence	73.0	346
Interest in understanding violence, irrespective of nursing duties, and wish to increase knowledge of the subject	69.4	329
Course attendance suggested by nursing managers	40.3	191
An increase in knowledge and skills in the management of violence felt to be necessary for clinical specialties in which they hoped to work in future	31.9	151
Colleagues had recommended the course as being helpful in the clinical area in which they were working at the time	27.8	132
Heard that the course was enjoyable	18.4	87
Thought that attending the course would improve promotion prospects	17.3	82
Course provided an opportunity for a break from work	14.6	69
Thought that course attendance would increase opportunities to move jobs	12.4	59
Took course in preparation for a post in a secure unit	4.9	23
Expected to attend the course before taking up a new post	0.8	4
Other	16.2	77
No answer	0.4	2

Community staff, however, were far less likely than hospital mental health staff to embark on the course with expectations of enhancing their knowledge [32.3 per cent (10) compared with 61.1 per cent (187), $p < 0.005$)]. Conversely, the former were more likely than the latter to start the course with the expectation of learning about the management of violence [64.5 per cent (20) compared with 51.0 per cent (166)] or the prevention of violence [48.4 per cent (15) compared with 36.6 per cent (112)]. (These two differences were not, however, significant at the 0.05 level.)

Differences between certain sub-groups were even more marked; for example, special hospital staff were far less likely than health visitors to hold expectations about management of violence [33.3 per cent compared with 73.3 per cent ($p < 0.05$)] and much more likely to hold expectations about increased knowledge [74.1 per cent compared with 33.3 per cent ($p < 0.025$)]. These findings may reflect the differing working conditions of these groups; for example, when staff in special hospitals experience violence, they are likely to be facing the situation with colleagues rather than alone. The management of violence, therefore,

Table 26.3 Members' expectations of Course 955

Expectations of course	Proportion of respondents (N=474)	
	%	n
To gain or enhance knowledge/understanding of violence	60.5	287
To learn about the management of violence	55.7	264
To learn about the prevention of violence	39.7	188
To make contact with other nursing and non-nursing personnel	20.7	98
To gain personal knowledge and/or enhance development	19.4	92
To develop observation and assessment skills	13.3	63
To further professional development and teaching skills	10.1	48
To obtain experience of other institutions and areas	7.0	33
To learn about legal aspects of violence	2.7	13
To gain experience of specific teaching methods	2.5	12
To learn about documentation and post-incident procedures	1.3	6
Miscellaneous	12.2	58

may be less of an issue for them than it is for health visitors, who may be less likely to be confronted with violence but are likely to be on their own when it does occur.

Forty-four per cent of the respondents said that all their expectations of the course had been met, a further 19 per cent said the same but added a qualifying statement, and 14 per cent said that more than half of their expectations had been met. When the analysis was focused on expectations rather than on the course members, it was found that those concerned with the management of violence were less likely to be met than those concerned with the enhancement of knowledge [48.9 per cent compared with 71.4 per cent ($p<0.0005$)]. Further analysis of these data by specialty showed that this difference was greatest for expectations held by community respondents.

Mixed clinical specialty membership on Course 955

Findings showed that the course had mixed clinical specialty membership, although hospital mental health nursing staff were in the majority. Although reasons for course attendance did not differ by specialty, differences in this respect were found in relation to expectations held and whether or not they were met, particularly those concerning the management of violence. Moreover, some community staff indicated that they had found the course too hospital orientated and thus not particularly relevant to their own work situation. On the other hand, many community staff, as well as those from other specialties, said that one of the main benefits of the course had been learning from the experience of people whose work situation and experiences of violence were very different from their own. This point was developed by the tutors, all of whom said that efforts were made to ensure a mixed clinical specialty membership because of the opportunity it afforded for sharing experience. This would be lost in single specialty courses but, as they all commented, it was important to plan the course so that individual needs could also be met.

Teaching techniques of physical restraint on Course 955

The exploratory and pilot phases of the research revealed a diversity of views as to whether techniques of physical restraint should be included in the syllabus for Course 955, so this issue was explored in some detail in the main study. Centres varied as to whether or not such sessions were included regularly in the course. At six centres a minority of respondents had attended such sessions; they had either been a member of one of the few courses held at the centre that had included a session, or they had had a session during a placement or visit to a secure unit. At two centres, sessions had been introduced after the course had been running for a few years, and at the other two they had been a regular feature of the course since its inception.

Taking the respondents as a whole, just under a quarter (111) said that the course they attended had included a session on physical restraint. A variety of views was expressed when they were asked in what ways, if any, they had found the session useful. Forty-two per cent (47) made only positive comments on the experience and these focused on building up confidence in facing violent situations and knowing how to restrain safely without causing harm to the patient or to the staff involved. A fifth said that they had found the session useful, but qualified this with reservations, while 22 per cent had only negative comments on the experience. Three main themes emerged from the statements made by the latter two groups of respondents: first, that the sessions were too short to be useful (most were half a day or less); second, that the techniques demonstrated were inapplicable to the respondent's particular work situation; third, that the techniques required regular practice if expertise in their deployment was to be developed and maintained.

Two-thirds of those respondents whose course had *not* included a physical restraint session said that they would have liked one. Reasons cited most frequently for having wanted a session were to increase confidence, to learn how to restrain safely and without causing injury and to explore what constitutes 'minimum force' – a phrase frequently used in guidelines on violence. Just under a third of those whose course had not included a physical restraint session said that they would not have liked one to have been included. Some of the reasons cited by this group for holding this view echoed those expressed by respondents who had had a session but had not found it useful, for example, the inappropriateness of physical restraint in nursing, encouraging its use as a first rather than a last line of action, the dangers of accusations of assault, and dangers of injury when holds are applied by inexperienced practitioners.

In summary, then, some nurses held the view that learning techniques of physical restraint might help them in coping with situations for which they had felt unprepared. On the other hand, the inclusion of these techniques in the nurses' repertoire of skills, particularly if taught within a short course such as the 955, were in the view of other respondents not without attendant problems. This project has only raised these issues in the context of one short course, but the findings do indicate that they need to be carefully considered by those responsible for continuing education in this area.

Visits and placements on Course 955

The ENB course outline specifies that participants should visit a psychiatric hospital or unit, an accident and emergency department and a forensic unit. As this aspect of the course can require a considerable commitment of time on the part of the course organisers and participants and the staff of the host institutions, it was explored in some detail. Three main findings emerged. First, 45.4 per cent (215) of participants spent a period of time working in another institution(s) or service as well as, or instead of, a short visit. Second, although less than 10 per cent of participants visited or undertook a placement in all three of the areas specified in the course outline, a much wider range of institutions was included in the visits and/or placements undertaken, such as prisons, police stations and courts. Third, respondents found placements in nearly all areas to be significantly more useful than visits, primarily because they provided the opportunity to work with staff rather than merely to observe them.

Post-course careers and experience

Feedback to colleagues

To maximise the investment of time and resources made in staff attending Course 955, it might have been expected that on return to work they would have been encouraged to discuss the relevance of course content and experience with their colleagues. However, this proved not to be the case for the majority of participants. Just under a third (32.2 per cent) said that they had had a specific session with a senior colleague to discuss the relevance of the course to their own nursing responsibilities, and only 28.1 per cent said that time had been specifically set aside to discuss course content with colleagues. In both cases, over three-quarters of respondents who had not had a feedback session said that they would have liked one. It seems regrettable that opportunities for new insights, knowledge and skills to be shared and perhaps developed with a wider audience were so limited.

Career since course completion

Nearly all respondents held a nursing, midwifery or health visiting post at the time of the survey and very few had left the profession. The majority had remained in the same specialty as the one they were working in at the time of course attendance: a total of 78.1 per cent of those from mental health nursing, 73.3 per cent of those from general nursing and midwifery in hospital and 74.2 per cent of those from the community. These findings accord with those of Rogers (1983), who found that staff taking Joint Board courses stayed in the profession and in a specialty to which the course was relevant.

Usefulness of course to career

Since course completion, the 474 respondents had held a total of 671 posts between them. The respondents were asked to rate the usefulness of the course to each of the posts they had held on a 1–5 scale (1 = of no use and 5 = very useful), and a total of 49.5 per cent of these posts were given a rating of 4 or 5. Differences between specialties were not significant. Sixty-one per cent of the respondents said that the course had increased their confidence. Some respondents said that they had been unable to put their new-found knowledge and

Table 26.4 In-service course provision on violence by district in 1984, 1985 and 1986

Course provision	Proportion of districts	
	%	n
Courses held in 1984 and 1985 and planned for 1986	35.7	55
Courses held in 1984 and 1985 but none planned for 1986	15.6	24
Courses not held in 1984 and 1985 but some planned for 1986	8.4	13
Courses not held in 1984 and 1985 and none planned for 1986	40.3	62
Total	100.0	154

skill to use; reasons for this included attitudes of staff with whom they worked, lack of encouragement and support from management, staff shortages, and being moved to an area of patient care to which the course content was not relevant.

In-service courses

Turning now to in-service course provision, Table 26.4 shows the findings from the 154 districts for which information was provided (this includes special hospitals and London postgraduate teaching hospitals).

The findings show that courses had been held in a total of 79 districts and were planned in a total of 68. In 40 per cent of districts, however, courses had neither been held nor planned. Respondents in six of these districts commented that receipt of our questionnaire had prompted them to ascertain whether staff felt a need for courses on this topic.

In these districts a total of 485 courses had been held in 1984/5 and 365 had been planned for 1986. Information on course length showed that two-thirds (304) of these lasted for half a day or less; the corresponding figure for courses planned was 47.4 per cent (173). The largest proportion of courses was designed for between 12 and 24 people (47 per cent of those held and 34.0 per cent of those planned), and the size of other courses ranged from fewer than 12 to 72 places. Demand in excess of places available had been a problem in relation to just 14 per cent of the courses held in 1984 and 1985.

The emphasis in the Course 955 membership on hospital nurses in the mental health field was reflected in findings on the intended audience for in-service courses on violence. Twenty per cent (98) of the courses held and 36 per cent (132) of those planned were open to staff from all clinical specialties. The majority (over 80 per cent) of the remainder were open to staff caring for the mentally ill, but this proportion dropped to less than half for accident and emergency staff and to less than 10 per cent for health visitors.

Findings on induction courses showed that 30 districts provided induction courses for nurses at district level that included a session on violence; the corresponding figure for nursing auxiliaries was 28 districts. Data on provision at unit level showed that 63 per cent (86) of districts provided courses for nurses, and 60 per cent (82) did so for nursing auxiliaries. Further information indicated that mental illness units were the most likely to include a session on violence in the programme.

Personnel who provided the data on in-service courses were asked to comment on whether difficulties were encountered in providing courses. Just over a third said that they had insufficient staff to organise and run courses, some also adding that it was difficult to find speakers on this topic. Other problems, each cited by less than a third of respondents, included difficulties in releasing staff to attend courses because of staff shortages, lack of funds to put on courses and lack of staff interest when they were provided.

CONCLUSION

Findings from this project showed that, by the end of 1985, over 700 staff had attended ENB Course 955, 60 per cent of districts had held and/or planned in-service courses on violence, and sessions on violence were included in a proportion of induction courses held at district and unit level. Although staff from a wide range of clinical specialties were included in the membership of all three types of provision, the emphasis was very much on those from mental health nursing. The project also identified a number of important issues, relevant to the provision of continuing education on the subject of violence: first, the needs of staff from different specialties and the advantages and disadvantages of mixed clinical specialty course membership; second, the perception of potential problems, as well as the potential benefits, involved in teaching techniques of physical restraint; third, the relative usefulness of placements and visits; fourth, the provision of opportunities for feedback to colleagues from course members; and fifth, obstacles that may prevent implementation of new-found knowledge and skills.

All of these issues need to be considered when providing continuing education for staff on the subject of violence. In addition, further work is needed to determine the views of nursing staff on the kinds of continuing education opportunities they would like on this complex and emotive subject, and to ascertain which are found to be most helpful.

ACKNOWLEDGEMENTS

We would like to thank the following: the Department of Health and Social Security for funding the research; all those who completed questionnaires, took part in interviews and helped us with arrangements to carry out the project; Keith Jacka for computing and statistical assistance; and Carolyn Dereky for administrative and secretarial assistance.

REFERENCES

Altschul A (1981) Issues in psychiatric nursing. In: *Current Issues in Nursing.* ed. Hockey L. Edinburgh: Churchill Livingstone.
Armitage P (1977) *Statistical Methods in Medical Research,* 4th edn. Oxford: Blackwell Scientific.
Burrows R (1984) Nurses and violence. *Nursing Times,* **80**(4): 50–58.
Campbell W and Mawson D (1978) Violence in a psychiatric unit. *Journal of Advanced Nursing,* **3**(3): 55–64.
Cardwell S (1984) Violence in accident and emergency departments. *Nursing Times,* **80**(14): 32–34.
Casseem M (1984) Violence on the wards. *Nursing Mirror,* **158**(21): 14–16.
Cobb J P and Gossop M R (1976) Locked doors in the management of disturbed psychiatric patients. *Journal of Advanced Nursing,* **1**(6): 469–480.
Confederation of Health Service Employees (1977) *The Management of Violent or Potentially Violent Patients.* Banstead, Essex: COHSE.
Department of Health and Social Security (1976) *The Management of Violent or Potentially Violent Hospital Patients.* HC(76)11. London: DHSS.

Dingwall R (1984) Who is to blame anyway? *Nursing Times*, **84**(15): 42-43.

Drinkwater J and Feldman P (1982) *Violent Incidents in a British Psychiatric Hospital: a Preliminary Study*. Unpublished manuscript, Department of Psychology, University of Birmingham. Cited in Hodgkinson et al, 1984 (op cit).

Fottrell E (1981) Violent behaviour by psychiatric patients. *British Journal of Hospital Medicine*, **25**(1): 28-38.

Frost M (1972) Violence in psychiatric patients. *Nursing Times*, **68**(24): 748-749.

Gosnold J K (1978) The violent patient in the accident and emergency department. *Royal Society of Health Journal*, **98**(4): 189-190.

Harrington J A (1972) Hospital violence. *Nursing Mirror*, **135**(3): 12-13, **135**(4): 32-33.

Hodgkinson P, Hills T and Russell D (1984) Assaults on staff in a psychiatric hospital (Part 3 of series on aggression management). *Nursing Times*, **80**(14): 44-46.

Holmes P (1985) Base control to sister. *Nursing Times*, **81**(49): 22.

James D J (1972) Practical care of the aggressive patient (mentally subnormal). *Nursing Times*, **68**(43): 1352-1353.

Joint Board of Clinical Nursing Studies (1978) *Short Course on the Care of the Violent or Potentially Violent Individual*. London: English National Board for Nursing, Midwifery and Health Visiting.

Leiba P A (1980) Management of violent patients. *Nursing Times*, Occasional Paper, **76**(23): 101-104.

Martin J P (1984) *Hospitals in Trouble*. Oxford: Basil Blackwell.

National Association for Mental Health (1971) *Guidelines for the Care of Patients who Exhibit Violent Behaviour in Mental and Mental Subnormality Hospitals - a Consultative Document*. London: National Association for Mental Health.

Packham H (1978) Managing the violent patient. *Nursing Mirror*, **146**(25): 17-20.

Rogers J (1983) *The Follow-Up Study, vol. 1. The Career Patterns of Nurses who have Completed a JBCNS Certificate*. DHSS Report. London: DHSS.

Rogers J and Lawrence J (1987) *Continuing Professional Education for Nurses, Midwives and Health Visitors*. London University: Institute of Education.

Royal College of Nursing and Royal College of Psychiatrists (1972) *The Care of the Violent Patient*. Royal College of Nursing, London and Royal College of Psychiatrists, London.

Strong P G (1973) Aggression in the general hospital. *Nursing Times*, Occasional Paper, **69**(6): 21-24.

Trick K L and Obcarskas S (1982) *Understanding Mental Illness and its Nursing*, 3rd edn. London: Pitman Books.

Weaver S M, Broome A K and Kat B J B (1987a) Some patterns of disturbed behaviour in a closed ward environment. *Journal of Advanced Nursing*, **3**(3): 251-263.

Weaver S M, Armstrong N E, Broome A K and Stewart L (1978b) Behavioural principles applied in a security ward. *Nursing Times*, **74**(1): 22-24.

Winterbottom S (1978) Violence in the accident and emergency department. *Nursing Mirror*, **146**(24): 21-23.

Section 4
Career Paths of Nurses and Midwives

Chapter 27

Career Intentions and Career Paths of Midwives

Sarah Robinson and Heather Owen

Recruitment and retention levels of nursing and midwifery staff are currently major issues of concern in the National Health Service. Changes in the demographic structure of the population mean a decrease in the pool of school-leavers from which potential recruits can be drawn, while at the same time wastage levels after qualification are high (Price Waterhouse, 1988).

Various studies have been undertaken to investigate nurses' and midwives' reasons for taking training and for subsequently remaining in or leaving the profession. Factors identified include those concerned with the nature of the work itself as well as those concerned with conditions and terms of employment; they include standards of care, levels of staffing, volume of work, role clarity, opportunities to use skills and knowledge appropriately, management support, career prospects, pay and flexible working hours (see, for example, Hockey, 1976; Mercer, 1979; Redfern and Spurgeon, 1980; Wallis and Cope, 1980; Moores et al, 1983; Mackay, 1988; Price Waterhouse, 1988).

Very few studies have been undertaken, however, that follow the careers of individual nurses and midwives, exploring the extent to which career intentions are translated into practice and the way in which certain factors or sets of circumstances may combine to influence career decisions in particular directions. Groups whose careers since qualification have been studied include nursing graduates and midwives. Graduates from nursing degree courses have been followed up by most of the university and polytechnic departments offering such programmes; these studies are briefly reviewed in chapter 29. Midwives are the subject of two longitudinal studies currently in progress: the first is following the careers of two groups trained in Scotland (Mander, 1987); the second is following the careers of two groups trained in England and Wales, and is the subject of this chapter. A third study investigated the careers of male midwives from qualification up until 1987 (Lewis, 1987, and chapter 28).

RECRUITMENT AND RETENTION IN MIDWIFERY

The impetus for the project described here came from two main areas of concern: the large numbers of nurses who take midwifery training for reasons other than wishing to practise midwifery - and the attendant waste of training facilities-and the high attrition rate from the profession in the years following qualification. Both of these are long-standing problems. The former has been an issue ever since the early 1900s, when the legislative and examination machinery for midwifery was first established (Central Midwives Board, 1913), and was not affected by lengthening the training in 1916 and again in 1926 or by dividing it into two parts in 1938.

The issue was addressed by the 1949 Working Party on Midwives set up to investigate the shortage of midwives prevailing in the 1940s. Research carried out for the working party showed that only 38 per cent of midwives qualifying in 1945 trained because they wanted to take up midwifery as a profession, whereas 51 per cent said that it was to obtain an additional qualification that might be useful in the future (Ministry of Health et al, 1949). The data also showed that 29 per cent of those qualifying in 1945 were not in midwifery practice by August 1947. The midwifery qualification was still required for many nursing posts and the working party recommended that employing authorities should no longer insist on this, as nurses would then be deterred from taking midwifery training solely for career purposes.

The working party also suggested there should be an increase in the proportion of older women recruited to the profession, as official returns and their own research showed that wastage after training was greatest among the younger age groups. They also paid considerable attention to factors that they identified as affecting job satisfaction and retention; these included conditions of employment, and the extent to which midwives' opportunities to exercise their skills and clinical judgment in the care of normal childbearing women were being reduced by the medical profession (Ministry of Health et al, 1949).

Figures published by the Central Midwives Board showed that the pattern of wastage continued throughout the 1950s and 1960s, with about half of those qualifying each year notifying their intention to practise and this proportion falling to a third by the second year after training. At the same time, concern was expressed throughout these two decades that the midwifery service was very understaffed (see, for example, Central Midwives Board, 1957; Ministry of Health, 1959; Royal College of Midwives, 1964). A 1963 study showed a continuation of the trend whereby only a minority of those entering midwifery training did so because they wanted to embark on a career in midwifery and that 53 per cent of those qualifying in 1961 were not practising midwifery 2 years later (Ramsden and Radwanski, 1963).

The final report published by the Central Midwives Board showed little proportional change in wastage after training during the 1970s (Central Midwives Board, 1983). During this period a shortage of midwives in the maternity services persisted and Robinson (1980) demonstrated a national shortage in all grades, particularly at staff midwife level. Evidence submitted annually by the Royal College of Midwives to the Pay Review Body indicates that staff shortages remain a major concern. The late 1970s also saw increasing concern about the erosion of the midwife's role by medical involvement in normal maternity care (see Robinson et al, 1983, and chapter 8), a development that, as the 1949 working party had commented, might well have deleterious effects on job satisfaction and retention.

Midwifery training was also the subject of concern in the 1970s. It was maintained that 12 months was insufficient time to cover the syllabus in depth and that not enough time was available for clinical experience (Central Midwives Board, 1977). The Board decided to extend the training to 18 months and, as Stewart (1981) comments, it was hoped that this extension would 'be used to develop clinical skills and to give opportunity for the student midwife to become confident and wish to practise as a midwife'. The latter was of particular importance to a profession so long dominated by concerns over recruitment and retention levels.

AIMS AND METHODS OF THE CAREER PATTERNS PROJECT

The decision to extend midwifery training for nurses from 12 to 18 months provided the initial impetus for the research described in this chapter, because if any judgments were to be made about the effects of the 18-month training on confidence and career intentions, comparable data had first to be obtained from those taking the 12-month course. Once this stage of the research was complete we had an ideal opportunity to explore the extent to which career intentions were realised, so a second stage of the study was initiated in which the careers of the two groups were followed up. The project has now been in progress at the Nursing Research Unit since 1978; its three main phases are shown in Figure 27.1.

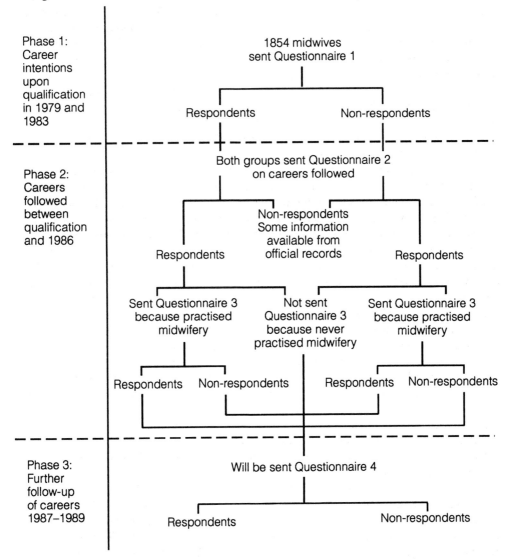

Fig. 27.1 The three phases of the midwives' career patterns project

Phase 1: career intentions and views of training at the time of qualification

Aims of this phase were:

1. To ascertain whether reasons for taking midwifery training and career intentions of a group of midwives who qualified after an 18-month course differed from a group who took a 12-month course.
2. To ascertain whether the group taking the longer course felt better prepared to practise midwifery than the group who had taken the shorter course.

A predominantly closed-item questionnaire, covering these issues and requesting various biographical details, was piloted with a group of midwives who qualified in 1978 (Golden, 1980). The revised questionnaire was then sent to 932 midwives, who qualified in 1979 after a 12-month course, approximately 1 month after qualifying; 83.9 per cent (782) responded. Four years later an identical questionnaire was sent to 931 midwives qualifying in 1983 after an 18-month course, and an 88.9 per cent (828) response rate was achieved. Findings relating to career intentions and their relationship to careers followed are included in this chapter (all the data from this phase of the research are available in Robinson 1986a, b, c).

Phase 2: careers followed since qualification

Aims of this phase are to determine:

1. the career paths followed by the two groups of midwives;
2. whether or not career intentions and patterns of those aged over 30 years at the time of qualification differ from those under 30 years;
3. the extent to which career intentions expressed at the time of qualification correlate with careers actually followed;
4. how well midwives feel their training prepared them for the responsibilities of midwifery practice;
5. the reasons midwives give for remaining in midwifery, for changing from one midwifery post to another and for leaving the profession for other occupations/activities. Particular attention was paid to factors that our earlier study had identified as germane to job satisfaction – namely opportunities for role fulfilment and adequate staffing levels – and to factors identified in other studies of recruitment and retention;
6. whether or not midwives experience difficulties when seeking to return to practice after a break and/or in combining work with child care.

Data on these topics were obtained from questionnaires sent in November 1986 to all those asked to take part in phase 1. The original plan was to send one questionnaire to each of these midwives, but this proved not to be feasible, as providing for all possible sequences of posts and activities entailed an extremely lengthy questionnaire, which would have militated against a high response rate. Consequently, a different strategy was adopted. A short questionnaire asking for a chronological list of activities and employment since qualification was sent to all members of the two groups. Those who had never practised midwifery were asked why this was, whether they intended to practise in the future and whether the training had been of any use to their subsequent work. Those who had practised as midwives were sent a second questionnaire, made up of blocks of questions that related to the career they had followed. Respondents were also asked about their career intentions and for their views on factors that cause midwives to leave the profession and those that might encourage them to return.

Contact with respondents was made via the UKCC, the Royal College of Midwives and the Health Visitors Association and by asking those who had replied if they knew of the whereabouts of midwives with whom they had trained, but who had not as yet replied. Through this combination of strategies the first questionnaire was returned by 58 per cent (536) of the 1979 group and by 68 per cent (629) of the 1983 group who had been sent a questionnaire at the time they qualified, and the second and more detailed questionnaire was returned by 80 per cent of these two groups of respondents. Questionnaires were returned from all parts of the United Kingdom, from Australia, New Zealand, Canada and North America and from many countries in Europe, Africa, the near East and the far East. At the time of writing, findings relating to the first three aims of the research are available, so are included in this chapter.

Phase 3: subsequent career progress

The third phase of the project involves a subsequent follow-up of the two groups of midwives, and questionnaires were sent out in March 1989 for an update of careers since November 1986.

Analysis

The data were analysed using the SPSS-X package; the main statistical test applied was the difference between proportions (Armitage, 1977).

FINDINGS

Reasons for deciding to take midwifery training

Earlier studies indicated that the majority of midwives took the training for purposes primarily concerned with a nursing career (Ministry of Health et al, 1949; Ramsden and Radwanski, 1963). Table 27.1 (below) shows that a similar situation pertained for those midwives qualifying in 1979 and in 1983, in that the two reasons cited most frequently were 'to broaden my experience' and 'as an additional qualification to improve my career prospects'. The 1983 group was, however, significantly less likely than the 1979 group to say that they thought their training was incomplete without midwifery ($p < 0.0001$) and were significantly more likely to say that they intended to work as a midwife after qualifying ($p < 0.00001$).

Career intentions expressed at time of qualification

The respondents were asked to recall what their career intentions had been before they embarked on midwifery training and immediately after they qualified. The findings for both groups are shown in Table 27.2 (below).

The first three options listed in Table 27.2 indicate an intention to practise as a midwife, even if only for a short time, and have been sub-totalled to show the overall proportion of respondents who expressed an intention to practise. The fourth and fifth options

Table 27.1   Reasons for deciding to take midwifery training: 1979 and 1983

Reasons	Midwives qualifying in:			
	1979 (12-month course) (N = 782)		1983 (18-month course) (N = 828)	
	%	n	%	n
To broaden my experience	57.7	451	62.7	519
As an additional qualification to improve my career prospects	49.1	384	52.8	437
I thought my training was incomplete without midwifery training	34.8	272	23.1	191
I intended to work as a midwife after qualifying	26.1	204	38.8	321
To see if I liked midwifery	14.5	113	17.3	143
I needed the qualification to work overseas	19.7	154	17.4	144
I wanted a change from nursing	7.5	59	10.7	89
Other reasons	12.1	95	19.4	161

have also been sub-totalled to show the overall proportion of respondents who did not express an intention to practise as a midwife.

The findings on career intentions before taking training show that the 18-month group were significantly more likely than the 12-month group to express an intention to practise midwifery once qualified: 77.7 per cent compared with 65.7 per cent ($p < 0.0001$). This difference may reflect a reluctance to embark on the longer 18-month training by some who formerly would have sought the midwifery qualification primarily as part of their nursing career.

The largest proportion of respondents in both groups said that they intended to practise midwifery after qualifying, but were not sure if this would be for a short time only or as a career; this was the case for career intentions at the beginning of training and after qualifying. There is, however, a small increase in the proportion who expressed a definite intention to make a career in midwifery having qualified: 24.0 per cent in 1983 compared with 17.4 per cent in 1979 (this is significant at the 0.005 level but not at the 0.001 level). It may be that changes in the length, content and structure of the course have led to an increase in the number of newly qualified midwives who feel sufficiently confident to practise. However, the relationship between a midwife's experience of training and her career intentions is complex, and further analyses are in progress to explore this in more depth.

Careers followed

Data obtained from the questionnaires sent out in 1986 revealed an immense variation, not only in the posts held and activities pursued since qualification, but also in the order in which they were undertaken. These diverse career paths were grouped into the broad categories shown in Table 27.3 (p. 272), so that overall trends could be demonstrated, for example the proportion who practised midwifery continuously and the proportion who held midwifery posts and then returned to nursing.

Table 27.2 Career intentions before taking training and after qualifying: 1979 and 1983

Career intentions	Midwives qualifying in							
	1979 (12-month course)				1983 (18-month course)			
	Before taking training		After qualifying		Before taking training		After qualifying	
	%	n	%	n	%	n	%	n
Intending to make a career in midwifery	13.4	105	17.4	136	16.2	134	24.0	199
Intending to practise midwifery, but not sure whether for a short time or for a career	38.4	300	39.6	310	47.7	395	48.7	403
Intending to practise for some time as a midwife, but not to make midwifery a career	13.9	109	16.2	127	13.8	114	12.3	102
Total expressing an intention to practise	65.7	514	73.3	573	77.7	643	85.0	704
Not sure whether want to practise at all as a midwife	26.3	206	14.7	115	16.5	137	7.0	58
Not intending to practise midwifery after qualifying	7.9	62	11.6	91	3.3	27	5.6	46
Total not expressing an intention to practise	34.3	268	26.3	206	19.8	164	12.6	104
No answer	–	–	0.4	3	2.5	21	2.4	20
Total	100	782	100	782	100	828	100	828

One of the objectives of the project is to compare the career paths of those who qualified in 1979 after a 12-month course with those who qualified in 1983 after an 18-month course. By November 1986, when the follow-up questionnaires were sent out, the former group had been qualified for 7 years and the latter for 3 years. In order to provide comparable data on the two groups, a summary was also made of the careers followed by the 1979 group from qualification up until November 1982 (i.e. 3 years after qualification). In Table 27.3, the first column shows data for the 1983 respondents in the 3 years between qualification and November 1986, the second column shows data for the 1979 respondents between qualification and November 1982 (thus enabling a comparison to be made between the two groups) and the third column shows data for the 1979 group for the 7 years between qualification and November 1986.

The findings show that, 3 years after qualification, the 1983 respondents were more likely than the 1979 respondents to be practising midwifery (55.8 per cent compared with 48.3 per cent, $p < 0.025$) and to have practised continuously since qualifying (36.6 per cent compared with 29.3 per cent, $p < 0.025$). Conversely, the 1979 group were more likely than the 1983 group never to have practised midwifery (20.0 per cent compared with 9.7 per cent, $p < 0.00001$). Approximately one-third of both groups had practised midwifery but were

Table 27.3 Careers followed since qualification

Career followed since qualification	3 years after qualification				7 years after qualification	
	1983 group in 1986		1979 group in 1982		1979 group in 1986	
	%	n	%	n	%	n
A Practising midwifery now						
1 Continuous practice since qualification	36.6	230	29.3	157	17.4	93
2 Midwifery practice broken only by maternity leave	9.7	61	5.6	30	10.6	57
3 Midwifery practice broken only by maternity leave *and* other posts	1.1	7	1.3	7	6.2	33
4 Midwifery practice broken only by other posts	8.4	53	12.1	65	10.8	58
Total in midwifery practice	55.8	351	48.3	259	45.0	241
B Not practising midwifery but have done so since qualification						
5 On maternity leave, having practised midwifery only since qualification	10.3	65	6.7	36	4.5	24
6 On maternity leave, having practised midwifery *and* held other posts since qualification	3.3	21	4.7	25	6.7	36
7 Now nursing, have practised midwifery	10.8	68	11.2	60	13.1	70
8 Now on health visitor's course	1.9	12	2.2	12	0.4	2
9 Now health visiting	4.9	31	3.9	21	6.9	37
10 Now in a health care related post	1.1	7	0.7	4	1.9	10
11 Now in a non health care related post	2.1	13	2.2	12	2.8	15
Total who have practised midwifery since qualification but not doing so now	40.5	217	31.7	170	36.2	194
C Never practised midwifery since qualifying						
12 On maternity leave	1.7	11	2.6	14	3.9	21
13 Nursing	5.2	33	12.7	68	10.1	54
14 On a health visitor's course	0.5	3	-	-	-	-
15 Health visiting	1.3	8	3.5	19	3.2	17
16 In a health care related post	0.3	2	0.4	2	0.6	3
17 In a non health care related post or activity	0.6	4	0.7	4	0.9	5
Total who never practised midwifery	9.7	61	20.0	107	18.7	100
No answer	-	-	-	-	0.2	1
Total	100	629	100	536	100	536

in other occupations or activities 3 years after qualification. Of those who practised midwifery and then left, the largest group were practising as nurses, and the same is the case for those who never practised midwifery. Findings for the 1979 group indicated that the proportion of respondents in the three main categories (practising midwifery, have practised midwifery but not at present, and never practised) changed little between 3 and 7 years after qualification.

Data on whether non-respondents had practised was obtained in the course of tracing their whereabouts, and, when combined with data from the respondents, they showed that a total of 29 per cent of the 1979 group had never practised midwifery since qualifying compared with 22 per cent of the 1983 group ($p < 0.0005$). The latter figure could only decrease with time, so it appears that those who took the 18-month training were more likely to practise than those who took the shorter course, albeit with a relatively small proportional difference.

Relationship of career intentions to careers followed

The majority of those who completed the follow-up questionnaire in 1986 had also returned a questionnaire at the time of qualification: 490 members of the 1979 group (63 per cent) and 581 (70 per cent) of the 1983 group. Data from the two questionnaires demonstrated the extent to which career intentions were translated into practice, and this is shown in Table 27.4 (below).

The main finding was that the majority of respondents who had definite intentions in relation to practising midwifery fulfilled these in the years following qualification. Three years after qualification a total of 75 per cent of the 1983 group and 65 per cent of the 1979 group who said that they intended to make a career in midwifery had in fact done so. The figures for the 1979 group were not significantly different between the 3-year and the 7-year period. Similarly, over 70 per cent who said they did not intend to practise midwifery at all had not done so in the 3-year period since qualification, this figure dropping slightly for the 7-year period.

Findings from the other three groups present a more complex picture. Of the 1983 respondents who said that they intended to practise midwifery for a short time but not to make it a career, 36.1 per cent were in fact practising midwifery 3 years after qualification, and a further 16.4 per cent were on maternity leave. The largest group (44.3 per cent) had practised for a short time and were now in another occupation or post. The corresponding figures for the 1979 group showed slight but not significant differences, and the same was true for this group 7 years after qualification.

Two groups of respondents were unsure about their career plans in relation to midwifery. Of those who said that they intended to practise but were not sure whether this would be for a short time or for a career, the majority were in fact practising midwifery 3 years after qualification: a total of 61.8 per cent of the 1983 group and 63.9 per cent of the 1979 group. This latter figure dropped only slightly to 59.7 per cent for the 7-year period. Just over one-fifth of both groups had practised for a short time, but had subsequently taken up other activities or posts.

The majority of those who were uncertain as to whether they would practise at all had in fact not done so in the 3-year period after qualification (63.6 per cent and 56.2 per cent of the 1983 and 1979 groups respectively), a situation that differed little for the 7-year period. Nonetheless, 36 per cent of the 1979 group and 44 per cent of the 1983 group had practised midwifery, approximately half of whom were in practice 3 years after qualification, and 7 years after in the case of the 1979 group.

Table 27.4 Career intentions by careers followed

Career followed since qualification	Career intentions at the time of qualifying as a midwife									
	3 years after qualification									
	1983 group in 1986									
	Intend to make a career in midwifery		Intend to practise midwifery for a short time but not to make it a career		Intend to practise midwifery but not sure whether for a short time or for a career		Not sure whether will practise at all		Intend not to practise midwifery at all	
	%	n	%	n	%	n	%	n	%	n
Practising midwifery having:										
1 Practised midwifery continuously since qualification	54.5	79	19.7	12	40.9	121	3.0	1	–	–
2 Practised midwifery since qualification with breaks for maternity leave only	13.1	19	8.2	5	9.1	27	6.1	2	–	–
3 Practised midwifery since qualification with breaks for maternity leave and other posts, or other posts only	6.9	10	8.2	5	11.8	35	9.1	3	9.4	3
On maternity leave having:										
1 Practised midwifery only since qualification	11.7	17	11.5	7	11.5	34	–	–	–	–
2 Practised midwifery and held other posts since qualification	2.1	3	4.9	3	3.4	10	3.0	1	3.1	1
In post/activity *other* than midwifery but have practised midwifery since qualification	10.3	15	44.3	27	21.6	64	15.2	5	15.6	5
In post/activity *other* than midwifery and never practised midwifery	1.4	2	3.3	2	1.7	5	63.6	21	71.9	23
Total	100.0	145	100.0	61	100.0	296	100.0	33	100.0	32

Table **27.4** (continued)

Career intentions at the time of qualifying as a midwife																			
3 years after qualification										7 years after qualification									
1979 group in 1982										1979 group in 1986									
Intend to make a career in midwifery		Intend to practise midwifery for a short time but not to make it a career		Intend to practise midwifery but not sure whether for a short time or for a career		Not sure whether will practise at all		Intend not to practise midwifery at all		Intend to make a career in midwifery		Intend to practise midwifery for a short time but not to make it a career		Intend to practise midwifery but not sure whether for a short time or for a career		Not sure whether will practise at all		Intend not to practise midwifery at all	
%	n	%	n	%	n	%	n	%	n	%	n	%	n	%	n	%	n	%	n
51.1	45	28.6	21	37.2	71	4.1	3	1.7	1	31.8	28	21.5	17	19.4	37	-	-	-	-
5.7	5	5.1	4	8.9	17	2.7	2	-	-	17.0	15	6.3	5	16.8	32	2.7	2	-	-
8.0	7	13.9	11	17.8	34	17.8	13	3.4	2	10.2	9	16.5	13	23.6	45	19.2	14	6.9	4
18.2	16	3.8	3	7.9	15	-	-	-	-	13.6	12	3.8	3	2.6	5	-	-	-	-
1.1	1	11.4	9	2.1	4	6.8	5	5.2	3	3.4	3	10.1	8	6.8	13	8.2	6	3.4	2
11.4	10	32.9	26	21.5	41	12.3	9	15.5	9	19.3	17	36.7	29	26.7	51	16.4	12	19.0	11
4.5	4	6.3	5	4.7	9	56.2	41	74.1	43	4.5	4	5.1	4	3.7	7	53.4	39	70.7	41
100.0	88	100.0	79	100.0	191	100.0	73	100.0	58	100.0	88	100.0	79	100.0	191	100.0	73	100.0	58

Overall, these findings suggest that career intentions stated at the time of qualification are a relatively good predictor of career paths followed. In a review of the literature on motivation for career development, Law and Ward (1981) drew attention to a paucity of studies that have looked at the relationship between career choices and subsequent work patterns. Those that do exist are primarily in the field of school leavers' aspirations and subsequent careers, and do suggest a relationship between the two (e.g. Stern, 1961; Maizels, 1970). Findings from this study appear, therefore, to complement earlier work on career development.

Mature entrants and midwifery practice

Another of the study's objectives was to ascertain whether some groups of midwives were more likely than others to remain in the profession; mature entrants were of particular interest in this respect. At the time of qualification, 90 per cent of midwives in both groups were aged 30 years or younger. Analysis of career intentions after qualifying by age group demonstrated that those who were aged 31 years or over were significantly more likely than those aged 30 years or under to express an intention to make a career in midwifery. For the 1979 group, 15.6 per cent (110) of those who were 30 years or younger said that they intended to make a career in midwifery, compared with 36.6 per cent (26) of those aged 31 years or over ($p < 0.00001$). The corresponding figures for the 1983 group were 22.3 per cent (166) and 41.7 per cent (30) ($p < 0.0005$). Table 27.5 shows the extent to which these differences were maintained 3 years after qualification for both groups and 7 years after qualification for the 1979 group.

The findings show that 3 years after qualification, 71.2 per cent of the 1983 group and 66 per cent of the 1979 group who were over 30 years at the time of qualification were practising midwifery, compared with 55.1 per cent and 46.5 per cent of the under 30s ($p < 0.03$ and $p < 0.015$ respectively). This difference is maintained 7 years after qualification for the 1979 group ($p < 0.04$). For both 1979 and 1983 respondents, differences between the two age groups were even more marked for those who have been in continuous practice as a midwife since qualification. This is not unexpected as the younger group are more likely than the older group to break the early years of their career with maternity leave.

The finding that those aged over 30 years at the time they qualified were more likely to express an intention to make a career in midwifery and were more likely to do so than those in younger age groups is not surprising. It may be that commitment to a lengthy training at this age is more likely to be followed by putting the training to use. Information as to whether these differences are maintained in succeeding years will be provided by subsequent stages of this longitudinal project. Findings to date do seem to suggest that mature entrants to midwifery may well be a better investment in terms of their long-term contribution to the profession than those from younger groups, and that active consideration should be given to recruiting from older groups of women. As noted in the introduction, the same findings were obtained and the same conclusions reached 40 years ago by the 1949 Working Party on Midwives.

FUTURE WORK ON CAREER PATHS

Data available so far from this longitudinal study of midwives have shown that those who took the 18-month course are more likely than those who took the shorter course to express

Table 27.5 Careers followed since qualifying as a midwife by age group

Career followed since qualification	3 years after qualifying								7 years after qualifying			
	1983 group in 1986				1979 group in 1982				1979 group in 1986			
	At time of qualification % of respondents aged:											
	30 yrs or under		31 yrs or over		30 yrs or under		31 yrs or over		30 yrs or under		31 yrs or over	
	%	n	%	n	%	n	%	n	%	n	%	n
1. Continuous midwifery practice since qualification	34.4	180	63.5	33	27.4	121	42.6	20	14.5	64	38.3	18
2. Practising midwifery, having practised since qualification with breaks only for maternity leave	10.5	55	1.9	1	5.9	26	4.3	2	11.8	52	4.3	2
3. Practising midwifery, having practised since qualification with breaks for maternity leave and other posts or other posts only	10.1	53	5.8	3	13.2	58	19.1	9	17.5	77	17.0	8
Total in practice in Nov 1986	55.1	288	71.2	37	46.5	205	66.0	31	43.8	193	59.6	28
4. Practised midwifery since qualification, now on maternity leave	11.1	58	-	-	7.3	32	4.3	2	4.5	20	-	-
5. Practised midwifery since qualification, now in another occupation/activity	24.1	126	17.3	9	25.2	111	12.8	6	32.0	141	23.4	11
6. Never practised midwifery after qualifying	9.8	51	11.5	6	21.1	93	17.0	8	19.5	86	17.0	8
No answer	-	-	-	-	-	-	-	-	0.2	1	-	-
Total	100	523	100	52	100	441	100	47	100	441	100	47

an intention to practise midwifery. The data also showed that they were more likely to practise in the 3 years after qualification. To this extent, lengthening the training appears to have achieved at least one of its objectives, namely increasing the proportion of midwives who remain in practice after qualifying. However, this difference cannot necessarily be attributed to the extended length of training but may be related to other factors, such as changing employment opportunities. Analysis of data from the second and more detailed questionnaire, currently in progress, will provide information on reasons for career choices. The third phase of the project, in which all respondents will be sent another questionnaire, will provide information on subsequent careers. Of particular interest will be the proportion of each group still in midwifery, whether the differences between the two groups have been maintained, and whether some of those who had left midwifery by 1986, or were on maternity leave, have returned.

Longitudinal studies of this kind provide essential information for those responsible for ensuring adequate recruitment and retention levels of health service staff. They identify those groups of staff most likely to remain (in this study those aged over 30 years at the time of qualification) and those circumstances most likely to lead to high attrition rates, some of which may well be amenable to remedial action.

Few such studies exist however, partly no doubt because they require a considerable commitment of resources over a long time span. Nonetheless, investment in such work is needed if information is to be available upon which workforce planning can be based and realistic strategies developed for recruitment and retention of staff. A number of further studies on the careers of nurses and midwives are, therefore, being developed as part of the programme of work at King's College.

ACKNOWLEDGEMENTS

We wish to record our thanks to the following: Josephine Golden, who was responsible for many of the ideas and much of the work involved in the first phase of the project; DHSS for funding the research; the midwives who kindly completed our questionnaires; Keith Jacka for computing and statistical assistance, and Carolyn Dereky and Bee Ogilvie for administrative and secretarial assistance.

REFERENCES

Armitage P (1977) *Statistical Methods in Medical Research*. Oxford: Blackwell Scientific.
Central Midwives Board (1913) *Annual Report for the Year Ending 31 March 1913*.
Central Midwives Board (1957) *Annual Report of the Board for the Year Ending 31 March 1957*. Suffolk: Hymns Ancient and Modern Ltd.
Central Midwives Board (1977) *Letter from Board to midwifery training schools, regional and area nursing officers, regarding the decision to extend the 12 month training to 18 months, June 1977*. London: Central Midwives Board.
Central Midwives Board (1983) *Final Report on the Work of the Board*. Suffolk: Hymns Ancient and Modern Ltd.
Golden J (1980) Midwifery training: the views of newly qualified midwives. *Midwives Chronicle and Nursing Notes*, **93**(1109): 190-194.
Hockey L (1976) *Women in Nursing*. Sevenoaks: Hodder and Stoughton.

Law B and Ward R (1981) Is career development motivated? In: *Career Development in Britain*, eds. Watts A, Super D and Kidd J. Cambridge: Published for CRAC by Hobsons Press.

Lewis P (1987) *Ten Years on: a Study of the Uptake of Midwifery Training by Men in the United Kingdom and the Careers of Male Midwives.* Dissertation for BSc Nursing Studies degree, King's College, London University.

Mackay L (1988a) Career women. *Nursing Times*, **84**(10): 42-44.

Mackay L (1988b) No time to care. *Nursing Times*, **84**(11): 33-34.

Maizels J (1970) *Adolescent Needs and the Transition from School to Work.* London: Athlone.

Mander R (1987) Change in employment plans. *Midwifery*, **3**(2): 62-71.

Mercer G M (1979) *The Employment of Nurses.* London: Croom Helm.

Ministry of Health, Department of Health for Scotland, Ministry of Labour and National Service (1949) *Report of the Working Party on Midwives* (Chairman: Mrs M Stocks). London: HMSO.

Ministry of Health (1959) *Report of the Maternity Services Committee* (Chairman: The Earl of Cranbrook). London: HMSO.

Moores, B, Singh B B and Tun A (1983) An analysis of the factors which impinge on a nurse's decision to enter, stay in, leave or re-enter the nursing profession. *Journal of Advanced Nursing*, **8**: 227-235.

Price Waterhouse (1988) *Nurse Retention and Recruitment: a Matter of Priority.* Bristol: Price Waterhouse.

Ramsden D and Radwanski P (1963) Some Aspects of the Work of the Midwife. London: Dan Mason Nursing Research Committee of the National Florence Nightingale Memorial Committee.

Redfern S J and Spurgeon P (1980) Job satisfaction and withdrawal of hospital sisters in the UK. In: *Changes in Working Life*, eds. Duncan K, Gruneberg M and Wallis D. Chichester: Wiley.

Robinson S (1980) Are there enough midwives? *Nursing Times*, **76**(17): 726-730.

Robinson S (1986a) The 18 month training: what difference has it made? *Midwives Chronicle*, **99** (1177): 22-29.

Robinson S (1986b) Career intentions of newly qualified midwives. *Midwifery*, **2**(1): 25-37.

Robinson S (1986c) Midwifery training: The views of newly qualified midwives. *Nurse Education Today*, **6**(2): 49-59.

Robinson S, Golden J and Bradley S (1983) *A Study of the Role and Responsibilities of the Midwife.* NERU Report No. 1. Chelsea College, London University: Nursing Research Unit.

Royal College of Midwives (1964) *Statement of Policy on the Maternity Services.* London: Royal College of Midwives.

Stern H H (1961) A follow-up study of adolescents' views of their personal and vocational future. *Journal of Educational Psychology*, vol. 31.

Stewart A (1981) The present state of midwifery training. *Midwife, Health Visitor and Community Nurse*, **17**(7): 270-272.

Wallis D and Cope D (1980) Pay off conditions for organizational change in the hospital service. In: *Changes in Working Life*, eds. Duncan K, Gruneberg M and Wallis D. Chichester: Wiley.

Chapter 28

Male Midwives: Reasons for Training and Subsequent Career Paths

Paul Lewis

BACKGROUND

The phenomenon of the modern day male midwife is a different entity from the 'man-midwife' of old, for he enters the profession with a background in nursing and not as a 'doctor substitute'. The discussions and controversies that have surrounded the training and practice of men as midwives are, therefore, concerned not with the possibility of a new breed of practitioner, but with the encroachment of men into an all-female profession and the effects this might have for better or worse on the women for whom they care.

Midwifery has traditionally been synonymous with the care of pregnant women by women, during and after childbirth. However, from the sixteenth century, history began to record an increasing interest and involvement by men in this previously exclusive female preserve. Donnison (1977) asserts that, by that time, 'enough men were involved in midwifery, for the term "Man-Midwife" to be included in the English language'. Nevertheless, women remained the principle practitioners of the art up until the eighteenth century (Donnison, 1977).

The subsequent rise of the 'man-midwife' in the years that followed provoked bitter interprofessional rivalry, for their practice was often at odds with that of female practitioners, and as the social and professional status of these men rose, so that of the midwife fell (Towler and Bramall, 1986). The passing of the Medical Acts (1858, 1886) further consolidated the position of the 'man-midwife', who emerged as the forerunner of the modern day obstetric specialist.

Female practitioners of midwifery were not to gain similar legal recognition until 1902, with the passing of the Midwives Act. Yet while this prohibited the practice of midwifery to unqualified females, unqualified men could continue to practise as midwives until the penal ban of 1926 closed this loophole (Donnison, 1973).

Accordingly, a system of maternity care developed within the UK, in which a predominantly male medical profession and an exclusively female midwifery profession became the sole providers of care to pregnant, parturient and post-partum women. This position was further strengthened with the Midwives Act (1952), which prohibited men from training and practising as midwives.

However, in the late 1960s and early 1970s a small number of male nurses vocalised their dissatisfaction at the exclusion of men from midwifery and campaigned for legal change. This challenge to the exclusion of men received some support from the efforts of the Government of the day, who were attempting to introduce an Act of Parliament to prevent sex discrimination and provide equal opportunities in employment.

In 1975, against a background of professional and mixed public opposition to men becoming midwives, the Bill to abolish sex discrimination in employment became law, and in August of that year an amendment to the Act removed the barriers to men entering the midwifery profession. However, transitional restrictions on their entry were imposed (Speak and Aitken-Swan, 1982).

These restrictions confined the training and employment of men as midwives to those courses and hospitals approved by the Secretary of State. Following wide consultation, only two training schools were selected, in which closely monitored experimental schemes were established in order to determine the suitability of men as midwives and their acceptability to women.

In 1977, the first men entered the experimental training scheme at the Islington School of Midwifery, while in Scotland, owing to a lack of suitable candidates, the scheme commenced the following year at the Forth Valley Midwifery School. At its conclusion in 1979, only a small number of male candidates had been accepted and qualified as midwives. Nevertheless, the report of the experimental scheme concluded that 'male midwives were generally acceptable to mothers, husbands, midwifery and medical staff' (Speak and Aitken-Swan, 1982).

The report suggested that candidates for training needed to be carefully selected and that the issue of chaperonage required further consideration. The existence of professional and individual prejudice from midwives and medical men was also identified as a potential difficulty in the harmonious assimilation of men into midwifery. Speak and Aitken-Swan (1982) suggested that it would be interesting to learn what motivated male nurses to apply for midwifery training and recommended that follow-up studies be undertaken should more men enter the profession.

On 16 March 1983 the Secretary of State announced that the barriers contained within the Sex Discrimination Act (1975), which had restricted the training of men in midwifery, were to be lifted. Thus the amendment contained in Section 20 of the Act was removed and from 1 September 1983 it became unlawful to discriminate in the fields of midwifery training and employment on the grounds of sex (HC[83]15). Men were now free to train and practise as midwives on equal terms with women.

Some individuals and organisations called for further studies to investigate male midwifery training and practice; Ward (1984), for example, concluded that if there was an increased demand from men to pursue midwifery:

> 'the profession should make every effort to retain them and to assess their progress for the benefit of the maternity services.'

However, although many small-scale studies have looked at the male nurse within the maternity unit (Tagg, 1981; Newbold, 1984; Cooper, 1987), and the occasional article has detailed the experiences and perceptions of qualified male midwives (e.g. Tiller, 1981; Lewis, 1984), no in-depth evaluation of male midwifery training or assessment of the experiences of male midwives has been undertaken. Consequently, many questions about men in midwifery, such as their number, continuing acceptability, need for chaperonage, reasons for entering or leaving the profession and their subsequent career patterns, remain unanswered.

The aim of the study described in this chapter was to provide information on these topics; it was undertaken in 1987, exactly 10 years after men first entered midwifery training.

Although no previous research had been undertaken on male midwives apart from the Speak and Aitken-Swan study, a number of studies have explored the career intentions and career paths of other groups. A review of these studies identified a number of issues, which were explored in the current study. Those focusing on the careers of midwives include Robinson (1986), Robinson and Owen (chapter 27), Mander (1987) and Brookes et al (1987). Graduate nurses have been the focus of a number of follow-up studies and these are reviewed in chapter 29 on the King's College graduates.

A review of the literature on the careers of men in nursing provided important data for comparison with men in midwifery. It was found that male nursing students in one of the most comprehensive studies of men in that profession (Brown and Stones, 1973), when asked about their career intentions, planned to remain in nursing. The follow-up study of post-registered male nurses showed that the majority kept to these plans. These men also tended to have a greater expectation of promotion than did their female colleagues. This expectation was borne out in practice, for although they comprise only 9 per cent of the total nursing workforce, they have attained 50 per cent of the senior posts within the profession (Gaze, 1987). The reasons for this have been ascribed to a greater job mobility and the fact that, unlike women, men rarely take time out of the 'career ladder' (Davies and Rosser, 1986). Additional factors were also identified in a small study by Hardy (1987), who found not only a greater emphasis on men to perform and achieve well, but also that they received more support from senior nursing colleagues.

Several other studies have examined the factors and issues that have impinged on the career choices and decisions of nurses in general (Mercer and Mould, 1977; Moores et al, 1983; Waite, 1987). One key issue raised is the satisfaction, or lack of it, that nurses experience in their work. It was also seen that side-steps to undertake further training, as well as family commitments, were significant contributors to nurse turnover or wastage from the profession. Waite (1987) identified that job security, levels of pay, working atmosphere, the feeling of doing a worthwhile job and the opportunity of using their abilities to the full were also important issues that influenced nurses' decisions about whether to stay in or leave nursing.

AIMS AND METHODS

The study comprised three parts; the aims and methods of each were as follows.

Phase 1

The aims of the first phase of the project were:

1. To determine the interest shown by men eligible to undertake midwifery training in entering the profession.
2. To identify the total number of men who have entered, or intend to enter, midwifery training in the UK between May 1977 and September 1987.
3. To establish the numbers of men in training to become midwives, the number who have qualified and the number currently in practice as midwives.

4. To identify the numbers of men who have discontinued midwifery training and the reasons for this.
5. To obtain the names and addresses of qualified and student male midwives in order to proceed to the second phase of the study.

A short postal questionnaire was designed to obtain information on these five topics and was sent to the heads of all midwifery training schools within the UK, of which 171 process applications for midwifery training. A response rate of 100 per cent was achieved.

In order to contact the current students and qualified male midwives (n = 70), the schools in the survey had been asked to provide their names and addresses. This posed a dilemma over the need for confidentiality. However, 23 schools complied with our request, while eight agreed to forward the questionnaires on to those concerned. Information published in the *Nursing Times* and *Midwives Chronicle* resulted in eight respondents contacting this writer direct.

Phase 2

The aims of the second phase of the project were as follows:

1. To determine the academic standing of men entering midwifery training and their demographic details.
2. To ascertain the reasons why men had chosen to enter midwifery.
3. To investigate the problems or difficulties they encountered during training or practice, especially concerning their perceptions of the issues of acceptability and chaperonage.
4. To determine how the student and qualified male midwife perceived his role in relation to his female colleagues.
5. To establish the reasons given by qualified male midwives for either leaving the midwifery profession or remaining within it.

A questionnaire was sent to all those men identified in phase 1 as current students or qualified male midwives. This was developed with reference to the recommendations for follow-up studies made by Speak and Aitken-Swan (1982), as well as to the literature on the career patterns of midwives. Some of the issues addressed arose out of the personal experience of this writer as a midwife, together with those highlighted in the studies related to men in maternity care. The questionnaire sought to establish demographic details, the educational qualifications and professional experience of men entering training, factors related to entry, experiences of training and practice, the male midwife–mother relationship, post-qualification details and the career patterns of male midwives. A combination of closed-item and open-ended questions were included. Although the questionnaire was long and detailed, the time taken for its completion depended on the status of the respondent. Only currently practising male midwives were required to complete the whole questionnaire. The time estimated for this was 45 minutes and, therefore, relied heavily on the interest and commitment of the respondents to ensure a satisfactory response rate.

The questionnaire was piloted three times to maximise reliability and validity. On the first occasion it was discussed with two practising male midwives, and then postal versions were sent out on two occasions to a random sample of student and qualified male midwives.

In view of the small numbers of men identified in phase 1 as having entered midwifery, the total population of current students and male midwives was sent questionnaires – a total

Table 28.1 Overall response rate for male midwifery questionnaires

Status	Number of men in midwifery	Number of respondents	Response rate %
Student midwives	22	20	91.0
Qualified non-practising midwives	31	22	71.0
Practising midwives	17	16	94.1
Total	70	58	82.9

of 70 subjects. As a result of the number of questionnaires sent abroad to Australia and New Zealand, 6 weeks were allowed before follow-up; by this time a response rate of 60.0 per cent (n=42) had been achieved. In order to improve this a reminder letter was sent to non-responders, increasing the response rate to 75.7 per cent (n=53). Finally, after a further 3-week period, a second questionnaire and covering letter was sent to non-responders, achieving an overall response rate of 82.9 per cent (n=58) as shown in Table 28.1.

As Table 28.1 shows, a high response rate was achieved for the two groups currently involved in the profession.

Phase 3

In phase 3 of the study, face-to-face semi-structured interviews were carried out with six practising male midwives in an attempt to explore some of the relevant issues in greater depth than the questionnaire format permitted. The interviews were tape-recorded with permission of the subjects and a verbatim transcription of the responses carried out. These were subject to content analysis, the results of which were not available at the time of writing.

FINDINGS: PHASE 1

One hundred and thirty-nine (81.3 per cent) schools of midwifery had received enquiries from men interested in becoming midwives, while 32 (18.7 per cent) had not. Yet, of the former, only 31 (22.3 per cent) had trained, or were currently training, men, although a further 12 men were expected to take up training prior to September 1987. However, nine (6.5 per cent) schools did indicate that they had offered course places to 12 other candidates, who, for various reasons, either failed to accept the place offered or withdrew their applications.

Table 28.2 The status of men in midwifery up until February 1987

Status of men	n
Qualified as midwives	48
Currently in training	22
Failed on examination	1
Discontinued from training	19
Total	90

In total, 90 men had entered midwifery training between May 1977 and February 1987, and Table 28.2 shows their status at that time.

Of the 48 qualified male midwives shown in Table 28.2, only nine (18.8 per cent) were identified as currently practising.

Where men had been discontinued from training, the tutors' perceptions of the reasons for this had been sought and two principal reasons were cited: personal and family pressures, and an inability to meet the required academic standards.

FINDINGS: PHASE 2

A total of 64 of the 70 questionnaires sent to student and qualified midwives were returned, of which 58 were suitable for analysis. Twelve questionnaires indicated a change in the status of some respondents since the completion of phase 1 of the project, four students having successfully qualified as midwives, while eight previously identified in phase 1 as non-practising indicated that they were currently working as midwives. Table 28.3 shows the status of men in midwifery as of July 1987.

Of those 19 practising male midwives shown in Table 28.3, eight were working abroad and 11 within the UK.

The findings from phase 2 presented in this chapter include demographic details, reasons for training, and career intentions and career paths. Data on the experience of training have been published elsewhere (Lewis, 1987, 1988).

Demographic profile

Demographic details revealed that the majority of respondents were British, young, single, academically well qualified and had a good background in nursing. Nearly half (48.3 per cent) were aged between 25 and 29 years of age on commencing midwifery training, while a little more than a third (34.5 per cent) were younger. Seventeen per cent were aged 30 years or over. In comparison, other studies (Robinson, 1986; Mander, 1987) show female midwives to be younger on entering midwifery.

Only 32.8 per cent of the men in the study were married, and, of these, 27.4 per cent (13) had children primarily of pre-school age. These family commitments did not appear to have the same significance in terms of having to give up work as those identified in other studies for female nurses and midwives. This has important implications for the profession of midwifery, for if the careers of the men in its ranks are not hampered by 'fatherhood', then why should the careers of female midwives suffer as a consequence of motherhood?

Table 28.3 The current status of men in midwifery

Position in midwifery	n
Practising midwives	19
Qualified non-practising midwives	33
Current student midwives	18
Total	70

Although the majority of respondents were British, a surprising and unexpected finding revealed that over a third of the men who had entered midwifery training in this country held Australian or New Zealand nationality. While the reasons for this are unclear, several respondents indicated that midwifery training in Australia, where midwives are more akin to maternity nurses, would be an inadequate preparation for the career paths they wished to follow, such as working in the outback, with Voluntary Service Overseas, or in nurse practitioner positions.

Reasons for training as a midwife

The reasons that respondents gave for entering midwifery training were comparable with those found for female midwives in the studies by Mander (1987), Robinson (1986) and Robinson and Owen (chapter 27) with the majority of respondents citing reasons allied to nursing as their primary motive. It is of interest that 53.4 per cent entered training to fulfil a personal desire to become a midwife, while 22.4 per cent did so in order to work abroad, either in a developed or a developing country; 20.7 per cent of respondents, however, entered midwifery as a challenge to the previous exclusion of men from the profession.

In applying to train as midwives 34.5 per cent (20) of respondents claimed that they had encountered some difficulties, although these were primarily related to information, access and entry on to available courses. However, incidences were cited that indicated that applications for training had been ignored, replies to enquiries had been hostile and interviews had tended to overemphasise the problems of a man in a female-dominated profession. When accepted for training, respondents considered that the following factors were the most important in contributing to their acceptance: having applied to the hospital in which they had undertaken their maternity care experience; previous nursing experience, especially with women or children; determination to become a midwife; being married with a family; and the willingness of the midwifery tutors to train men as midwives.

Career intentions and career paths

Until this study was undertaken no information was available concerning the career intentions or patterns of employment of male midwives. Table 28.4 shows the career paths of the respondents who took part in this study.

The majority of students (50.5 per cent) indicated that they intended to practise as midwives on qualifying, if only for a short time, while a further quarter (25.0 per cent) intended to make careers in midwifery. These figures compare favourably with those found in Robinson's study (1986) and are substantially better than those for female midwifery students in the study by Mander (1987).

Data obtained for men who had qualified as midwives revealed a close association between intended and actual careers. As shown in Table 28.5, 89.4 per cent stated their intentions to practise as midwives if even for a short time, 82.4 per cent of whom fulfilled their intentions.

Although the number of men in this study is small, these figures compare very favourably with those for female midwives identified in other studies (Robinson, 1986; Mander, 1987), and this suggests that the investment in training men is well rewarded, as they are more likely to practise as a midwife, if even for a short time, than their female colleagues.

The reasons given by respondents for remaining in midwifery practice highlighted their enjoyment and satisfaction with the work involved, which they considered a challenge, and

Table 28.4 Career paths of respondents

Table 28.5 Intended and actual career paths of qualified male midwives

Career intention	Intend to make a career as a midwife		Intend to practise for some time but not make a career		Intend to practise for some time but not certain about career		Intend not to practise as a midwife		Uncertain about practising as a midwife	
	%	n	%	n	%	n	%	n	%	n
Prior to qualification	39.4	15	18.4	7	31.6	12	7.9	3	2.6	1
Actual career path										
Practised continuously	46.7	7	–		25.0	3	–		–	
Left midwifery but returned and now in practice	20.0	3	14.3	1	16.7	2	–		–	
Practised for a short time then left midwifery	20.0	3	71.4	5	33.3	4	–		–	
Left on qualifying	13.3	2	14.3	1	25.0	3	100.0	3	100.0	1
Total	100	15	100	7	100	12	100	3	100	1

incorporated the important elements of allowing them to take more of their own decisions. The preventative aspect of health care in their work was also seen to contribute towards job satisfaction and the desire to continue in practice.

Nevertheless, of those who had left on qualifying, or had subsequently left midwifery after a short period of practice, all had remained within the nursing profession, and the majority stated that they were unlikely to return to midwifery. The most common reason given for leaving midwifery was 'at the time of qualifying the law prevented practice outside of the experimental schemes', so it would be interesting to see if more men will be willing to enter the profession and remain in practice now that the legal barriers are removed.

CONCLUSION

Findings such as the high discontinuation rate may reflect sound ongoing assessment. Nonetheless, nearly a quarter of the men entering midwifery discontinued training, and although the reasons cited appear plausible, the wastage of time and resources should be carefully investigated.

It would also be interesting to know the criteria that are used to determine academic standards, when failure to meet these is given as a major reason for the discontinuation of men from training.

The large numbers of Australasian men who, while appearing to prefer a British midwifery training, subsequently return home also raises important implications in terms of cost/return benefit to the profession in this country. Nevertheless, these men have all appeared to make good use of their training, if not in midwifery then within the nursing profession; this highlights the issue of whether we train midwives to benefit local, national or international needs.

Similarly, the actual career paths of male midwives should possibly be considered for further study, for it remains important to assess the continuing contribution any group may make in the profession to which it belongs. The findings related to the career intentions and career paths of men suggest that they are a good investment and that the issues raised pertaining to reasons for leaving or remaining in midwifery are similar to those cited by female midwives in other studies. It is evident that men and women within the midwifery profession are faced with the same kinds of constraints, problems and difficulties. Male midwives, it appears, are midwives who happen to be 'male'.

ACKNOWLEDGEMENTS

I would like to thank Sarah Robinson who, as my research supervisor, has given me invaluable advice and support, together with the King Edward's Hospital Fund for London and the Iolanthe Trust for their generous financial support. I would also like to thank all the schools of midwifery and the men who participated in this study, whose help made this research possible.

REFERENCES

Brooks F, Long A and Rathwell S (1987) *Midwives' Perceptions on the Status of Midwifery*. Leeds University: Nuffield Centre for Health Service Studies.

Brown R and Stones R (1973) *Male Nurse*. Occasional Paper on Social Administration No. 52. London: Bell and Son.

Cooper M (1987) A suitable job for a man. *Nursing Times*, **83**(34): 49-50.

Davies C and Rosser J (1986) *Processes of Discrimination*. A report on a study of women working in the NHS. London: DHSS.

Donnison J (1977) *Midwives and Medical Men. A History of Interprofessional Rivalry and Women's Rights*. London: Heinemann.

Gaze H (1987) Man Appeal. *Nursing Times*, **82**(20): 24-27.

Lewis P (1984) The inside story. *Nursing Times*, **158**(12): 17-18.

Lewis P (1987) *Ten Years On: a Study to Investigate the Uptake of Male Midwifery Training within the United Kingdom and the Career Patterns of Male Midwives*. Unpublished BSc dissertation, Dept of Nursing Studies, King's College, London University.

Lewis P (1988) Men in midwifery. In: *Research and the Midwife Conference Proceedings for 1987*, eds. Robinson S and Thomson A. King's College, London University: Nursing Research Unit.

Mander R (1987) Change in employment plans. *Midwifery*, June, **3**(2): 62-71.

Mercer G and Mould C (1977) An investigation into the level and character of labour turnover amongst trained nurses. *Journal of Advanced Nursing*, **8**: 227-235.

Moores B, Singh B and Tun A (1983) *An Analysis of the Factors which Impinge on Nurses' Decisions to Enter, Stay in, Leave or Re-enter the Nursing Profession*. Leeds: Department of Sociology, Leeds University.

Newbold D (1984) The value of male nurses in maternity care. *Nursing Times*, **80**(42): 40-43.

Robinson S (1986) Career intentions of newly qualified midwives. *Midwifery*, **2**(1): 25-36.

Speak M and Aitken-Swan J (1982) *Male Midwives - a Report of Two Studies*. London: DHSS.

Tagg P (1981) Male nurses in midwifery. *Nursing Times*, **77**(43): 1851-1853.

Tiller A (1980) A man in a woman's world. *Woman's Realm*, 6 Sept, 10-12.

Towler J and Bramall J (1986) *Midwives in History and Society*. London: Croom Helm.

Waite R (1987) Waste not, want not. *Nursing Times*, **83**(27): 24-27.

Ward E (1984) Men in midwifery. *Maternal and Child Health*, **9**(2): 44-47.

Chapter 29

A Longitudinal Study of Nurse Graduates from King's College, London University

Julia Brooking, Christine Terrey, and Joanne Howard

INTRODUCTION

The Department of Nursing Studies was established at Chelsea College in 1977 and offers a 4-year full-time BSc (Hons) degree in Nursing Studies, with registration as a general nurse. Clinical work is carried out mainly in the Wandsworth Health Authority. The first intake graduated in 1981. In October 1985, King's, Chelsea and Queen Elizabeth Colleges amalgamated to form a new school of the University of London, known as King's College (KQC). In 1986, a 1-year full-time BSc (Hons) degree in Nursing Studies was introduced for holders of the University's extra mural Diploma in Nursing, but these graduates were not included in this research. The aims of the study reported in this chapter were as follows:

1. To chart the career paths of King's College nursing graduates.
2. To find out the graduates' future career plans.
3. To obtain graduates' opinions about the degree course, including its adequacy as preparation for a nursing career.
4. To obtain graduates' views of their role and contribution in nursing.
5. To assess graduates' satisfaction with nursing as a career.
6. To find out why some graduates leave nursing.

PREVIOUS STUDIES OF NURSING GRADUATES IN BRITAIN

The first nursing degree in Britain was established at Edinburgh University in 1960. Since then, more than 20 courses have developed at universities, polytechnics and other colleges. The majority offer a degree in nursing integrated with registration as a nurse; some offer a degree in a related discipline combined with nurse registration. Degrees in nursing for registered nurses are also available.

Studies of the career paths of nurse graduates reveal very similar patterns of career progression. Research in Edinburgh (Sinclair, 1984), Southampton (Martin and Gastrel, 1982),

Surrey (Montague and Herbert, 1982), Newcastle-upon-Tyne (O'Brien, 1984), Manchester (Marsh, 1976) and Ulster (Reid et al, 1987) has found that the great majority of graduates remain in nursing for at least several years after qualifying. Clinical posts are more popular in the early years, and there is some tendency to move into specialties that permit a high degree of autonomy and close contacts with patients (Sinclair, 1984). It appears that more graduates choose to progress into education and research than into management.

It generally appears that a high proportion of graduates take further nursing courses: more than half of Hull graduates within 2 years of graduation (Kemp, 1985), nearly two-thirds of Surrey graduates within 3 years (Montague and Herbert, 1982), and about a fifth of Edinburgh graduates every year (Sinclair, 1984). O'Brien (1984) claimed that most Newcastle-upon-Tyne graduates who took further professional courses did so to enter or to remain in a clinical specialty.

There have been few studies of job satisfaction in British nurses (Redfern, 1980), and few researchers have specifically considered nurse graduates. Studies at Southampton (Martin and Gastrel, 1982) and Ulster (Reid et al, 1987) found that graduates expected their degrees to give them broader insight, greater knowledge and more professional confidence. Attrition from nursing after graduation is relatively small and is mostly associated with marriage and motherhood (Sinclair, 1984; Reid et al, 1987), although Montague and Herbert (1982) also cited lack of academic stimulation, rigid attitudes and poor pay. Reid et al (1987) found a high level of job mobility in Ulster graduates early in their careers, which Redfern (1980) considers could be an indicator of dissatisfaction.

Discussing the contribution of graduates to nursing, Altschul (1983) expressed concern that 'graduates do not have career aspirations commensurate with their qualifications and that the profession still fails to find graduates to fill senior posts'. Sinclair (1987) observed the same phenomenon and recommended career guidance and encouragement for personal development. Summarising a conference on nursing degrees, Sladden (1987) claimed that there was widespread concern at the absence of clear policies for the utilisation of nurse graduates, and suggested that managers should intervene to create an atmosphere in which graduates could contribute more fully. McFarlane (1987), speaking at the same conference, argued that nurse graduates should contribute to shaping health service development, develop the knowledge base for practice, work in advanced clinical roles and contribute to education.

The role of graduates in nursing is inevitably influenced by the attitudes of the profession. McFarlane (1987) described how attitudes have moved from rejection in the early 1960s to a stage in which graduates are seen as irrelevant to the manpower needs of the health service. Several studies have found that graduates encounter scepticism and antagonism from colleagues (Martin and Gastrel, 1982; O'Brien, 1984; Reid et al, 1987).

THE KING'S COLLEGE (LONDON) FOLLOW-UP STUDY: AIMS AND METHODS

Work reported here is part of an ongoing longitudinal study using postal questionnaires completed by graduates of the 4-year BSc nursing course. This serves to maintain information on career patterns and to gain a systematic picture of subjects' views on nursing, their preparation for their posts and future aspirations. The questionnaire is initially mailed not less than 18 months after graduation and then at 2-yearly intervals, which seems to be frequent enough to reflect career and opinion change and yet sustain a high response rate.

Graduates are requested to inform the Department of Nursing Studies of any change of address, which they do very conscientiously, and this obviously facilitates the study. We are very grateful for this and their willingness to participate in this research, although, of course, they are under no obligation to do so. The questionnaire consists of closed and open questions, and lengthy comments are often received, but in general the document is restricted to six pages in length. Questionnaires are also sent with an accompanying letter providing news of the department and an expression of gratitude for their help with this study. As this is a continuing study, three researchers have been responsible for data collection and analysis to date.

Earlier follow-up of the first three sets of graduates from years 1981, 1982 and 1983 has already been reported (Howard, 1985; Howard and Brooking, 1987). This work laid the foundation for further mailings by testing the main questionnaire format, which also contained questions previously used in follow-up studies by other colleges. Subsequently, the next two sets of graduates (1984 and 1985) received and (most) responded to their first questionnaires. This was then analysed by Brooking. In all, this rendered a sample of 101 graduates, 88 of whom replied, providing an 87 per cent response rate.

Second questionnaires were then sent by Terrey to the first 4 years of graduates from 1981 to 1984 in order to trace their career moves, professional activities, job satisfaction and views on nursing as well as comments on the degree course in relation to their careers. Seventy-nine graduates were mailed and 61 replied, providing a response rate of 77 per cent. As with other studies, response rates tend to fall for subsequent follow-ups, in part due to unrecorded change of address and possibly also a drop in motivation. It may also be the case that a greater proportion of non-respondents had left nursing, although informal contacts would not support this. Results from the initial and follow-up studies are summarised below.

FINDINGS

Career patterns and plans

There were only two males amongst the first samples of 88 graduates. Eighty-five still lived in Britain, 28 were married and seven had children. On graduation, only eight subjects did not take up a nursing position, while the majority (70) worked as hospital staff nurses. The remainder (10) joined nursing agencies prior to deciding on an appointment, went into research or undertook further nursing courses. After 1 year, 78 of the 88 (89 per cent) graduates were in nursing posts, and at 2 years this had dropped to 76 per cent. The majority were still working in hospital but most had taken or were enrolled for specialist courses in such areas as psychiatric nursing, health visiting or midwifery.

Longer-term (3–6 years after graduation) follow-up of the first four sets of respondents (reported by Terrey, 1987) revealed that 43 of the 61 (70 per cent) were in nursing posts. These included four senior nurses and nine sisters, six in research posts, six health visitors, four midwives and a nurse practitioner. Most popular specialties included psychiatric nursing, health visiting, midwifery and care of the elderly. Seventy-nine per cent had taken a specialist course, seven had masters' degrees and three had completed or were working for a doctorate. Graduates changed their posts for a variety of reasons, the most usual being 'to widen their experience', to 'take another course' or to seek a more convenient location or working arrangement to suit their domestic situation. Promotion was cited by 16 respondents and

13 said they had changed posts having completed their contractual period. Only nine gave negative reasons such as boredom or frustration.

When replying to questions on professional activities undertaken since qualifying, 74 per cent of these graduates mentioned some contribution. These included publishing articles, presenting conference papers, giving lectures and introducing change or innovation in practice.

Future career plans were commented on at length by many graduates, several mentioning further specialist qualifications they sought; 10 were intending to undertake higher degrees. Eighty per cent of this sample fully intended to remain in nursing, giving a broad range of areas for their future work, although few mentioned nurse management.

Job satisfaction

For this longer-term follow-up sample, questions on their work experience revealed a great mixture of responses. Initially these subjects had been attracted by nursing in order to help people and to gain a varied, responsible and secure job. Factors that were raised as having little or no influence on the decision to become a nurse were salary, work schedules and conditions. Since working as a nurse these graduates found several aspects 'very satisfying'. For over a quarter of respondents these included opportunities to use communication skills, teach, change poor practice, obtain wide experience in different specialties, have a secure job and see good career prospects. Areas providing most satisfaction were given as psychiatry (7), community nursing (6), intensive care (3), terminal care and oncology (3), midwifery (2), research (2) and nursing education (2). Factors that attracted these replies included being able to practise individualised care, the degree of autonomy possible, a variety of work and an ability to use specialised skills.

When asked about changes that would possibly increase job satisfaction, there was a marked consistency among respondents, higher salaries and better staffing levels being mentioned by nearly half. More educational opportunities and support from managers and other colleagues were also considered to be important by a sizeable minority. A better career structure and more scope to implement change were also included in these comments. In contrast to earlier motivations, dissatisfaction among these graduates was focused on their salary and the fact that no recognition was afforded to their degree qualification. More than half were unhappy about their conditions of work, the hours and poor management. Low morale among other nurses and general apathy increased their dissatisfaction. These reasons were included in those given for leaving by 16 graduates no longer in nursing, and by eight more who had considered this action.

Of those who had left the profession, that is 21 out of the 88 respondents (24 per cent), only four had never held a post since qualifying. As a group they had a wide range of jobs; some had been unemployed and nine had taken other professional qualifications. Four had gone into social work, two into teaching and two into retail management. A significantly higher proportion of these respondents than of those still in nursing were earning in excess of £11 000.

Comments on the nursing degree course

By far the most numerous comments on the degree course were positive – three-quarters of the graduates were 'very' or 'moderately' satisfied with the academic components. The range and depth of subjects were seen as good, and the formal sessions were of a high standard and academically stimulating. Many gave very favourable comments on being able to choose 'optional', non-nursing course units. Negative comments tended to be quite specific, including a relative lack of input on disease and pathology, practical and medical procedures and management (subsequently many of these comments have been used to modify some courses).

A majority of subjects rated themselves as moderately satisfied with the clinical components of the degree. Most common among the positive comments were those that highlighted the balance and integration between 'theory' and practice. Clinical experience was seen to be well structured, varied and interesting. Clinical teaching by lecturers was also seen to be of a high standard. However, some considered that their clinical experience was somewhat fragmented, especially in the first year of the course. Respondents also frequently mentioned problems in relationships with ward staff who sometimes saw them as 'different', which was not appreciated by students.

More than three-quarters of the respondents considered that the degree course had prepared them well for the role of staff nurse. Initial lack of confidence was soon overcome and one-third specifically mentioned that they had maintained a questioning approach, had a good knowledge base and had an ability to find additional sources of information when necessary. In contrast, a minority considered that no course could prepare them for the frustrations of nursing, such as resistance to change among staff and poor pay or shift work.

When asked to consider advantages of a degree in nursing rather than a conventional 3-year course, graduates mentioned greater knowledge, better intellectual and research skills, increased job opportunities, greater personal development, increased status and respect from others and greater understanding of current knowledge on which to base practice. However, 10 per cent said they could not see any advantages.

Disadvantages of graduate training in nursing were few; however, where cited, they tended to pertain to other nurses' attitudes reflecting resentment and suspicion. A few mentioned that it was frustrating having knowledge and yet too few opportunities to put this into practice.

In all, 84 per cent of this sample from 5 years of graduates said that they would select the same course again because it satisfied their intellectual and caring aspirations. It was thought to provide graduates with more skills, particularly in research, and a majority considered that they had the ability to improve standards of clinical care. Despite some negative comments on aspects of the course, in general the graduates seemed to value the educational experience and to be using this in their careers.

DISCUSSION

These findings support those of other studies reviewed in that the majority of graduates selected careers in nursing immediately after graduating and up to 6 years after graduating. As in other studies, the majority chose clinical posts in the early years, although there was some movement into research, management and teaching. Contrary to popular misconception, very few climbed the career ladder unusually quickly, confirming Altschul's (1983) concern that career aspirations may not be commensurate with qualifications.

The main reasons for changing jobs were to broaden experience or take a course. Four-fifths undertook further nursing courses, confirming previous findings (Sinclair, 1984; Kemp, 1985; Montague and Herbert, 1985). Although a few studied for higher degrees, the vast majority took further clinical training, most commonly in psychiatric nursing, health visiting, midwifery and intensive care. Several complained that they had to repeat previous work, often at a lower level, supporting Andrew's (1984) criticisms about the lack of relevance of conventional post-basic clinical courses to graduate nurses. It is reasonable to speculate, as did Sinclair (1984), that the most popular clinical specialties are those that allow a high degree of autonomy and in which the nursing contribution is clearly central to ensuring high standards of care.

The level of general professional contributions among the graduates was very high, with three-quarters having been involved in professional activities outside their day-to-day work. Although no comparative data are available, it is likely that this is a higher proportion than would be expected from a comparable group of conventionally trained nurses.

Most respondents had originally entered nursing because of a desire to care for people and the expectation of a sense of achievement from nursing. Salary and conditions of work had little influenced the original career choice. Nevertheless, as qualified nurses, their major sources of dissatisfaction were low salaries (particularly because of lack of reward for additional qualifications), unsocial shift work, lack of autonomy and inadequate recognition for their work from managers and medical colleagues. Many would consider leaving nursing if staffing levels were further reduced.

Despite these problems, more than two-thirds of the respondents were still in nursing, which indicates general satisfaction with the profession. They expressed satisfaction with many intrinsic aspects of the work, including autonomy, responsibility, variety, opportunities to use their skills in research, teaching and communication and being able to improve poor practices. These findings supported those of Redfern (1980) with hospital sisters.

About a quarter of the graduates had left nursing, mainly because of staff shortages and excessive demands of the job, shift work, poor pay and inability to use their knowledge and skills. Some were employed in other 'caring professions', such as teaching and social work, others in a variety of occupations, many earning more than their nursing contemporaries. Graduates appear to be attractive to employers and none have been unemployed, although some chose full-time motherhood.

In evaluating the degree course, most were positive. The main strengths of the degree were seen as academic rigour and breadth, research training and experience and encouragement to think critically. The main weaknesses of the degree were seen as the short duration and fragmentation of clinical placements, and the difficulties of implementing the ideal standards taught. One major area of difficulty was the attitude towards them of some non-graduate nurses, including resentment, suspicion and, sometimes, unrealistic expectations. Some respondents became reluctant to admit to having a nursing degree. Nevertheless, 84 per cent indicated that they would choose this course again if starting their nursing careers afresh.

This group clearly considered that graduates can make a major contribution to the future development of nursing. Most saw their main contributions in developing and using research, raising standards of care, acting as agents of change and improving the status of nursing.

These findings have a number of implications for nursing practice and policy. This group of graduates appears to have received little support from other members of their profession. Given the working conditions and poor salaries about which they complain, it is surprising that so few have left nursing for other more rewarding careers. If the nursing profession is serious about improving standards of education and standards of patient care, graduate nurses should be rewarded at a similar level to other graduates and should be nurtured and developed by managers, and their knowledge and skills should be utilised more fully.

The work reported here is just one approach to evaluating nursing degree courses. Important questions about the clinical effectiveness of graduates compared with conventionally prepared nurses remain unanswered, but should be tackled.

REFERENCES

Altschul A T (1983) Nursing and higher education. *International Journal of Nursing Studies*, **30**: 123–130.
Andrew S H (1984) The relevance of post-basic courses to graduate nurses. *Journal of Advanced Nursing*, **9**: 89–93.
Howard J M (1985) *A Follow-up Study of Graduates in Nursing Studies from Chelsea College, University of London*. Dissertation submitted for BSc (Hons) Nursing Studies, Chelsea College, University of London.
Howard J M and Brooking J I (1987) The career paths of nursing graduates from Chelsea College, University of London. *International Journal of Nursing Studies*, **24**: 181–189.
Kemp J (1985) The graduates' progress. *Nursing Times*, **81**: 42–43.
Marsh N (1976) Summary report of a study of the career patterns of graduates of the undergraduate nursing course in the University of Manchester, England. *Journal of Advanced Nursing*, **1**: 539–543.
Martin J P and Gastrel P (1982) An experiment in nurse education at Southampton University. *Nursing Times*, **78**: 30 June, 73–76; July 77–78.
McFarlane J K (1987) The role of nurse graduates in the health service in the year 2000. *Nurse Education Today*, **7**: 38–41.
Montague S E and Herbert R A (1982) Career paths of graduates of a degree-linked nursing course. *Journal of Advanced Nursing*, **7**: 359–370.
O'Brien D (1984) Evaluation of an undergraduate nursing course. *Journal of Advanced Nursing*, **9**: 401–406.
Redfern S J (1980) Hospital sisters: work attitudes, perceptions and wastage. *Journal of Advanced Nursing*, **5**: 451–466.
Reid N G, Nellis P and Boore J (1987) Graduate nurses in Northern Ireland: their career paths, aspirations and problems. *International Journal of Nursing Studies*, **24**: 215–225.
Sinclair, H (1984) The careers of nurse graduates. *Nursing Times*, **80**(7): 56–59.
Sinclair H (1987) Graduate nurses in the United Kingdom: myth and reality. *Nurse Education Today*, **7**: 24–29.
Sladden S (1987) Some issues discussed. *Nurse Education Today*, **7**: 42–46.
Terrey C (1987) *An Investigation into Job Satisfaction and Dissatisfaction with Nursing as Experienced by Chelsea College, University of London, graduates of the BSc RGN degree in Nursing Studies, 1981–1984 inclusive*. Dissertation submitted for BA (Hons) Combined Studies, Polytechnic of North London.

Index